RN Pharmacology for Nursing Review Module Edition 5.0

Contributors

Audrey Knippa, MS, MPH, RN, CNE
Nursing Education Coordinator and Content Project Leader

Sheryl Sommer, PhD, MSN, RN
Director, Nursing Curriculum and Education Services

Brenda Ball, MEd, BSN, RN
Nursing Education Specialist

Lois Churchill, MN, RN
Nursing Education Specialist

Carrie B. Elkins, DHSc, MSN, PHCNS, BC
Nursing Education Specialist

Mary Jane Janowski, MA, BSN, RN
Nursing Resource Specialist

Karin Roberts, PhD, MSN, RN, CNE
Nursing Education Coordinator

Mendy G. Wright, DNP, MSN, RN
Nursing Education Specialist

Derek Prater, MS Journalism
Lead Product Developer and Editorial Project Leader

Erika A. Archer, BS Education, Foreign Language
Product Developer

Johanna Barnes, BA Journalism
Product Developer

Chris Crawford, BS Journalism
Product Developer

Hilary E. Groninger, BS Journalism
Product Developer

Megan E. Herre, BS Journalism
Product Developer

Amanda Lehman, BA English
Product Developer

Joanna Shindler, BA Journalism
Product Developer

Brant L. Stacy, BS Journalism, BA English
Product Developer

Consultants

Susan Adcock, MS, RN

Tracey Bousquet, BSN, RN

Joyce Campbell, MSN, CCRN, FNP-BC

Pam Forsythe, MSN, RN

Deb Johnson-Schuh, MSN, RN

INTELLECTUAL PROPERTY NOTICE

IMPORTANT NOTICE TO THE READER

Assessment Technologies Institute®, LLC is the publisher of this publication. The publisher reserves the right to modify, change, or update the content of this publication at any time. The content of this publication, such as text, graphics, images, information obtained from the publisher's licensors, and other material contained in this publication are for informational purposes only. The content is not providing medical advice and is not intended to be a substitute for professional medical advice, diagnosis, or treatment. Always seek the advice of your primary care provider or other qualified health provider for any questions you may have regarding a medical condition. Never disregard professional medical advice or delay in seeking it because of something you have read in this publication. If you think you may have a medical emergency, go to your local emergency department or call 911 immediately.

The publisher does not recommend or endorse any specific tests, primary care providers, products, procedures, processes, opinions, or other information that may be mentioned in this publication. Reliance on any information provided by the publisher, the publisher's employees, or others contributing to the content at the invitation of the publisher is solely at your own risk. Health care professionals need to use their own clinical judgment in interpreting the content of this publication, and details such as medications, dosages, and laboratory tests and results should always be confirmed with other resources.

This publication may contain health- or medical-related materials that are sexually explicit. If you find these materials offensive, you may not want to use this publication.

The publishers, editors, advisors, and reviewers make no representations or warranties of any kind or nature, including, but not limited to, the accuracy, reliability, completeness, currentness, timeliness, or the warranties of fitness for a particular purpose or merchantability, nor are any such representations implied with respect to the content herein (with such content to include text and graphics), and the publishers, editors, advisors, and reviewers take no responsibility with respect to such content. The publishers, editors, advisors, and reviewers shall not be liable for any actual, incidental, special, consequential, punitive, or exemplary damages (or any other type of damages) resulting, in whole or in part, from the reader's use of, or reliance upon, such content.

USER'S GUIDE

Welcome to the Assessment Technologies Institute® RN Pharmacology for Nursing Review Module Edition 5.0. The mission of ATI's Content Mastery Series® review modules is to provide user-friendly compendiums of nursing knowledge that will:

- Help you locate important information quickly.
- Assist in your remediation efforts.
- Provide exercises for applying your nursing knowledge.
- Facilitate your entry into the nursing profession as a newly licensed RN.

Organization

This review module is organized into units covering pharmacological principles (Unit 1) and medications affecting the body systems and physiological processes (Units 2 to 12). Chapters within these units conform to one of two organizing principles for presenting the content:

- Nursing concepts
- Medications

Nursing concepts chapters begin with an overview describing the central concept and its relevance to nursing. Subordinate themes are covered in outline form to demonstrate relationships and present the information in a clear, succinct manner.

Medications chapters include an overview describing a disorder or group of disorders. Medications used to treat these disorders are grouped according to classification. A specific medication may be selected as a prototype or example of the characteristics of medications in this classification. These sections include information about how the medication works, its therapeutic uses, and routes of administration. Next, you will find information about complications, contraindications, and medication and food interactions, as well as nursing interventions and client education to help prevent and/or manage these issues. Finally, the chapter includes information on nursing administration of the medication and evaluation of the medication's effectiveness.

Application Exercises

Questions are provided at the end of each chapter so you can practice applying your knowledge. The Application Exercises include both NCLEX-style questions, such as multiple-choice and multiple-select items, and questions that ask you to apply your knowledge in other formats, such as short-answer and matching items. After the Application Exercises, an answer key is provided, along with rationales for the answers.

NCLEX® Connections

To prepare for the NCLEX-RN, it is important for you to understand how the content in this review module is connected to the NCLEX-RN test plan. You can find information on the detailed test plan at the National Council of State Boards of Nursing's Web site: https://www.ncsbn.org/. When reviewing content in this review module, regularly ask yourself, "How does this content fit into the test plan, and what types of questions related to this content should I expect?"

To help you in this process, we've included NCLEX Connections at the beginning of each unit and with each question in the Application Exercises Answer Keys. The NCLEX Connections at the beginning of each unit will point out areas of the detailed test plan that relate to the content within that unit. The NCLEX Connections attached to the Application Exercises Answer Keys will demonstrate how each exercise fits within the detailed content outline.

These NCLEX Connections will help you understand how the detailed content outline is organized, starting with major client needs categories and subcategories and followed by related content areas and tasks. The major client needs categories are:

- Safe and Effective Care Environment
  - Management of Care
  - Safety and Infection Control
- Health Promotion and Maintenance
- Psychosocial Integrity
- Physiological Integrity
  - Basic Care and Comfort
  - Pharmacological and Parenteral Therapies
  - Reduction of Risk Potential
  - Physiological Adaptation

An NCLEX Connection might, for example, alert you that content within a unit is related to:

- Pharmacological and Parenteral Therapies
  - Adverse Effects/Contraindications/Side Effects/Interactions
    - Identify a contraindication to the administration of a medication to the client.

Icons

Icons are used throughout the review module to draw your attention to particular areas. Keep an eye out for these icons:

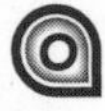

This icon indicates an Overview, or introduction, to a particular subject matter. Descriptions and categories will typically be found in an Overview.

This icon is used for the Application Exercises and the Application Exercises Answer Keys.

This icon is used for NCLEX connections.

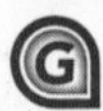

This icon is used for gerontological content. When you see this icon, take note of information that is specific to aging or the care of older adult clients.

This icon is used for content related to safety. When you see this icon, take note of safety concerns or steps that nurses can take to ensure client safety and a safe environment.

This icon is used for examples of how to apply math concepts, such as in dosage calculation.

Feedback

ATI welcomes feedback regarding this review module. Please provide comments to: comments@atitesting.com.

Table of Contents

Unit 6 Medications Affecting the Gastrointestinal System and Nutrition

Unit 7 Medications Affecting the Reproductive System

Unit 10 Medications Affecting the Endocrine System

Unit 11 Medications Affecting the Immune System

Unit 12 Medications for Infection

UNIT 1: PHARMACOLOGICAL PRINCIPLES

- Pharmacokinetics and Routes of Administration
- Safe Medication Administration and Error Reduction
- Dosage Calculation
- Intravenous Therapy
- Adverse Effects, Interactions, and Contraindications
- Individual Considerations of Medication Administration

NCLEX® CONNECTIONS

When reviewing the chapters in this unit, keep in mind the relevant sections of the NCLEX® outline, in particular:

CLIENT NEEDS: SAFETY AND INFECTION CONTROL

Relevant topics/tasks include:

- Error Prevention
  - Assess for client allergies/sensitivities and intervene as needed.
- Reporting of Incident/Event/Irregular Occurrence/Variance
  - Identify need/situation where reporting of incident/event/irregular occurrence/variance is appropriate.

CLIENT NEEDS: PHARMACOLOGICAL AND PARENTERAL THERAPIES

Relevant topics/tasks include:

- Adverse Effects/Contraindications/Side Effects/Interactions
  - Identify a contraindication to the administration of a medication to the client.
- Dosage Calculation
  - Perform calculations needed for medication administration.
- Medication Administration
  - Prepare and administer medications, using the rights of medication administration.

UNIT 1 PHARMACOLOGICAL PRINCIPLES

Chapter 1 Pharmacokinetics and Routes of Administration

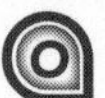

Overview

- Pharmacokinetics refers to how medications travel through the body. Medications undergo a variety of biochemical processes that result in absorption, distribution, metabolism, and excretion.

Phases of Pharmacokinetics

- Absorption is the transmission of medications from the location of administration (Gastrointestinal [GI] tract, muscle, skin, or subcutaneous tissue) to the bloodstream. The most common routes of administration are enteral (through the GI tract) and parenteral (by injection). Each of these routes will have a unique pattern of absorption.
  - The rate of medication absorption determines how soon the medication will take effect.
  - The amount of medication absorbed determines its intensity.
  - The route of administration affects the rate and amount of absorption.

ROUTES AND ABSORPTION		
ROUTE	BARRIERS TO ABSORPTION	ABSORPTION PATTERN
Oral	Medications must pass through the layer of epithelial cells that line the GI tract.	Varies greatly due to the following variables: • Stability and solubility of the medication • GI pH and emptying time • Presence of food in the stomach or intestines • Other medications currently being administered • Forms of medications (enteric-coated pills, liquids)

ROUTES AND ABSORPTION		
ROUTE	BARRIERS TO ABSORPTION	ABSORPTION PATTERN
Subcutaneous and intramuscular	The capillary wall has large spaces between cells; therefore, there is no significant barrier.	The rate of absorption is determined by: • Solubility of the medication in water ○ Highly soluble medications will be absorbed in 10 to 30 min. ○ Poorly soluble medications will be absorbed more slowly. • Blood perfusion at the site of injection ○ Sites with high blood perfusion will have rapid absorption. ○ Sites with low blood perfusion will have slow absorption.
Intravenous	No barriers	• Immediate – administered directly into blood • Complete – all of it reaches the blood

- Distribution is the transportation of medications to sites of action by bodily fluids. Distribution may be influenced by the ability to:
  - Travel to the site of action through the bloodstream (peripheral vascular or cardiac disease may delay medication distribution).
  - Leave the bloodstream by traveling between the capillaries' cells
    - Plasma protein binding: Medications compete for protein binding sites within the bloodstream, primarily albumin. The ability of a medication to bind to a protein can affect how much of the medication will leave and travel to target tissues. Two medications can compete for the same binding sites, resulting in toxicity.
    - Barriers: Medications that are lipid soluble or have a transport system can cross the blood brain barrier or the placenta.
- Metabolism (biotransformation) changes medications into less active or inactive forms by the action of enzymes. This occurs primarily in the liver, but also takes place in the kidneys, lungs, bowel, and blood.
  - Factors influencing the rate of medication metabolism include:

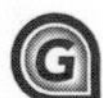

    - Age – Infants have limited medication-metabolizing capacity. The aging process can also influence medication metabolism, but varies by individual. In general, hepatic medication metabolism tends to decline with age.

        - An increase in certain medication-metabolizing enzymes – This can cause that particular medication to be metabolized sooner, requiring an increase in dosage of that medication to maintain a therapeutic level. It can also cause an increase in the metabolism of other medications that are being used concurrently.
        - First-pass effect – Some medications are inactivated on their first pass through the liver and must be given by a nonenteral route because of their high first-pass effect. These medications are usually given by alternate routes such as SL or IV.
        - Similar metabolic pathways – When two medications are metabolized by the same pathway they can interfere with the metabolism of one or both of the medications. In this way, the rate of metabolism can be decreased for one or both of the medications leading to medication accumulation.
        - Nutritional status – A malnourished client may be deficient in the factors that are necessary to produce specific medication-metabolizing enzymes. Consequently, medication metabolism may be impaired.
    - Outcomes of metabolism include:
        - Increased renal excretion of medication
        - Inactivation of medications
        - Increased therapeutic effect
        - Activation of pro-medications into active forms
        - Decreased toxicity when active forms of medications are converted to inactive forms
        - Increased toxicity when inactive forms of medications are converted to active forms
- Excretion is the elimination of medications from the body primarily through the kidneys. Elimination also takes place through the liver, lungs, bowel, and exocrine glands. Renal dysfunction may lead to an increase in duration and intensity of medication response.
- Medication responses – Plasma medication levels can be regulated to control medication responses. Medication dosing attempts to maintain plasma levels between the minimum effective concentration (MEC) and the toxic concentration. A plasma medication level is in the therapeutic range when it is effective and not toxic. Therapeutic levels are well established for many medications, and these levels can be used to monitor a client's response.
- Therapeutic index (TI) – Medications with a high TI have a wide safety margin. Therefore, there is no need for routine serum medication level monitoring. Medications with a low TI should have serum medication levels monitored closely. Monitor peak levels based on the route of administration. For example, an oral medication may have a peak of 1 to 3 hr after administration. If the medication is given intravenously, the peak time might occur within 10 min. *(Refer to a drug reference or pharmacist for specific medication peak times.)* For trough levels, blood is drawn immediately before the next medication dose regardless of the route of administration.

- Half-life (t½) refers to the period of time needed for the medication to be reduced by 50% in the body. Half-life may be affected by liver and kidney function. It usually takes four half-lives to achieve a steady state of serum concentration (medication intake = medication metabolism and excretion).

SHORT HALF-LIFE	LONG HALF-LIFE
• Medications leave the body quickly (4 to 8 hr).	• Medications leave the body more slowly (24+ hr). There is a greater risk for medication accumulation and toxicity.
• Short-dosing interval or minimum effective concentration (MEC) will drop between doses.	• Medications are given at longer intervals without loss of therapeutic effects. • Medications take a longer time to reach a steady state.

- Pharmacodynamics (mechanism of action) describes the interactions between medications and target cells, body systems, and organs to produce effects. These interactions result in functional changes that are considered the mechanism of action of the medication. Medications interact with cells in one of two ways.
    - An agonist is a medication that can mimic the receptor activity regulated by endogenous compounds. For example, morphine sulfate is classified as an agonist because it activates the receptors that produce analgesia, sedation, constipation, and other effects.
    - An antagonist is a medication that can block normal receptor activity regulated by endogenous compounds or receptor activity caused by other medications. For example, losartan (Cozaar), an angiotensin II receptor blocker, is classified as an antagonist. Losartan works by blocking angiotensin II receptors on blood vessels, which prevents vasoconstriction.
    - Partial agonists may act as an agonist/antagonist and have limited affinity to receptor sites. For example, nalbuphine (Nubain) acts as an antagonist at mu receptors and an agonist at kappa receptors, causing analgesia with minimal respiratory depression at low doses.

Routes of Administration

ROUTE OF ADMINISTRATION	NURSING IMPLICATIONS
Oral or enteral (tablets, capsules, liquids, suspensions, elixirs)	• Contraindications for oral medication administration include vomiting, absence of gag reflex, difficulty swallowing, and decreased level of consciousness. • Have the client sitting upright, in Fowler's or semi-Fowler's position to facilitate swallowing. • Administer irritating medications with small amounts of food. • Do not mix with large amounts of food or beverages in case the client is unable to consume the entire quantity. • Avoid administration with contraindicated foods or beverages such as grapefruit juice. • In general, administer oral medications on an empty stomach (1 hr before meals, 2 hr after meals). • Follow the manufacturer's directions for crushing, cutting, and diluting medications. A complete list can be found at the Institute for Safe Medication Practice's Web site (http://www.ismp.org/Tools/DoNotCrush.pdf). • Enteric-coated or time-release medications must be swallowed whole. • Time-release medications must be swallowed whole to prevent faster absorption. • Use a liquid form of the medication to facilitate swallowing whenever possible.
Sublingual (under the tongue) and buccal (between the cheek and the gum)	• Instruct clients to keep the medication in place until it is absorbed. • Clients should not eat or drink while the tablet is in place.
Liquids, suspensions, elixirs	• Follow directions for dilution and shaking. • When administering the medication, the base of the meniscus (lowest fluid line) is at the level of the desired dose.
Transdermal (medication stored in a skin patch and absorbed through the skin, producing systemic effects)	Instructions to clients should include: • Apply patches as provided to ensure proper dosing. • Wash skin with soap and water, and dry thoroughly before applying a new patch. • Place the patch on a hairless area of the skin and rotate sites to prevent skin irritation.
Topical	• Apply with a glove, tongue blade, or cotton-tipped applicator. • Never apply with a bare hand.

ROUTE OF ADMINISTRATION	NURSING IMPLICATIONS
Instillation (drops, ointments, sprays; generally used for eyes, ears, and nose)	• Eyes ○ Use surgical aseptic technique when instilling medications in eyes. ○ Have the client sit upright or lie supine with the head tilted slightly and looking up at the ceiling. ○ Rest the dominant hand on the client's forehead, hold dropper above the conjunctival sac approximately 1 to 2 cm, drop the medication into the center of sac and have the client close the eye gently. ○ Apply gentle pressure with the finger and a clean tissue on the nasolacrimal duct for 30 to 60 sec to prevent systemic absorption of the medication. • Ears ○ Use medical aseptic technique when administering medications into the ears. ○ Have the client sit upright or maintain a side-lying position. ○ Straighten the ear canal by pulling the auricle upward and outward for adults or down and back for children. Hold the dropper 1 cm above the ear canal, install the medication, and then gently apply pressure with finger to the tragus of the ear. • Nose ○ Use medical aseptic technique when administering medications into the nose. ○ Place the client supine with the head positioned to allow medication to enter the appropriate nasal passage. ○ Use the dominant hand to instill drops, supporting the head with the nondominant hand. ○ Instruct the client to breathe through the mouth, stay in a supine position, and avoid blowing his or her nose for 5 min after drop insertion.

ROUTE OF ADMINISTRATION	NURSING IMPLICATIONS
Inhalation (medications usually administered through metered dose inhalers [MDI] or dry powder inhalers [DPI])	• For an MDI, instruct the client to: o Remove the cap from the inhaler. o Shake the inhaler five to six times. o Hold the inhaler with the mouthpiece at the bottom. o Hold the inhaler with the thumb near the mouthpiece and index and middle fingers at the top. o Hold the inhaler approximately 2 to 4 cm (1 to 2 inches) away from the front of the mouth. o Take a deep breath and then exhale. o Tilt the head back slightly, and press the inhaler. While pressing the inhaler, begin a slow, deep breath that should last for 3 to 5 seconds to facilitate delivery to the air passages. o Hold breath for 10 seconds to allow medication to deposit in the airways. o Take the inhaler out of the mouth and slowly exhale through pursed lips. o Resume normal breathing. • A spacer may be used to keep the medication in the device longer thereby increasing the amount of medication delivered to the lungs and decreasing the amount of the medication in the oropharynx. If a spacer is used, instruct the client to: o Remove the covers from the mouthpieces of the inhaler and the spacer o Insert the MDI into the end of the spacer. o Shake the inhaler five to six times. o Exhale completely and then close the mouth around the spacer mouthpiece. Continue as with an MDI.

ROUTE OF ADMINISTRATION	NURSING IMPLICATIONS
Inhalation (medications usually administered through metered dose inhalers [MDI] or dry powder inhalers [DPI])	• For a DPI, instruct the client to: ○ Avoid shaking the device. ○ Take the cover off the mouthpiece. ○ Follow the directions of the manufacturer for preparing the medication, such as turning the wheel of the inhaler. ○ Exhale completely. ○ Place the mouthpiece between the lips and take a deep breath through the mouth. ○ Hold breath for 5 to 10 seconds. ○ Take the inhaler out of the mouth and slowly exhale through pursed lips. ○ Resume normal breathing. ○ If more than one puff is ordered, wait the length of time directed before administering the second puff. ○ Remove the canister and rinse the inhaler, cap, and spacer once a day with warm running water and dry completely before using again
Nasogastric and gastrostomy tubes	• Check for proper tube placement. • Use a syringe and allow the medication to flow in by gravity, or push in with the plunger of the syringe. • General guidelines ○ Use liquid forms of medications. ○ Do not give sublingual medications. ○ Do not crush specially prepared oral medications (extended/time-release, fluid-filled, enteric coated). ○ Check the compatibility of medications before mixing. ○ Do not mix medications with enteral feedings. • To prevent clogging, flush the tubing before and after each medication with 5 to 30 mL of warm water. When administration of medications is complete, flush with 30 to 60 mL of warm water.

ROUTE OF ADMINISTRATION	NURSING IMPLICATIONS
Suppositories	• Follow the manufacturer's directions for storage. • Wear gloves for the procedure. • Remove the foil wrapper and lubricate the suppository if necessary. • Rectal suppositories ○ Position the client in left lateral position. ○ Insert just beyond the internal sphincter. ○ Instruct the client to retain the medication 20 to 30 min for stimulation of defecation and 60 min for systemic absorption. • Vaginal suppositories ○ Position the client supine with knees bent, feet flat on the bed and close to hips (modified lithotomy position). ○ Suppositories are generally inserted with an applicator. ○ Instruct the client to remain in the position for a prescribed amount of time.
Parenteral	General considerations for parenteral medications include: • The vastus lateralis site is usually the recommended site for infants and children < 2 years of age. • After age 2, the ventral gluteal site can be used. Both of these sites can accommodate fluid up to 2 mL. The deltoid site has a smaller muscle mass and only can accommodate up to 1 mL of fluid. • Use a needle size and length appropriate to the type of injection and client size. Syringe size should approximate the volume of medication. • Use a tuberculin syringe for solution volume < 0.5 mL. • Rotate injection sites to enhance medication absorption, and document each site used. • Do not use injection sites that are edematous, inflamed, or have moles, birthmarks, or scars. • If medication is given intravenously, immediately monitor the client for therapeutic and side/adverse effects. • Discard all sharps (broken ampule bottles, needle) in designated containers. Containers should be leak- and puncture-proof.

ROUTE OF ADMINISTRATION	NURSING IMPLICATIONS
Intradermal	• This route is usually used for tuberculin testing or checking for medication/allergy sensitivities. • It may be used for some cancer immunotherapy. • Use small amounts of solution (0.01 to 0.1 mL) in a tuberculin syringe with a fine-gauge needle (26 to 27) in lightly pigmented, thin-skinned, hairless sites (inner surface of mid-forearm or scapular area of back) at a 10 to 15° angle.
Subcutaneous	• This route is appropriate for small doses of nonirritating, water-soluble medications and is commonly used for insulin and heparin. • Use a 3/8- to 5/8-inch, 25- to 27-gauge needle, or an insulin syringe of 28- to 31-gauge. Inject no more than 1.5 mL solution. For an average-size client, pinch up skin and inject at a 45 to 90° angle. For an obese client, use a 90° angle. • Sites are selected for adequate fat-pad size (abdomen, upper hips, lateral upper arms, thighs).
Intramuscular	• This route is appropriate for irritating medications, solutions in oils, and aqueous suspensions. • Most common sites include ventrogluteal, dorsogluteal, deltoid, and vastus lateralis (pediatric). • Use needle size 18 to 27 (usually 22- to 25-gauge), 1 to 1½ inches long, and inject at a 90° angle. Volume injected is usually 1 to 3 mL. If a greater amount is required, divide into two syringes and use two sites.
Z-Track	• Z-track is a type of IM injection that prevents medication from leaking back into subcutaneous tissue. • It is often used for medications that cause visible and/or permanent skin stains such as certain iron preparations.
Intravenous	• This route is appropriate for administration of medications, fluid, and blood products. • Vascular access devices can be for short-term use (catheters) or long-term use (infusion ports). Use 16-gauge for trauma clients, 18-gauge for surgical clients, and 22- to 24-gauge for children, older adults, medical clients, and stable postoperative clients. • Preferred sites are peripheral veins in the arm or hand. Ask the client which site he or she prefers. In neonates, veins of the head, lower legs, and feet may be used. After administration, immediately monitor for therapeutic and side/adverse effects.

ROUTE OF ADMINISTRATION	NURSING IMPLICATIONS
Epidural	• Administration of intravenous opioid analgesia (morphine [Duramorph] or fentanyl [Sublimaze]). • A catheter is advanced through a needle that is inserted into the epidural space at the level of the fourth or fifth vertebrae. • Infusion pumps are necessary to administer medication.

- Advantages and Disadvantages of Different Routes

ROUTE	ADVANTAGES	DISADVANTAGES
Oral	• The oral route is safe, inexpensive, easy and convenient.	• Oral medications have a highly variable absorption. • Inactivation can occur by GI tract or first-pass effect. • The client must be cooperative and conscious. • Contraindications include nausea and vomiting.
Subcutaneous and intramuscular	• These routes are used for poorly soluble medications. • These routes are appropriate for administering medications that are absorbed slowly for an extended period of time (depot preparations).	• Intramuscular (IM) injections are associated with a higher cost. • IM injections are inconvenient. • There can be pain with the risk for local tissue damage and nerve damage. • There is a risk for infection at the injection site.
Intravenous	• Onset is rapid, and absorption of the medication into the blood is immediate, which provides an immediate response. • This route allows control over the precise amount of medication given. • This route allows for administration of large volumes of fluid. • Irritating medications can be given with free-flowing IV fluid.	• Intravenous (IV) injections are associated with an even higher cost. • IV injections are more inconvenient. • Immediate absorption of the medication into the blood can be potentially dangerous if the wrong amount, or the wrong medication, is given. • There is an increased risk for infection or embolism with IV injections.

CHAPTER 1: PHARMACOKINETICS AND ROUTES OF ADMINISTRATION

 Application Exercises

1. Identify several factors that can influence individual differences in medication response.

2. A client is prescribed phenobarbital sodium (Luminal) for a seizure disorder. Phenobarbital has a long half-life of 4 days. Based on the half-life of phenobarbital, it will most likely be prescribed

   A. once a day.

   B. twice a day.

   C. three times a day.

   D. four times a day.

3. An order has been written to "draw peak and trough levels" for a particular medication. When should blood be drawn for each level?

4. A medication has to bind to a __________ in a cell to produce an effect.

5. Medication dosages may need to be decreased for which of the following reasons? (Select all that apply.)

   _____ Increased renal excretion

   _____ Increased medication-metabolizing enzymes

   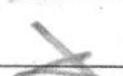 Liver failure

   _____ Peripheral vascular disease

   _____ Concurrent use of medication metabolized by the same pathway

6. Proper administration of eye drops should include which of the following nursing interventions? (Select all that apply.)

   _____ Using medical aseptic technique

   _____ Asking the client to look up at the ceiling

   _____ Having the client lie in a side-lying position

   _____ Dropping medication into the center of the client's conjunctival sac

   _____ Instructing the client to close the eye gently

CHAPTER 1: PHARMACOKINETICS AND ROUTES OF ADMINISTRATION

Application Exercises Answer Key

1. Identify several factors that can influence individual differences in medication response.

Influential factors include body weight, age, gender, genetics, biorhythmic cycles, tolerance, accumulation, psychological factors, and medical conditions.

NCLEX® Connection: Pharmacological and Parenteral Therapies: Expected Actions/ Outcomes

2. A client is prescribed phenobarbital sodium (Luminal) for a seizure disorder. Phenobarbital has a long half-life of 4 days. Based on the half-life of phenobarbital, it will most likely be prescribed

A. once a day.

B. twice a day.

C. three times a day.

D. four times a day.

Medications with long half-lives remain at their therapeutic levels between doses for long periods of time. Therefore, this medication can be administered once a day.

NCLEX® Connection: Pharmacological and Parenteral Therapies: Medication Administration

3. An order has been written to "draw peak and trough levels" for a particular medication. When should blood be drawn for each level?

Peak blood draw depends on the route of administration. Oral medications take longer to peak than medications given by the intravenous route. Trough blood draw should be done immediately before the next medication dose.

NCLEX® Connection: Pharmacological and Parenteral Therapies: Expected Actions/Outcomes

4. A medication has to bind to a __________ in a cell to produce an effect.

Receptor

For a medication (a chemical) to have an effect on the body, it must interact with other chemicals (the receptors).

NCLEX® Connection: Pharmacological and Parenteral Therapies: Expected Actions/Outcomes

5. Medication dosages may need to be decreased for which of the following reasons? (Select all that apply.)

   _____ Increased renal excretion

   _____ Increased medication-metabolizing enzymes

   __X__ **Liver failure**

   _____ Peripheral vascular disease

   __X__ **Concurrent use of medication metabolized by the same pathway**

   Liver failure can decrease metabolism and thus increase the concentration of a medication. When two medications are metabolized in the same way they may compete for metabolism, thereby increasing the concentration of one or both medications. Increased renal excretion may decrease concentration of the medication, requiring an increased dosage. Increased medication-metabolizing enzymes can decrease the concentration of the medication. The dose might need to be increased. Peripheral vascular disease may impair distribution, and more of the medication may be needed.

   NCLEX® Connection: Pharmacological and Parenteral Therapies: Expected Actions/ Outcomes

6. Proper administration of eye drops should include which of the following nursing interventions? (Select all that apply.)

   _____ Using medical aseptic technique

   __X__ **Asking the client to look up at the ceiling**

   _____ Having the client lie in a side-lying position

   __X__ **Dropping medication into the center of the client's conjunctival sac**

   __X__ **Instructing the client to close the eye gently**

   The client should be asked to look up at the ceiling, the medication should be dropped into the center of the conjunctival sac, and the client should be instructed to close the eye gently. Surgical aseptic technique is used to administer eye drops. The client should be sitting or in a supine position to facilitate proper administration of eye drops.

   NCLEX® Connection: Pharmacological and Parenteral Therapies: Medication Administration

UNIT 1 PHARMACOLOGICAL PRINCIPLES

Chapter 2 Safe Medication Administration and Error Reduction

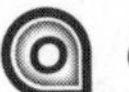

Overview

- The health care providers that are legally permitted to write prescriptions in the United States include physicians, advanced practice nurses, dentists, and physician assistants. These health care providers are responsible for:
  - Obtaining the client's medical history and physical examination
  - Diagnosing
  - Prescribing medications
  - Monitoring the response to therapy
  - Modifying medication orders as necessary

- Nurses are legally responsible for:
  - Having knowledge of federal, state (nurse practice act), and local laws, and health care facility policies that govern the prescribing, dispensing and administration of medications.
  - Preparing, administering, and evaluating client responses to medications.
  - Developing and maintaining an up-to-date knowledge base of medications administered, including uses, mechanisms of action, routes of administration, safe dosage range, side effects, adverse responses, precautions, and contraindications
  - Maintaining acceptable practice and skill competency
  - Determining accuracy of medication orders
  - Reporting all medication errors
  - Safeguarding and storing medications

Medication Category and Classification

- Nomenclature
  - Chemical name is the name of the medication determined by its chemical composition.
  - Generic name is the official or nonproprietary name that is given by the United States Adopted Names Council. Each medication has only one generic name.
  - Trade name is the brand or proprietary name given by the company that manufacturers the medication. One medication may have multiple trade names.

- Prescription medications are administered under the supervision of providers. These medications may be habit-forming, have potential harmful effects, and/or require supervision.
    - Uncontrolled substances require monitoring by a provider, but do not pose risk of abuse and/or addiction. Antibiotics are an example of uncontrolled prescription medications.
    - Controlled substances have a potential for abuse and dependence and are categorized into schedules. Heroin is a medication in Schedule I and has no medical use in the United States. Medications categorized in Schedules II through V all have approved applications. Each level has decreasing risk of abuse and dependence. For example, morphine sulfate (Duramorph) is a Schedule II medication that has a greater risk of abuse and dependence than phenobarbital (Luminal), which is a Schedule IV medication.

KNOWLEDGE REQUIRED PRIOR TO MEDICATION ADMINISTRATION	
Medication category/class	Medications may be organized according to pharmacological action, therapeutic use, body system, chemical makeup, and safe use during pregnancy. • For example, lisinopril (Zestril) is classified as an angiotensin-converting enzyme inhibitor (pharmacological action) and an antihypertensive (therapeutic use).
Mechanism of action	This is how the medication produces the desired therapeutic effect. • For example, glipizide (Glucotrol) is an oral hypoglycemic agent that lowers blood glucose levels primarily by stimulating pancreatic islet cells to release insulin.
Therapeutic effect	This is the preferred and expected effect for which the medication is administered to a specific client. One medication may have more than one therapeutic effect. • For example, one client is administered acetaminophen (Tylenol) to lower fever, whereas another client may be administered this medication to relieve pain.
Side effects	These are usually expected and inevitable when a medication is given at a therapeutic dose. • For example, morphine sulfate given for pain relief usually results in constipation. Side effects are usually identified according to body system.
Adverse effects	These are undesired, inadvertent and unexpected dangerous effects of the medication. Adverse effects are usually identified according to body system.
Toxic effects	Medications can have specific risks and manifestations of toxicity. • For example, clients taking digoxin (Lanoxin) should be monitored closely for dysrhythmias, a sign of cardiotoxicity. Hypokalemia places these clients at greater risk for digoxin toxicity.

KNOWLEDGE REQUIRED PRIOR TO MEDICATION ADMINISTRATION	
Medication interactions	Medications can interact with each other resulting in desired or undesired effects. • For example, a desired interaction is the beta-blocker atenolol (Tenormin) used concurrently with the calcium channel blocker nifedipine (Procardia) to prevent reflex tachycardia. Take complete medication history and be knowledgeable of clinically significant interactions.
Precautions/ Contraindications	Medications may be contraindicated for a client with a specific disease or condition. • For example, tetracyclines can stain developing teeth and should not be administered to children under 8 years of age. Some medications should only be used cautiously. • For example, vancomycin (Vancocin) is excreted unchanged in the kidneys and should be used cautiously in clients with renal impairment.
Preparation, dosage, administration	It is important to know any special considerations for preparation, recommended dosages, and how to administer the medication. • For example, morphine sulfate is available in 10 formulations. Oral doses of morphine are generally higher than parenteral doses due to extensive first-pass effect. Clients with chronic, severe pain, as seen with cancer, are generally given oral doses of morphine.
Nursing implications	Know how to monitor therapeutic effects, prevent and treat adverse effects, provide for comfort, and instruct clients in the safe use of medications.

Medication Prescriptions

- Each facility has written policies related to medication orders. Policies include which health care providers can write, receive, and transcribe medication orders.
- Types of medication orders include:
  - Routine order/standard order
    - A routine/standard order is an order that identifies medications that are given on a regular schedule. It may or may not have a termination date. Without a specified termination date, the order will be in effect until the provider discontinues it or the client is discharged.
    - Certain medications such as opioids and antibiotics must be reordered within a specified amount of time or will automatically be discontinued.
  - Single/one-time order
    - A single/one-time order is to be given once at a specified time or as soon as possible. For example, a one-time order instructs the nurse to give warfarin (Coumadin) 5 mg PO at 1700.

- Stat order
  - A stat order is only given once, and it is given immediately. For example, a stat order instructs the nurse to give digoxin 0.125 mg IV bolus stat.
- PRN order
  - A PRN order stipulates at what dosage, what frequency, and under what conditions a medication may be given. The nurse uses clinical judgment to determine the client's need for the medication. For example, a PRN order instructs the nurse to give morphine sulfate 2 mg IV bolus q 1 hr PRN for chest pain.
- Standing orders
  - Standing orders may be written for specific circumstances and/or for specific units. For example, the critical care unit has standing orders to treat a client with asystole.

- Components of a medication order include:
  - The client's name
  - Date and time of order
  - Name of medication (may be generic or brand)
  - Dosage of medication
  - Route of administration
  - Time and frequency of medication administration – exact times or number of times per day (dictated by facility policy or specific qualities of the medication).
  - Signature of prescribing provider.
- Communicating Medication Prescriptions
  - Origination of Medication Prescriptions
    - Medication prescriptions are written on the client's medical record by the provider or a nurse who takes a verbal or telephone prescription from a provider. If the nurse writes a medication prescription on the client's medical record facility policy specifies how much time the provider has in which to sign the prescription (usually 24 hr). Medication prescriptions are transcribed to the medication administration record (MAR) by a nurse or other health care provider.
  - Taking a telephone order:
    - If possible, have a second nurse listen on an extension.
    - Ensure that the prescription is complete and correct by reading back to the provider: the client's name, the name of the medication, the dosage, the time to be given, frequency, and route.
    - Remind the provider that the prescription must be signed within the specified amount of time.
    - Write the prescription in the client's medical record

- Medication Reconciliation
  - The Joint Commission requires policies and procedures for medication reconciliation. The nurse should compile a list of current medications ensuring that all medications are included, with correct dosages and frequency. This list should be compared with new prescriptions and reconciled to resolve any discrepancies. This list becomes the current list from which medications should be administered. This process should take place on admission, when transferring between units or facilities and at discharge.

Preassessment for Medication Therapy

- The following information should be obtained prior to the initiation of medication therapy, and updated as necessary.
  - Health History
    - Age
    - Diagnosed health problems and current reason for seeking care
    - All medications currently being taken (prescription and nonprescription): name, dose, route, and frequency of each medication
    - Any symptoms possibly related to medication therapy
    - Use of herbal or "natural" products for medicinal purposes
    - Use of caffeine, tobacco, alcohol, and/or street drugs
    - Client's understanding of the purpose of the medications
    - All known medication and food allergies
  - Physical Examination
    - A systemic physical examination provides a baseline to evaluate therapeutic effects of medication therapy and detect possible side and adverse medication effects.

Six Rights of Safe Medication Administration

- Right Client
  - Verify the client's identification each time a medication is given. The Joint Commission requires that two client identifiers be used when administering medications.
    - Acceptable identifiers include the client's name, an assigned identification number, telephone number, birth date, or another person-specific identifier.
    - Check identification bands for name, identification number, and/or photograph.
    - Check for allergies by asking the client, looking for an allergy bracelet, and reviewing the medication administration record.
    - Bar code scanners may be used to identify clients.

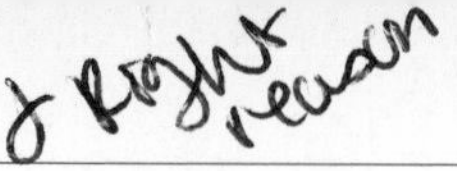

- Right Medication
  - Correctly interpret the medication order (verify completeness and clarity).
    - Read the label three times: when the container is selected, when removing the dose from container, and when the container is replaced.
    - Leave unit-dose medication in its package until administration.
- Right Dose
  - Calculate the correct medication dose.
  - Check a drug reference to ensure the dose is within the usual range.
- Right Time
  - Give medication on time to maintain consistent therapeutic blood level.
    - It is generally acceptable to give the medication ½ hr before or after the scheduled time. However, refer to the drug reference or institution policy for exceptions.
- Right Route
  - Most common routes of administration are oral, topical, subcutaneous, intramuscular (IM), and intravenous (IV).
  - Select the correct preparation for the ordered route (for example, otic vs ophthalmic topical ointment or drops).
  - Know how to administer medication safely and correctly.
- Right Documentation
  - Immediately record pertinent information, including the client's response to the medication.

Additional Considerations

- Assessment
  - Collect appropriate data before administering medication (for example, checking apical heart rate before giving digitalis preparations). Assess the client for physical and psychosocial factors that may affect medication response.
- Education
  - As part of informed consent, provide accurate information about the medication therapy and its implications (therapeutic response, side/adverse effects). To individualize the teaching, determine what the client already knows about the medication, needs to know about the medication, and wants to know about the medication.
- Evaluation
  - Determine the effectiveness of the medication based on the client's response, as well as the occurrence of side/adverse effects.

- Medication Refusal
  - Clients have the right to refuse to take a medication. Determine the reason for refusal, provide information regarding the risk of refusal, notify the appropriate health care personnel, and document refusal and actions taken.
- Resources for medication information
  - Nursing drug handbooks
  - Pharmacology textbooks
  - Professional journals
  - *Physicians' Desk Reference* (PDR)
  - Professional Web sites

Medication Error Prevention

- Common medication errors include:
  - Wrong medication or IV fluid
  - Incorrect dose or IV rate
  - Wrong client, route, or time
  - Administration of known allergic medication
  - Omission of dose
  - Incorrect discontinuation of medication or IV fluid
- Use the nursing process to prevent medication errors
  - Assessment
    - Ensure knowledge of the medication to be administered. Use appropriate resources
      - Health care providers including nurses, physicians and pharmacists
      - Poison control centers
      - Sales representatives from drug companies
      - Nursing pharmacology textbooks and drug handbooks
      - Physicians' Desk Reference
      - Newsletters including *The Medical Letter on Drugs and Therapeutics* (bimonthly) and *Prescriber's Letter* (monthly)
      - Professional journals
      - Professional Web sites

- Obtain information about the client's medical diagnoses and conditions related to medication administration such as ability to swallow, allergies, and heart, liver, and/or kidney disorders).
  - Identify client allergies.
  - Obtain necessary preadministration data (heart rate, blood pressure).
  - Omit or delay doses as indicated by the client's condition.
- Determine if the medication prescription is complete – to include name of client, date and time, name of medication, dosage, route of administration, time, frequency, and signature of prescribing provider.
- Interpret the medication prescription accurately.
  - The Institute for Safe Medication Practices is a nonprofit organization working to educate health care providers and consumers regarding safe medication practices. Tools have been developed to decrease the risk of medication errors. Go to http://www.ismp.org/ for a complete list.
    - Error-Prone Abbreviation List – Abbreviations that have been associated with a high number of medication errors
    - Confused Medication Name List – Soundalike and lookalike medication names
    - High-Alert Medication List – medications that, if given in error, have a high risk for resulting in significant patient harm
- Question the provider if the prescription is unclear or seems inappropriate for the client's condition. Refuse to give a medication if it is believed to be unsafe. Notify the charge nurse or supervisor.
- Dosage changes are usually made gradually. Question the provider if abrupt and excessive changes in dosages are made.

- Planning
  - Identify client outcomes for medication administration.
  - Set priorities.
- Implementation
  - Avoid distractions during medication preparation (poor lighting, ringing phones). Interruptions may increase the risk of error.
  - Check the labels for the medication name and concentration. Read labels carefully. Measure doses accurately and double-check high-alert medications, such as insulin and heparin, with a colleague.
  - Doses are usually 1 to 2 tablets or one single-dose vial. Question multiple tablets or vials for a single dose.
  - Follow the Six Rights of Medication Administration consistently. Take the medication administration record (MAR) to the bedside.
  - Do not give medications that were prepared by someone else.

- Encourage clients to become part of the safety net, teaching them about medications and the importance of proper identification before medications are administered. Omit or delay a dose if the client questions the size of a dose or appearance of a medication.
- Follow correct procedures for all routes of administration.
- Communicate clearly both verbally and in writing.
- Use verbal orders only for emergencies and follow facility protocol for telephone orders.
- Omit or delay doses as indicated by the client's condition, and document and report appropriately.
- Follow all laws and regulations regarding controlled substances when preparing and administering medications. Keep controlled substances in a locked area. Discarding of an excess of a controlled substances should be witnessed by a licensed health care provider.
- Only leave medication at the bedside if allowed by facility policy (for example, topical medication).

- Evaluation
  - Evaluate client response to a medication and document and report appropriately.
  - Recognize side/adverse effects and document and report appropriately.
  - Report all errors and implement corrective measures immediately.
    - Complete an unusual occurrence report within the specified time frame, usually 24 hr. This report should include:
      - The client's identification
      - The time and place of the incident
      - An accurate account of the event
      - Who was notified
      - What actions were taken
      - The signature of the person completing the report
    - This report does not become a part of the client's permanent record and the report should not be referenced in another part of the record.

CHAPTER 2: SAFE MEDICATION ADMINISTRATION & ERROR REDUCTION

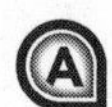

Application Exercises

1. A nurse is preparing a client's medications. Which of the following are legal responsibilities of the nurse? Select all that apply.

   ______ Maintaining skill competency
   ______ Determining the dosage
   ______ Monitoring for adverse effects
   ______ Safeguarding medications
   ______ Identifying the client's diagnosis

2. What is the nurse's responsibility when a client refuses to take a medication?

3. When preparing a medication, a nurse notes that the prescriber has doubled the previous dose of the medication. The nurse should

   A. administer the medication as prescribed.
   B. check the prescription with another nurse before giving the medication.
   C. check with the prescriber regarding the dose prescribed.
   D. record that a doubled dose was prescribed.

4. A nurse on a busy medical unit is administering 0600 medications. He enters the client's room, gently shakes the client awake, and calls her name. She awakens slowly and seems groggy. The nurse explains that he has her 0600 medication, which the client quickly takes before falling back to sleep. Outside the room, the nurse looks at the room number and realizes that he just gave the medication to the wrong client. Explain how this medication error could have been prevented.

5. Match the terms with their definitions.

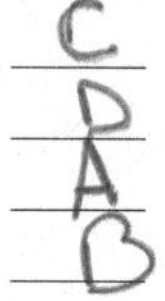

	Term	Definition
______	Contraindications	A. How the medication produces the desired therapeutic effect
______	Toxicity	B. Primary action for which the medication is prescribed
______	Mechanism of action	C. Indications for why a medication should not be given
______	Therapeutic effect	D. A serious adverse effect usually caused by excessive dosing

6. A health care provider prescribes lisinopril (Zestril) 10 mg PO every day. The nurse should recognize this as which of the following types of order?

   A. Single order
   B. Stat order
   C. Routine order
   D. Standing order

CHAPTER 2: SAFE MEDICATION ADMINISTRATION & ERROR REDUCTION

Application Exercises Answer Key

1. A nurse is preparing a client's medications. Which of the following are legal responsibilities of the nurse? Select all that apply.

   __X__ **Maintaining skill competency**

   _____ Determining the dosage

   __X__ **Monitoring for adverse effects**

   __X__ **Safeguarding medications**

   _____ Identifying the client's diagnosis

   The nurse is responsible for maintaining skill competency, monitoring for adverse effects and safeguarding medications. The prescribing provider is responsible for determining the dosage and identifying the client's diagnosis. However, the nurse is responsible for calculating correct medication dosage and checking the drug reference to ensure that the dose is within the usual range. The nurse should obtain information about the client's medical diagnoses and conditions and be familiar with why the medications are being given.

 **NCLEX® Connection: Pharmacological and Parenteral Therapies, Medication Administration**

2. What is the nurse's responsibility when a client refuses to take a medication?

   Determine the reason for the refusal, provide information regarding risk of refusal, notify the provider, and document the refusal and actions taken.

 **NCLEX® Connection: Pharmacological and Parenteral Therapies, Medication Administration**

3. When preparing a medication, a nurse notes that the prescriber has doubled the previous dose of the medication. The nurse should

   A. administer the medication as prescribed.

   B. check the prescription with another nurse before giving the medication.

   C. check with the prescriber regarding the dose prescribed.

   D. record that a doubled dose was prescribed.

   Increases in dosages are usually made gradually. Check with the provider first to determine if the new dosage is correct.

 **NCLEX® Connection: Pharmacological and Parenteral Therapies, Medication Administration**

4. A nurse on a busy medical unit is administering 0600 medications. He enters the client's room, gently shakes the client awake, and calls her name. She awakens slowly and seems groggy. The nurse explains that he has her 0600 medication, which the client quickly takes before falling back to sleep. Outside the room, the nurse looks at the room number and realizes that he just gave the medication to the wrong client. Explain how this medication error could have been prevented.

   The nurse did not use two acceptable client identifiers. The nurse relied on the client to respond to her name. Because the client had been asleep, she may have simply responded to being awakened. The nurse should have verified the client's identification by checking the identification band name, identification number, and/or photograph. The nurse should also check for allergies by asking the client, looking for an allergy bracelet, and reviewing the medical administration record.

 **NCLEX® Connection: Pharmacological and Parenteral Therapies, Medication Administration**

5. Match the terms with their definitions.

C	Contraindications	A. How the medication produces the desired therapeutic effect
D	Toxicity	B. Primary action for which the medication is prescribed
A	Mechanism of action	C. Indications for why a medication should not be given
B	Therapeutic effect	D. A serious adverse effect usually caused by excessive dosing

 **NCLEX® Connection: Pharmacological and Parenteral Therapies, Adverse Effects/Contraindications/Side Effects/Interactions**

6. A health care provider prescribes lisinopril (Zestril) 10 mg PO every day. The nurse should recognize this as which of the following types of order?

   A. Single order

   B. Stat order

   C. Routine order

   D. Standing order

   A routine order identifies a medication that should be given on a regular schedule. This medication should be given every day until discontinued. A single order is to be given once at a specified time or as soon as possible. A stat order is only given once, and it is given immediately. A standing order is written for specific circumstances or a specific unit.

 **NCLEX® Connection: Pharmacological and Parenteral Therapies, Medication Administration**

UNIT 1 PHARMACOLOGICAL PRINCIPLES

Chapter 3 Dosage Calculation

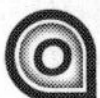

Overview

- Basic medication dose conversion and calculation skills are essential to the provision of safe nursing care.
- Regardless of the dosage calculation method used, knowledge of standard conversions and recognition of availability data are used to solve a clinical problem.
- Nurses are responsible for administering the correct amount of medication by calculating the appropriate amount of medication to give. Types of calculations required include:
    - Solid oral medication
    - Liquid oral medication
    - Injectable medication
    - Correct dose based on the client's weight
    - IV infusion
- Three methods for dosage calculation are presented. These include ratio and proportion, desired over have, and dimensional analysis.
- Standard conversion factors are as follows:
    - 1 mg = 1,000 mcg
    - 1 g = 1,000 mg
    - 1 kg = 1,000 g
    - 1 oz = 30 mL
    - 1 L = 1,000 mL
    - 1 tsp = 5 mL
    - 1 tbsp = 15 mL
    - 1 tbsp = 3 tsp
    - 1 kg = 2.2 lb
    - 1 gr = 60 mg

- General Rounding Guidelines
    - If the number to the right is equal to or greater than 5, round up by adding 1 to the number on the left.
    - If the number to the right is less than 5, round down by subtracting 1 from the number on the left.
    - For dosages less than 1.0, round to the nearest hundredth.
        - For example: The calculated dose is 0.746 mL. Look at the number in the thousandths place (6). Six is greater than 5. To round to hundredths, add 1 to 4 and drop the 6. The rounded dose is 0.75 mL.
    - For dosages greater than 1.0, round to the nearest tenth.

DOSAGE CALCULATIONS USING RATIO AND PROPORTION

- Process for calculating solid, liquid and injectable dosage using ratio and proportion

STEP 1: What is the dose needed? Dose needed = Desired

STEP 2: What is the dose available? Dose available = Have

STEP 3: Do the units of measurement need to be converted? Convert the unit of measurement of what is desired to the unit of measurement of what is available.

STEP 4: Determine the quantity of the dose available. This refers to how the medication is provided, such as 2 mL or 3 tablets.

STEP 5: Set up an equation using knowledge about basic equivalents and solve for X.

$$\frac{\text{Have}}{\text{Quantity}} = \frac{\text{Desire}}{X}$$

STEP 6: Reassess to determine if the amount to be given makes sense.

Solid dosage

Example: The provider prescribes phenytoin (Dilantin) 0.2 g PO, TID. The amount available is 200 mg/capsule. How many capsules should the nurse give?

- Follow the steps:

STEP 1: What is the dose needed? Dose needed = Desired

0.2 g

STEP 2: What is the dose available? Dose available = Have

200 mg

STEP 3: Do the units of measurement need to be converted?

Yes (g ≠ mg)

Convert the unit of measurement of what is desired to the unit of measurement of what is available.

Desire: g

Have: mg

0.2 g = X mg

Equivalents:

1 g = 1,000 mg (1 • 1,000)

Therefore:

0.2 g = 200 mg (0.2 • 1,000)

STEP 4: What is the quantity of the dose available?

1 capsule

STEP 5: Set up an equation and solve:

$$\frac{\text{Have}}{\text{Quantity}} = \frac{\text{Desire}}{\text{X}}$$

$$\frac{200 \text{ mg}}{1 \text{ capsule}} = \frac{200 \text{ mg}}{\text{X}}$$

Cross multiply and solve for X:

200X = 200

Isolate X by dividing both sides by 200:

$$\frac{200\text{X}}{200} = \frac{200}{200}$$

X = 1 capsules

STEP 6: Reassess to determine if the amount to be given makes sense. If there are 200 mg/capsule and the prescribed amount is 0.2 g or 200 mg, it makes sense to give 1 capsule.

The nurse should administer phenytoin 1 capsule PO 3 times per day.

Liquid dosage

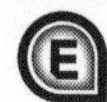 Example: The provider prescribes erythromycin estolate (Ilosone) oral suspension 0.25 g, PO, TID. The amount available is erythromycin oral suspension, 250 mg/mL. How many mL should the nurse administer with each dose?

- Follow the steps:

STEP 1: What is the dose needed? Dose needed = Desired

0.25 g

STEP 2: What is the dose available? Dose available = Have

250 mg

STEP 3: Do the units of measurement need to be converted?

Yes (g ≠ mg)

Convert the unit of measurement of what is desired to the unit of measurement of what is available.

Desire: g

Have: mg

0.25 g = X mg

Equivalents

1 g = 1,000 mg (1 • 1,000)

Therefore:

0.25 g = 250 mg (0.25 • 1,000)

STEP 4: What is the quantity of the dose available?

1 mL

STEP 5: Set up an equation and solve:

$$\frac{\text{Have}}{\text{Quantity}} = \frac{\text{Desire}}{\text{X}}$$

$$\frac{250 \text{ mg}}{1 \text{ mL}} = \frac{250 \text{ mg}}{\text{X}}$$

Cross multiply and solve for X:

250X = 250

Isolate X by dividing both sides by 250:

$$\frac{250X}{250} = \frac{250}{250}$$

$X = 1$ mL

STEP 6: Reassess to determine if the amount to be given makes sense. If there are 250 mg/mL and the prescribed amount is 0.25 g, it makes sense to give 1 mL.

The nurse should administer erythromycin estolate 1 mL PO 3 times a day.

Injectable Dosage

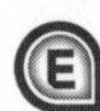

Example: The provider prescribes heparin 8,000 units subcutaneously, Q12 hr. The amount available is 5,000 units/mL. How many mL should the nurse administer?

- Follow the steps:

STEP 1: What is the dose needed? Dose needed = Desired

8,000 units

STEP 2: What is the dose available? Dose available = Have

5,000 units

STEP 3: Do the units of measurement need to be converted?

No (units = units)

STEP 4: What is the quantity of the dose available?

1 mL

STEP 5: Set up an equation and solve:

$$\frac{\text{Have}}{\text{Quantity}} = \frac{\text{Desire}}{X}$$

$$\frac{5{,}000 \text{ units}}{1 \text{ mL}} = \frac{8{,}000 \text{ units}}{X}$$

Cross multiply and solve for X:

$5{,}000X = 8{,}000$

Isolate X by dividing both sides by 5,000.

$$\frac{5{,}000X}{5{,}000} = \frac{8{,}000}{5{,}000}$$

$X = 1.6$ mL

STEP 6: Reassess to determine if the amount to be given makes sense. If there are 5,000 units/mL and the prescribed amount is 8,000 units, it makes sense to give 1.6 mL.

The nurse should administer heparin 1.6 mL subcutaneously every 12 hr.

Dosages by Weight

- Process for calculating dosage by weight using ratio and proportion
- Medications may be prescribed in daily amounts per kg of body weight such as "5 mg/kg/day," which is then divided into doses given throughout the day. The same process as for calculating oral dosages is used, but first the nurse must determine the client's weight in kg, the total daily dose, and the amount per dose.

Example: The provider prescribes cefixime (Suprax) 8 mg/kg/day PO to be given in 2 divided doses. The client weighs 22 lb. The amount available is 100 mg/5 mL suspension. How many mL should the nurse administer per dose?

STEP 1: What is the client's weight in kg?

2.2 lb = 1 kg

Client's weight in lb = X kg

Set up an equation:

$$\frac{2.2 \text{ lb}}{1 \text{ kg}} = \frac{\text{Client's weight in lb}}{\text{X kg}}$$

$$\frac{2.2 \text{ lb}}{1 \text{ kg}} = \frac{22 \text{ lb}}{\text{X kg}}$$

Cross multiply and solve for X:

2.2X = 22

X = 10 kg

STEP 2: What is the total daily dose?

Amount prescribed • kg weight (mg • kg) = total daily dose

8 mg/kg • 10 kg = 80 mg

STEP 3: What is the amount per dose?

$$\frac{\text{Total daily dose}}{\text{Number of doses prescribed per day}} = \text{Amount per dose}$$

$$\frac{80 \text{ mg}}{2 \text{ doses}} = 40 \text{ mg/dose}$$

STEP 4: What is the dose needed? Dose needed = Desired

Desired = 40 mg

STEP 5: What is the dose available? Dose available = Have

Have = 100 mg

STEP 6: Do the units of measurement need to be converted?

No (mg = mg)

STEP 7: What is the quantity of the dose available?

Quantity = 5 mL

STEP 8: Set up an equation using knowledge about basic equivalents.

$$\frac{\text{Have}}{\text{Quantity}} = \frac{\text{Desire}}{\text{X}}$$

$$\frac{100 \text{ mg}}{5 \text{ mL}} = \frac{40 \text{ mg}}{\text{X}}$$

Cross multiply and solve for X:

$$100\text{X} = 200$$

Isolate X by dividing each side by 100.

$$\frac{100\text{X}}{100} = \frac{200}{100}$$

$$\text{X} = 2 \text{ mL}$$

STEP 9: Reassess to determine if the amount to be given makes sense. If there are 100 mg/5 mL and the prescribed dose is 40 mg, it makes sense for the nurse to give 2 mL.

The nurse should administer cefixime 2 mL PO with each dose.

IV flow rates

- IV flow rates must be calculated for either:
  - Electronic IV Pumps
    - Flow rates on IV infusion pumps are set in whole mL/hr. The pump regulates the number of gtt/min based on this mL/hr setting.
    - While IV infusion pumps are usually programmed for whole numbers, most pumps are able to accept decimal flow rates. This option is usually reserved for use in the critical care setting or for pediatric clients where precise dosing is essential.

- Manual IV Infusions
  - The flow rate for Manual IV infusions is based on drops per minute.
    - Drops per minute is expressed as gtt/min.
  - Flow rate is calculated using “drop factors” found on each manufacturer’s IV tubing.
    - The drop factor is the number of drops per mL of liquid that an IV tubing set will drip into its drip chamber. Drops per mL is expressed as gtt/mL.

- Rounding
  - If a calculation results in a remaining decimal, round to the nearest whole number.
    - If the remaining decimal is less than 0.5, round down to the nearest whole number.
      - For example: Round 16.3 mL/hr to 16 mL/hr.
    - If the remaining decimal is 0.5 or greater, round up to the nearest whole number.
      - For example: Round 16.6 mL/hr to 17 mL/hr.
- When the time in hr is known, use the following formula:

$$\frac{\text{Volume (mL)}}{\text{Time (hr)}} = \text{IV flow rate (mL/hr)}$$

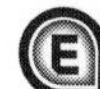

Example: The provider prescribes dextrose 5% in water 500 mL IV to infuse over the next 4 hr. The nurse should set the IV infusion pump to deliver how many mL/hr?

STEP 1: What is the volume to be infused? Volume to be infused = Volume (mL)

500 mL

STEP 2: What is the time for the infusion? Time of infusion = Time (hr)

4 hr

STEP 3: Set up an equation and solve:

$$\frac{\text{Volume (mL)}}{\text{Time (hr)}} = \text{IV flow rate (mL/hr)}$$

$$\frac{500 \text{ mL}}{4 \text{ hr}} = 125 \text{ mL/hr}$$

STEP 4: Reassess to determine if the IV flow rate makes sense. If 500 mL are to be infused in 4 hr, it makes sense to administer 125 mL/hr.

The nurse should set the IV pump to deliver 125 mL/hr.

- When the time in minutes is known, ratio and proportion may be used to find the flow rate (mL/hr):

STEP 1: What is the volume to be infused? Volume to be infused = Volume (mL)

STEP 2: What is the time for the infusion? Time of infusion = Time (min)

STEP 3: Set up an equation and solve:

$$\frac{\text{Volume (mL)}}{\text{Time (min)}} = \frac{\text{X mL}}{\text{60 min}}$$

Cross multiply and solve for X:

Time (min) • X mL = Volume (mL) • 60 min

STEP 4: Reassess to determine if the IV flow rate makes sense.

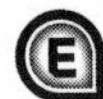

Example: The provider prescribes cefotaxime (Claforan) 1 g by intermittent IV bolus. The amount available is cefotaxime 1 g to be added to 100 mL of 0.9% sodium chloride, to infuse over 45 min. The nurse should set the IV infusion pump to deliver how many mL/hr?

- Follow these steps:

STEP 1: What is the volume to be infused? Volume to be infused = Volume (mL)

100 mL

STEP 2: What is the time for the infusion? Time of infusion = Time (min)

45 min

STEP 3: Set up an equation and solve:

$$\frac{\text{Volume (mL)}}{\text{Time (min)}} = \frac{\text{X mL}}{\text{60 min}}$$

$$\frac{\text{100 mL}}{\text{45 min}} = \frac{\text{X mL}}{\text{60 min}}$$

Cross multiply and solve for X:

45X = 6,000

X = 133.3 or 133

STEP 4: Reassess to determine if the IV flow rate makes sense. If 100 mL are to be infused in 45 min, it makes sense to administer 133 mL/hr.

The nurse should set the IV pump to deliver 133 mL/hr.

- Flow rates for manual IV infusions can easily be calculated using this simple formula:

$$\frac{\text{Volume to be infused}}{\text{Time (min)}} \cdot \text{Drop factor (gtt/mL)} = \text{IV flow rate (gtt/min)}$$

STEP 1: What is the volume to be infused? Volume to be infused = Volume (mL)

STEP 2: What is the time for the infusion? Time of infusion = Time (min)

Convert hr to min:

$$\frac{1\text{ hr}}{60\text{ min}} = \frac{\text{Prescribed hr}}{\text{X min}}$$

STEP 3: What is the drop factor on the IV tubing?

STEP 4: Set up an equation and solve:

$$\frac{\text{Volume to be infused}}{\text{Time (min)}} \cdot \text{Drop factor (gtt/mL)} = \text{IV flow rate (gtt/min)}$$

STEP 5: Reassess to determine if the IV flow rate makes sense.

Example: The provider prescribes lactated Ringer's IV 250 mL to infuse at 75 mL/hr. The drop factor on the manual IV tubing is 20 gtt/mL. The nurse should set the IV flow rate to deliver how many gtt/min?

- Follow these steps:

STEP 1: What is the volume to be infused? Volume to be infused = Volume (mL)

75 mL

STEP 2: What is the time for the infusion? Time of infusion = Time (min)

Convert hr to min:

$$\frac{1\text{ hr}}{60\text{ min}} = \frac{\text{Prescribed hr}}{\text{X min}}$$

1 hr = 60 min

STEP 3: What is the drop factor on the IV tubing?

20 gtt/mL

STEP 4: Set up an equation.

$$\frac{\text{Volume to be infused}}{\text{Time (min)}} \cdot \text{Drop factor (gtt/mL)} = \text{IV flow rate (gtt/min)}$$

$$\frac{75\text{ mL}}{60\text{ min}} \cdot 20\text{ gtt/mL} = \frac{1{,}500\text{ gtt}}{60\text{ min}} = 25\text{ gtt/min}$$

STEP 5: Reassess to determine if the IV flow rate makes sense.

The nurse should set the manual IV flow rate at 25 gtt/min.

Example: The provider prescribes ranitidine (Zantac) 150 mg by intermittent IV bolus. The amount available is dextrose 5% in water 100 mL to infuse over 30 min. The drop factor on the manual IV tubing is 10 gtt/mL. The nurse should set the IV flow rate to deliver how many gtt/min?

- Follow these steps:

  STEP 1: What is the volume to be infused? Volume to be infused = Volume (mL)

  100 mL

  STEP 2: What is the time for the infusion? Time of infusion = Time (min)

  30 min

  STEP 3: What is the drop factor on the IV tubing?

  10 gtt/mL

  STEP 4: Set up an equation.

  $$\frac{\text{Volume to be infused}}{\text{Time (min)}} \cdot \text{Drop factor (gtt/mL)} = \text{IV flow rate (gtt/min)}$$

  $$\frac{100 \text{ mL}}{30 \text{ min}} \cdot 10 \text{ gtt/mL} = \frac{1{,}000 \text{ gtt}}{30 \text{ min}} = 33.3 \text{ or } 33 \text{ gtt/min}$$

  STEP 5: Reassess to determine if the IV flow rate makes sense.

  The nurse should set the manual IV flow rate at 33 gtt/min.

DOSAGE CALCULATIONS USING THE DESIRED OVER HAVE METHOD

- Process of calculating solid, liquid and injectable dosage using the desired over have method

  STEP 1: What is the dose needed? Dose needed = Desired

  STEP 2: What is the dose available? Dose available = Have

  STEP 3: Do the units of measurement need to be converted? Convert the unit of measurement of what is desired to the unit of measurement of what is available.

  STEP 4: Determine the quantity of the dose available. Quantity of the available dose refers to how the medication is provided, such as 2 mL or 3 tablets.

  STEP 5: Set up an equation and solve:

  $$\frac{\text{Desired} \cdot \text{Quantity}}{\text{Have}} = \text{Amount to be given}$$

  STEP 6: Reassess to determine if the amount to be given makes sense.

Solid Dosages

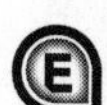

Example: The provider prescribes phenytoin (Dilantin) 0.2 g PO, TID. The amount available is 200 mg/capsule. How many capsules should the nurse give?

- Follow the steps:

STEP 1: What is the dose needed? Dose needed = Desired

0.2 g

STEP 2: What is the dose available? Dose available = Have

200 mg

STEP 3: Do the units of measurement need to be converted?

Yes (g ≠ mg)

Convert the unit of measurement of what is desired to the unit of measurement of what is available.

Desire: g

Have: mg

0.2 g = X mg

Equivalents:

1 g = 1,000 mg (1 • 1,000)

Therefore:

0.2 g = 200 mg (0.2 • 1,000)

STEP 4: What is the quantity of the dose available?

1 capsule

STEP 5: Set up an equation and solve:

$$\frac{\text{Desired} \cdot \text{Quantity}}{\text{Have}} = \text{Amount to be given}$$

$$\frac{200 \text{ mg} \cdot 1 \text{ capsule}}{200 \text{ mg}} = \text{X capsules}$$

$$\frac{200 \cdot 1}{200} = \frac{200}{200} = \text{X capsules}$$

X = 1 capsule

STEP 6: Reassess to determine if the amount to be given makes sense. If there are 200 mg/capsule and the prescribed amount is 0.2 g or 200 mg, it makes sense to give 1 capsule.

The nurse should administer phenytoin 1 capsule PO 3 times per day.

Liquid dosage

Example: The provider prescribes erythromycin estolate (Ilosone) oral suspension 0.25 g, PO, TID. The amount available is erythromycin oral suspension, 250 mg/mL. How many mL should the nurse administer with each dose?

- Follow these steps

STEP 1: What is the dose needed? Dose needed = Desired

0.25 g

STEP 2: What is the dose available? Dose available = Have

250 mg

STEP 3: Do the units of measurement need to be converted?

Yes (g ≠ mg)

Convert the unit of measurement of what is desired to the unit of measurement of what is available.

Desire: g

Have: mg

0.25 g = X mg

Equivalents

1 g = 1,000 mg (1 • 1,000)

Therefore:

0.25 g = 250 mg (0.25 • 1,000)

STEP 4: What is the quantity of the dose available?

1 mL

STEP 5: Set up an equation and solve:

$$\frac{\text{Desired} \cdot \text{Quantity}}{\text{Have}} = \text{Amount to be given}$$

$$\frac{250 \text{ mg} \cdot 1 \text{ mL}}{250 \text{ mg}} = \text{X mL}$$

$$\frac{250 \cdot 1}{250} = \frac{250}{250} = X \text{ mL}$$

X = 1 mL

STEP 6: Reassess to determine if the amount to be given makes sense. If there are 250 mg/mL and the prescribed amount is 250 mg, it makes sense to give 1 mL.

The nurse should administer erythromycin estolate 1 mL PO 3 times a day.

Injectable Dosage

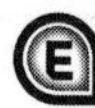

Example: The provider prescribes heparin 8,000 units subcutaneously, every 12 hr. The amount available is 5,000 units/mL. How many mL should the nurse administer?

- Follow the steps:

STEP 1: What is the dose needed? Dose needed = Desired

8,000 units

STEP 2: What is the dose available? Dose available = Have

5,000 units

STEP 3: Do the units of measurement need to be converted?

No (units = units)

STEP 4: What is the quantity of the dose available?

1 mL

STEP 5: Set up an equation and solve:

$$\frac{\text{Desired} \cdot \text{Quantity}}{\text{Have}} = \text{Amount to be given}$$

$$\frac{8{,}000 \text{ units} \cdot 1 \text{ mL}}{5{,}000 \text{ units}} = X \text{ mL}$$

$$\frac{8{,}000 \cdot 1}{5{,}000} = \frac{8{,}000}{5{,}000} = X \text{ mL}$$

X = 1.6 mL

STEP 6: Reassess to determine if the amount to be given makes sense. If there are 5,000 units/mL and the prescribed amount is 8,000 units, it makes sense to give 1.6 mL.

The nurse should administer heparin 1.6 mL subcutaneously every 12 hr.

Dosages by Weight

- Process for calculating dosage by weight using the desired over have method
  - Medications may be prescribed in daily amounts per kg of body weight such as "5 mg/kg/day" which is then divided into doses given throughout the day. The same process as for calculating oral dosages is used, but first the nurse must determine the client's weight in kg, the total daily dose, and the amount per dose.

Example: The provider prescribes cefixime (Suprax) 8 mg/kg/day PO to be given in 2 divided doses. The client weighs 22 lb. The amount available is 100 mg/5 mL suspension. How many mL should the nurse administer per dose?

STEP 1: What is the client's weight in kg?

2.2 lb = 1 kg

Client's weight in lb = X kg

Set up an equation:

$$\frac{2.2 \text{ lb}}{1 \text{ kg}} = \frac{\text{Client's weight in lb}}{\text{X kg}}$$

$$\frac{2.2 \text{ lb}}{1 \text{ kg}} = \frac{22 \text{ lb}}{\text{X}}$$

Cross multiply and solve for X:

2.2X = 22

X = 10 kg

STEP 2: What is the total daily dose?

Amount prescribed • kg weight (mg • kg) = total daily dose

8 mg/kg • 10 kg = 80 mg

STEP 3: What is the amount per dose?

$$\frac{\text{Total daily dose}}{\text{Number of doses prescribed per day}} = \text{Amount per dose}$$

$$\frac{80 \text{ mg}}{2 \text{ doses}} = 40 \text{ mg/dose}$$

STEP 4: What is the dose needed? Dose needed = Desired

Desired = 40 mg

STEP 5: What is the dose available? Dose available = Have

Have = 100 mg

STEP 6: Do the units of measurement need to be converted?

No (mg = mg)

STEP 7: What is the quantity of the dose available?

Quantity = 5 mL

STEP 8: Set up an equation:

$$\frac{\text{Desired} \bullet \text{Quantity}}{\text{Have}} = \text{Amount to be given}$$

$$\frac{40 \text{ mg} \bullet 5 \text{ mL}}{100 \text{ mg}} = \text{X mL}$$

$$\frac{40 \bullet 5}{100 \text{ mg}} = \text{X mL}$$

$$\frac{40 \bullet 5}{100} = \frac{200}{100} = \text{X mL}$$

X = 2 mL

STEP 9: Reassess to determine if the amount to be given makes sense. If there are 100 mg/5 mL and the prescribed dose is 40 mg, it makes sense for the nurse to give 2 mL.

The nurse should administer cefixime 2 mL PO with each dose.

DOSAGE CALCULATIONS USING DIMENSIONAL ANALYSIS

- Dimensional analysis is a method of calculation in which a series of ratios or factors, organized in the form of fractions, are multiplied.
  - Factors are two quantities that are related, such as 30 mg in 2 mL.
  - In dimensional analysis factors are expressed as fractions.
  - 30 mg in 2 mL may be expressed as:

$$\frac{30 \text{ mg}}{2 \text{ mL}} \text{ or } \frac{2 \text{ mL}}{30 \text{ mg}}$$

- One unit of measurement is converted to another unit of measurement by means of conversion factors or unit equivalence. A conversion factor is a unit equivalence such as 2.2 lb = 1 kg or 1,000 mcg = 1 mg.
  - Conversion factors link units of measurement of what is desired with units of measurement of what is available.

- Conversion factors are arranged in the form of a fraction.
- 1,000 mcg = 1 mg may be expressed as:

$$\frac{1{,}000\text{ mcg}}{1\text{ mg}} \text{ or } \frac{1\text{ mg}}{1{,}000\text{ mcg}}$$

- To create an equation using dimensional analysis:
  - Start with the unit of measurement that is to be calculated:
    - For example, when converting mcg to mg, mg are desired, so start with:

      mg =
  - Find the quantity with the same unit of measurement or the conversion factor with the same unit of measurement as what is desired (1 mg = 1,000 mcg) and place this (mg) in the numerator.

$$\text{mg} = \frac{1\text{ mg}}{1{,}000\text{ mcg}}$$

    - Remember, fractions are set up as the numerator over the denominator:

$$\frac{\text{numerator}}{\text{denominator}}$$

  - The fractions are arranged so that unwanted units cancel out and desired units remain.
    - A single quantity not associated with a related quantity is expressed as a fraction by placing it in the numerator and placing 1 in the denominator.

$$\frac{\text{X mcg}}{1}$$

  - If mcg are available and mg are desired, arrange the conversion factor so that mcg may be cancelled out to leave mg remaining:

$$\text{mg} = \frac{1\text{ mg}}{1{,}000\text{ mcg}} \bullet \frac{\text{X mcg}}{1}$$

    Cross out the identical units that are across and diagonal:

$$\text{mg} = \frac{1\text{ mg}}{1{,}000\ \cancel{\text{mcg}}} \bullet \frac{\text{X}\ \cancel{\text{mcg}}}{1}$$

  - In dimensional analysis, fractions are multiplied. To multiply fractions, first multiply across the numerator, and then multiply across the denominator. Finally, divide the numerator by the denominator.
  - Equations involving multiple factors are arranged so that the unit of measurement in the denominator of one factor is placed in the numerator of the following factor and so on. Unwanted units are then cancelled.

- Remember:
    - A single quantity not associated with a related quantity is expressed as a fraction by placing it in the numerator and placing 1 in the denominator.
    - Factors are two quantities that are related. Related quantities are arranged as fractions.
- Process of calculating dosage using dimensional analysis:

STEP 1: What is to be calculated?

What is the unit of measurement that is to be calculated?

STEP 2: What quantities are needed? Needed = desired

The quantity needed may be the prescribed dosage.

STEP 3: What quantities are available? Available = have

STEP 4: Are conversion factors needed to find the units that are to be calculated?

Conversion factors link units of measurement of what is available with units of measurement of what is to be calculated.

STEP 5: Set up an equation of factors using needed and available quantities and the conversion factors.

STEP 6: Multiply the numerator.

Multiply the denominator.

Divide the numerator by the denominator.

STEP 7: Reassess to determine if the amount makes sense.

Solid dosages

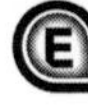

Example: The provider prescribes phenytoin (Dilantin) 0.2 g PO, TID. The amount available is 200 mg/capsule. How many capsules should the nurse give?

- Follow the steps:

STEP 1: What is to be calculated?

What is the unit of measurement that is to be calculated?

capsule

STEP 2: What quantities are needed? Needed = desired

The quantity needed may be the prescribed dosage.

0.2 g/1

STEP 3: What quantities are available? Available = have

200 mg/capsule

STEP 4: Are conversion factors needed to find what is desired?

Conversion factors link units of measurement of what is available with units of measurement of what is desired.

1,000 mg = 1 g

STEP 5: Set up an equation of factors using needed and available quantities and the conversion factors.

$$\text{capsule} = \frac{1\text{ capsule}}{200\text{ mg}} \bullet \frac{1{,}000\text{ mg}}{1\text{ g}} \bullet \frac{0.2\text{ g}}{1}$$

Cancel out identical units:

$$\text{capsule} = \frac{1\text{ capsule}}{200\text{ }\cancel{\text{mg}}} \bullet \frac{1{,}000\text{ }\cancel{\text{mg}}}{1\text{ }\cancel{\text{g}}} \bullet \frac{0.2\text{ }\cancel{\text{g}}}{1}$$

STEP 6: Multiply the numerator.

Multiply the denominator.

Divide the numerator by the denominator.

$$\text{capsule} = \frac{200\text{ capsule}}{200} = 1\text{ capsule}$$

STEP 7: Reassess to determine if the amount to be given makes sense. If there are 200 mg/capsule and the prescribed amount is 0.2 g or 200 mg, it makes sense to give 1 capsule.

The nurse should administer phenytoin 1 capsule PO 3 times per day.

Liquid dosage

Example: The provider prescribes erythromycin estolate (Ilosone) oral suspension 0.25 g, PO, TID. The amount available is erythromycin oral suspension, 250 mg/mL. How many mL should the nurse administer with each dose?

- Follow the steps:

STEP 1: What is to be calculated?

What is the unit of measurement that is to be calculated?

mL

STEP 2: What quantities are needed? Needed = desired

The quantity needed may be the prescribed dosage.

0.25g/1

STEP 3: What quantities are available? Available = have

250 mg/mL

STEP 4: Are conversion factors needed to find what is desired?

Conversion factors link units of measurement of what is available with units of measurement of what is desired.

1 g = 1,000 mg

STEP 5: Set up an equation of factors using needed and available quantities and the conversion factors.

$$\text{mL} = \frac{1\text{ mL}}{250\text{ mg}} \bullet \frac{1{,}000\text{ mg}}{1\text{ g}} \bullet \frac{0.25\text{ g}}{1}$$

Cancel out identical units:

$$\text{mL} = \frac{1\text{ mL}}{250\text{ }\cancel{\text{mg}}} \bullet \frac{1{,}000\text{ }\cancel{\text{mg}}}{1\text{ }\cancel{\text{g}}} \bullet \frac{0.25\text{ }\cancel{\text{g}}}{1}$$

STEP 6: Multiply the numerator.

Multiply the denominator.

Divide the numerator by the denominator.

$$\text{mL} = \frac{250\text{ mL}}{250} = 1\text{ mL}$$

STEP 7: Reassess to determine if the amount to be given makes sense. If there are 250 mg/mL and the prescribed amount is 250 mg, it makes sense to give 1 mL.

The nurse should administer erythromycin estolate 1 mL PO 3 times a day.

Injectable Dosage

Example: The provider prescribes heparin 8,000 units subcutaneously, every 12 hr. The amount available is 5,000 units/mL. How many mL should the nurse administer?

- Follow the steps:

STEP 1: What is to be calculated?

What is the unit of measurement that is to be calculated?

mL

STEP 2: What quantities are needed? Needed = desired

The quantity needed may be the prescribed dosage.

8,000 units/1

STEP 3: What quantities are available? Available = have

5,000 units /mL

STEP 4: Are conversion factors needed to find what is desired?

Conversion factors link units of measurement of what is available with units of measurement of what is desired.

No

STEP 5: Set up an equation of factors using needed and available quantities and the conversion factors.

$$\text{mL} = \frac{1\ \text{mL}}{5{,}000\ \text{units}} \bullet \frac{8{,}000\ \text{units}}{1}$$

Cancel out identical units:

$$\text{mL} = \frac{1\ \text{mL}}{5{,}000\ \cancel{\text{units}}} \bullet \frac{8{,}000\ \cancel{\text{units}}}{1}$$

STEP 6: Multiply the numerator.

Multiply the denominator.

Divide the numerator by the denominator.

$$\text{mL} = \frac{8{,}000\ \text{mL}}{5{,}000} = 1.6\ \text{mL}$$

STEP 7: Reassess to determine if the amount to be given makes sense. If there are 5,000 units in 1 mL and the prescribed amount is 8,000 units, it makes sense to give 1.6 mL.

The nurse should administer heparin 1.6 mL subcutaneously every 12 hr.

Dosages by Weight

- Process for calculating dosage by weight using dimensional analysis
  - Medications may be prescribed in daily amounts per kg of body weight such as "5 mg/kg/day," which is then divided into doses given throughout the day. Use the same process as for calculating oral dosages.

Example: The provider prescribes cefixime (Suprax) 8 mg/kg/day PO to be given in 2 divided doses. The client weighs 22 lb. The amount available is 100 mg/5 mL suspension. How many mL should the nurse administer per dose?

- Follow these steps:

STEP 1: What is to be calculated?

What is the unit of measurement that is to be calculated?

mL/dose

STEP 2: What quantities are needed? Needed = desired

The quantity needed may be the prescribed dosage.

8 mg/kg/day

STEP 3: What quantities are available? Available = have

2 doses/day

22 lb/1

100 mg/5 mL

STEP 4: Are conversion factors needed to find the units that are wanted?

Conversion factors link units of measurement of what is available with units of measurement of what is to be calculated.

2.2 lb = 1 kg

STEP 5: Set up an equation of factors using needed and available quantities and the conversion factors.

$$\text{mL/dose} = \frac{5\ \text{mL}}{100\ \text{mg}} \bullet \frac{8\ \text{mg}}{\text{kg/day}} \bullet \frac{1\ \text{kg}}{2.2\ \text{lb}} \bullet \frac{22\ \text{lb}}{1} \bullet \frac{1\ \text{day}}{2\ \text{doses}}$$

Cancel out identical units:

$$\text{mL/dose} = \frac{5\ \text{mL}}{100\ \cancel{\text{mg}}} \bullet \frac{8\ \cancel{\text{mg}}}{\cancel{\text{kg/day}}} \bullet \frac{1\ \cancel{\text{kg}}}{2.2\ \cancel{\text{lb}}} \bullet \frac{22\ \cancel{\text{lb}}}{1} \bullet \frac{1\ \cancel{\text{day}}}{2\ \text{doses}}$$

STEP 6: Multiply the numerator.

Multiply the denominator.

Divide the numerator by the denominator.

$$\text{mL/dose} = \frac{5\ \text{mL} \bullet 8 \bullet 22}{100 \bullet 2.2 \bullet 2\ \text{dose}} \bullet \frac{880\ \text{mL}}{440\ \text{dose}} = 2\ \text{mL/dose}$$

STEP 7: Reassess to determine if the amount to be given makes sense.

The nurse should administer cefixime 2 mL PO with each dose.

IV Flow Rates

- To determine mL/hr when administering fluid via an IV pump, the process is the same as the ratio and proportion/desired over have methods.
- When calculating gtt/min, follow these steps:

STEP 1: What is to be calculated?

What is the unit of measurement that is to be calculated?

gtt/min

STEP 2: What quantities are needed? Needed = desired

The quantity needed may be the prescribed dosage.

Volume (mL)/infusion time (min or hr)

STEP 3: What quantities are available? Available = have

Drop factor (gtt/mL)

STEP 4: Are conversion factors needed to find what is desired?

Conversion factors link units of measurement of what is available with units of measurement of what is desired.

60 min = 1 hr

STEP 5: Set up an equation of factors using needed and available quantities and the conversion factors.

- If minutes are available, the process is the same as the ratio and proportion/desired over have methods.
- If hours are available:

$$\text{IV flow rate (gtt/min)} = \frac{\text{gtt}}{\text{mL}} \cdot \frac{\text{Volume (mL)}}{\text{Time (hr)}} \cdot \frac{1 \text{ hr}}{60 \text{ min}}$$

Cancel out identical units:

$$\text{IV flow rate (gtt/min)} = \frac{\text{gtt}}{\cancel{\text{mL}}} \cdot \frac{\text{Volume (}\cancel{\text{mL}}\text{)}}{\text{Time (}\cancel{\text{hr}}\text{)}} \cdot \frac{1 \cancel{\text{hr}}}{60 \text{ min}}$$

STEP 6: Multiply the numerator.

Multiply the denominator.

Divide the numerator by the denominator.

STEP 7: Reassess to determine if the amount makes sense.

Example: The provider prescribes lactated Ringer's 250 mL to infuse at 75 mL/hr. The drop factor on the manual IV tubing is 20 gtt/mL. The nurse should set the IV flow rate to deliver how many gtt/min?

STEP 1: What is to be calculated?

What is the unit of measurement that is to be calculated?

gtt/min

STEP 2: What quantities are needed? Needed = desired

The quantity needed may be the prescribed dosage.

75 mL/hr

STEP 3: What quantities are available? Available = have

20 gtt/mL

STEP 4: Are conversion factors needed to find what is desired?

Conversion factors link units of measurement of what is available with units of measurement of what is desired.

60 min = 1 hr

STEP 5: Set up an equation of factors using needed and available quantities and the conversion factors.

- Hours are available:

$$\text{IV flow rate (gtt/min)} = \frac{20\text{ gtt}}{1\text{ mL}} \bullet \frac{75\text{ mL}}{1\text{ hr}} \bullet \frac{1\text{ hr}}{60\text{ min}}$$

Cancel out identical units:

$$\text{IV flow rate (gtt/min)} = \frac{20\text{ gtt}}{1\text{ }\cancel{\text{mL}}} \bullet \frac{75\text{ }\cancel{\text{mL}}}{1\text{ }\cancel{\text{hr}}} \bullet \frac{1\text{ }\cancel{\text{hr}}}{60\text{ min}}$$

STEP 6: Multiply the numerator.

Multiply the denominator.

Divide the numerator by the denominator.

$$\text{IV flow rate (gtt/min)} = \frac{1{,}500\text{ gtt}}{60\text{ min}} = 25\text{ gtt/min}$$

STEP 7: Reassess to determine if the amount makes sense.

The nurse should set the manual IV flow rate at 25 gtt/min.

CHAPTER 3: DOSAGE CALCULATION

Application Exercises

Directions: Solve each problem using ratio and proportion.

1. The provider prescribes cefotaxime sodium (Claforan) 500 mg by intermittent intravenous bolus every 12 hr. The amount available is cefotaxime 500 mg in dextrose 5% in water 100 mL to infuse over 45 min. The drop factor shown on the package of IV tubing is 10 gtt/mL. The nurse should set the IV to deliver how many gtt/min?

2. The provider prescribes clindamycin (Cleocin) 200 mg by intermittent IV bolus every 8 hr. The amount available is clindamycin 200 mg in 100 mL to infuse over 30 min. The nurse should set the IV pump to deliver how many mL/hr?

3. The provider prescribes 0.9% sodium chloride 1 L IV to infuse at 50 mL/hr. The drop factor on the manual IV tubing is 20 gtt/mL. The nurse should set the IV flow rate to deliver how many gtt/min?

Directions: Solve each problem using the desired over have method.

4. The provider prescribes furosemide (Lasix) oral solution 80 mg PO daily. The amount available is furosemide 40 mg/5 mL. How many mL should the nurse administer?

5. The provider prescribes dextrose 5% in water 750 mL IV to infuse over 6 hr. The nurse should set the IV pump to deliver how many mL/hr?

Directions: Solve each problem using dimensional analysis.

6. The provider prescribes haloperidol (Haldol) 2 mg, PO BID. The amount available is 1 mg/tablet. How many tablets should the nurse administer?

7. The provider prescribes amoxicillin (Amoxil) 20 mg/kg/day PO to be given in 2 divided doses. The client weighs 44 lb. The amount available is amoxicillin 250 mg/5 mL. How many mL should the nurse administer per dose?

CHAPTER 3: DOSAGE CALCULATION

Application Exercises Answer Key

Directions: Solve each problem using ratio and proportion.

1. The provider prescribes cefotaxime sodium (Claforan) 500 mg by intermittent intravenous bolus every 12 hr. The amount available is cefotaxime 500 mg in dextrose 5% in water 100 mL to infuse over 45 min. The drop factor shown on the package of IV tubing is 10 gtt/mL. The nurse should set the IV to deliver how many gtt/min?

STEP 1: What is the dose needed? Dose needed = Desired

100 mL

STEP 2: What is the time for the infusion? Time of infusion = Time (min)

45 min

STEP 3: What is the drop factor on the IV tubing?

10 gtt/mL

STEP 4: Set up an equation.

$$\frac{\text{Volume to be infused}}{\text{Time (min)}} \bullet \text{Drop factor (gtt/mL)} = \text{IV flow rate (gtt/min)}$$

$$\frac{100 \text{ mL}}{45 \text{ min}} \bullet 10 \text{ gtt/mL} = \frac{1{,}000 \text{ gtt}}{45 \text{ min}} = 22.2 \text{ or } 22 \text{ gtt/min}$$

STEP 5: Reassess to determine if the IV flow rate makes sense.

The nurse should set the manual IV flow rate at 22 gtt/min.

NCLEX® Connection: Pharmacological and Parenteral Therapies: Parenteral/Intravenous Therapy

2. The provider prescribes clindamycin (Cleocin) 200 mg by intermittent IV bolus every 8 hr. The amount available is clindamycin 200 mg in 100 mL to infuse over 30 min. The nurse should set the IV pump to deliver how many mL/hr?

STEP 1: What is the volume to be infused? Volume to be infused = Volume (mL)

100 mL

STEP 2: What is the time for the infusion? Time of infusion = Time (min)

30 min

STEP 3: Set up an equation and solve:

$$\frac{\text{Volume (mL)}}{\text{Time (min)}} = \frac{\text{X mL}}{\text{60 min}}$$

$$\frac{\text{100 mL}}{\text{30 min}} = \frac{\text{X mL}}{\text{60 min}}$$

Cross multiply and solve for X:

$30X = 6{,}000$

$X = 200$

STEP 4: Reassess to determine if the IV flow rate makes sense. If 100 mL are to be infused in 30 min, it makes sense to administer 200 mL/hr.

The nurse should set the IV pump to deliver 200 mL/hr.

NCLEX® Connection: Pharmacological and Parenteral Therapies: Parenteral/Intravenous Therapy

3. The provider prescribes 0.9% sodium chloride 1 L IV to infuse at 50 mL/hr. The drop factor on the manual IV tubing is 20 gtt/mL. The nurse should set the IV flow rate to deliver how many gtt/min?

STEP 1: What is the volume to be infused? Volume to be infused = Volume (mL)

50 mL

STEP 2: What is the time for the infusion? Time of infusion = Time (min)

Convert hr to min:

$$\frac{\text{60 min}}{\text{1 hr}} = \frac{\text{X min}}{\text{prescribed hr}}$$

60 min = 1 hr

STEP 3: What is the drop factor on the IV tubing?

20 gtt/mL

STEP 4: Set up an equation.

$$\frac{\text{Volume to be infused}}{\text{Time (min)}} \cdot \text{Drop factor (gtt/mL)} = \text{IV flow rate (gtt/min)}$$

$$\frac{\text{50 mL}}{\text{60 min}} \cdot \text{20 gtt/mL} = \frac{\text{1,000 gtt}}{\text{60 min}} = \text{16.6 or 17 gtt/min}$$

STEP 5: Reassess to determine if the IV flow rate makes sense.

The nurse should set the manual IV flow rate at 17 gtt/min.

NCLEX® Connection: Pharmacological and Parenteral Therapies: Parenteral/Intravenous Therapy

Directions: Solve each problem using the desired over have method.

4. The provider prescribes furosemide (Lasix) oral solution 80 mg PO daily. The amount available is furosemide 40 mg/5 mL. How many mL should the nurse administer?

STEP 1: What is the dose needed? Dose needed = Desired

80 mg

STEP 2: What is the dose available? Dose available = Have

40 mg

STEP 3: Do the units of measurement need to be converted?

No (mg = mg)

STEP 4: What is the quantity of the dose available?

5 mL

STEP 5: Set up an equation and solve:

$$\frac{\text{Desired} \cdot \text{Quantity}}{\text{Have}} = \text{Amount to be given}$$

$$\frac{80 \text{ mg} \cdot 5 \text{ mL}}{40 \text{ mg}} = \text{X mL}$$

$$\frac{80 \cdot 5}{40} = \frac{400}{40} = \text{X mL}$$

X = 10 mL

STEP 6: Reassess to determine if the amount to be given makes sense. If there are 40 mg/5 mL and the prescribed amount is 80 mg, it makes sense to give 10 mL.

The nurse should administer furosemide 10 mL PO daily.

NCLEX® Connection: Pharmacological and Parenteral Therapies: Dosage Calculation

5. The provider prescribes dextrose 5% in water 750 mL IV to infuse over 6 hr. The nurse should set the IV pump to deliver how many mL/hr?

STEP 1: What is the volume to be infused? Volume to be infused = Volume (mL)

750 mL

STEP 2: What is the time for the infusion? Time of infusion = Time (hr)

6 hr

STEP 3: Set up an equation and solve:

$$\frac{\text{Volume (mL)}}{\text{Time (hr)}} = \text{IV flow rate (mL/hr)}$$

$$\frac{750 \text{ mL}}{6 \text{ hr}} = 125 \text{ mL/hr}$$

STEP 4: Reassess to determine if the IV flow rate makes sense. If 750 mL are to be infused in 6 hr it makes sense to administer 125 mL/hr.

The nurse should set the IV pump to deliver 125 mL/hr.

NCLEX® Connection: Pharmacological and Parenteral Therapies: Dosage Calculation

Directions: Solve each problem using dimensional analysis.

6. The provider prescribes haloperidol (Haldol) 2 mg, PO BID. The amount available is 1 mg/tablet. How many tablets should the nurse administer?

STEP 1: What is to be calculated?

What is the unit of measurement that is to be calculated?

tablets

STEP 2: What quantities are needed? Needed = desired

The quantity needed may be the prescribed dosage.

2 mg/1

STEP 3: What quantities are available? Available = have

1 mg/tablet

STEP 4: Are conversion factors needed to find what is desired?

Conversion factors link units of measurement of what is available with units of measurement of what is desired.

No

STEP 5: Set up an equation of factors using needed and available quantities and the conversion factors.

$$\text{tablet} = \frac{1\ \text{tablet}}{1\ \text{mg}} \bullet \frac{2\ \text{mg}}{1}$$

Cancel out identical units:

$$\text{tablet} = \frac{1\ \text{tablet}}{1\ \cancel{\text{mg}}} \bullet \frac{2\ \cancel{\text{mg}}}{1}$$

STEP 6: Multiply the numerator.

Multiply the denominator.

Divide the numerator by the denominator.

$$\text{tablet} = \frac{1\ \text{tablet} \bullet 2}{1} = 2\ \text{tablets}$$

STEP 7: Reassess to determine if the amount to be given makes sense. If there is 1 mg/tablet and the prescribed amount is 2 mg, it makes sense to give 2 tablets.

The nurse should administer haloperidol 2 tablets PO 2 times per day.

NCLEX® Connection: Pharmacological and Parenteral Therapies: Dosage Calculation

7. The provider prescribes amoxicillin (Amoxil) 20 mg/kg/day PO to be given in 2 divided doses. The client weighs 44 lb. The amount available is amoxicillin 250 mg/5 mL. How many mL should the nurse administer per dose?

STEP 1: What is to be calculated?

What is the unit of measurement that is to be calculated?

mL/dose

STEP 2: What quantities are needed? Needed = desired

The quantity needed may be the prescribed dosage.

20 mg/kg/day

STEP 3: What quantities are available? Available = have

2 doses/day

44 lb/1

250 mg/5 mL

STEP 4: Are conversion factors needed to find what is desired?

Conversion factors link units of measurement of what is available with units of measurement of what is desired.

2.2 lb = 1 kg

STEP 5: Set up an equation of factors using needed and available quantities and the conversion factors.

$$\text{mL/dose} = \frac{5\text{ mL}}{250\text{ mg}} \bullet \frac{20\text{ mg}}{\text{kg/day}} \bullet \frac{1\text{ kg}}{2.2\text{ lb}} \bullet \frac{44\text{ lb}}{1} \bullet \frac{1\text{ day}}{2\text{ doses}}$$

Cancel out identical units:

$$\text{mL/dose} = \frac{5\text{ mL}}{250\ \cancel{\text{mg}}} \bullet \frac{20\ \cancel{\text{mg}}}{\cancel{\text{kg/day}}} \bullet \frac{1\ \cancel{\text{kg}}}{2.2\ \cancel{\text{lb}}} \bullet \frac{44\ \cancel{\text{lb}}}{1} \bullet \frac{1\ \cancel{\text{day}}}{2\text{ doses}}$$

STEP 6: Multiply the numerator.

Multiply the denominator.

Divide the numerator by the denominator.

$$\text{mL/dose} = \frac{5\text{ mL} \bullet 20 \bullet 44}{100 \bullet 2.2 \bullet 2 \bullet \text{dose}} \bullet \frac{4{,}400\text{ mL}}{1{,}100\text{ dose}} = 4\text{ mL/dose}$$

STEP 7: Reassess to determine if the amount to be given makes sense.

The nurse should administer amoxicillin 4 mL PO with each dose.

NCLEX® Connection: Pharmacological and Parenteral Therapies: Dosage Calculation

UNIT 1 PHARMACOLOGICAL PRINCIPLES

Chapter 4 Intravenous Therapy

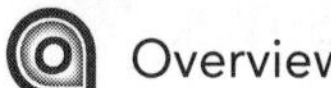

Overview

- Intravenous therapy involves administering fluids via an intravenous catheter for the purpose of providing medications, supplementing fluid intake, or giving fluid replacement, electrolytes, or nutrients.
- Large-volume IV infusions are administered on a continuous basis.
- An IV medication infusion may be mixed in a large volume of fluid and given as a continuous IV infusion or mixed in a small amount of solution and given intermittently. It can also be administered as an IV bolus: The medication is given in a small amount of solution, concentrated or diluted, and injected over a short time (1 to 2 min).

Indications and Risk Factors

- Advantages and Disadvantages of IV Therapy

ADVANTAGES	DISADVANTAGES
• Fast absorption and onset of action • Less discomfort after initial insertion • Maintains constant therapeutic blood levels • Less irritation to subcutaneous and muscle tissue	• Circulatory fluid overload is possible if the infusion is large and/or too rapid. • Immediate absorption leaves no time to correct errors. • IV administration can cause irritation to the lining of the vein. • Failure to maintain surgical asepsis can lead to local infection and septicemia.

Description of Procedure

- The provider prescribes the type of IV fluid, volume to be infused, and either the rate at which the IV fluid should be infused or the total amount of time it should take for the fluid to be infused. The nurse regulates the IV infusion to insure the appropriate amount is administered. This can be done with an IV pump or manually.
- Large-volume IV infusions are administered on a continuous basis such as 0.9% sodium chloride IV to infuse at 100 mL/hr or 0.9% sodium chloride 1,000 mL to be given IV over 3 hr.
- A fluid bolus is a large amount of IV fluid given in a short period of time, usually less than an hour. It is given to rapidly replace fluid loss that could be caused by dehydration, shock, hemorrhage, burns, or trauma.
  - A large-gauge angiocatheter (18 gauge or larger) is needed to maintain the rapid rate necessary to give a fluid bolus to an adult.

- IV medication infusions may be administered in the following ways:
  - The medication may be mixed in a large volume of fluid (500 to 1,000 mL) and given as continuous IV infusion. Potassium chloride may be administered this way.
  - The medication can be found in premixed solution bags or can be added to the IV bag by the pharmacist or the nurse.
  - Volume-controlled infusions
    - Some medications, such as antibiotics, are given intermittently in a small amount of solution (25 to 250 mL) through a continuous IV system, or with saline or heparin lock systems.
    - The medications infuse for short periods of time and are given on a scheduled basis.
    - These infusions can be administered by a piggyback IV bag or bottle or tandem setup, volume-control administration set, or mini-infusion pump.
  - IV bolus dose administration
    - The medications are typically in small amounts of solution, concentrated or diluted, that can be injected over a short time (1 to 2 min) in emergent and nonemergent situations.
    - Some medications, such as pain medications, are given directly into the peripheral IV or access port to achieve an immediate medication level in the bloodstream.
    - Make sure medications are prepared according to recommended concentration and administered according to the safe recommended rate.
    - Use extreme caution and observe for signs and symptoms of complications (redness, burning, or increasing pain).
- Types of IV Access
  - Intravenous access can be via a peripheral or central vein (central venous access device).
  - Central venous access devices can be peripherally inserted or directly inserted into the jugular or subclavian vein.

Guidelines for Safe IV Medication Administration

- Certain medications, such as potassium chloride, can cause serious adverse reactions and should be infused on an IV pump for accurate dosage control and never given by IV bolus.
- Add medication to a new IV fluid container, not to an IV container that is already hanging.
- Never administer IV medication through tubing that is infusing blood, blood products, or parenteral nutritional solutions.
- Verify compatibility of medications before infusing a medication through tubing that is infusing another medication.

- Needlestick Prevention
    - Be familiar with IV insertion equipment.
    - Avoid using needles when needleless systems are available.
    - Use protective safety devices when available.
    - Dispose of needles immediately in designated puncture-resistant receptacles.
    - Do not break, bend, or recap needles.
- Special Considerations

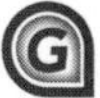

    - Older adult clients, clients taking anticoagulants, or clients with fragile veins:
        - Avoid tourniquets.
        - Use a blood pressure cuff instead.
        - Do not slap the extremity to visualize veins.
    - Edema in extremities:
        - Apply digital pressure over the selected vein to displace edema.
        - Apply pressure with an alcohol pad.
        - Cannulation must be quick.
    - Obese clients may require the use of anatomical landmarks to find veins.

- Preventing IV Infections
    - Use standard precautions.
    - Change IV sites according to facility/agency policy (usually 72 hr).
    - Remove catheters as soon as they are no longer clinically indicated.
    - Change catheter if any break in surgical aseptic technique is suspected, such as emergency insertions.
    - Use sterile needle/catheter for each insertion attempt.
    - Avoid writing on IV bags with pens or markers, because ink could contaminate the solution.
    - Change tubing immediately if contamination is known or suspected.
    - Fluids should not hang more than 24 hr unless it is a closed system (pressure bags for hemodynamic monitoring).
    - Wipe all ports with alcohol or an antiseptic swab before connecting IV lines or inserting a syringe to prevent the introduction of micro-organisms into the system.
    - Never disconnect tubing for convenience or to position the client.
    - Do not allow ports to remain exposed to air.
    - Perform hand hygiene before and after handling the IV system.

Preprocedure

- Equipment
    - Correct size catheter:
        - 16 gauge for trauma clients, rapid fluid volume
        - 18 gauge for surgical clients, rapid blood administration
        - 22 to 24 gauge all other clients (adults)
    - Correct tubing
    - Infusion pump, if indicated
    - Clean gloves
    - Scissors or electric shaver for hair removal
- Nursing Actions
    - Check the provider's order (e.g., solution, rate).
    - Assess the client for allergies to products used in initiating and maintaining IV therapy (latex, tape, iodine).
    - Follow the Six Rights of medication administration (including compatibilities of all IV solutions).
    - Perform hand hygiene.
    - Examine the solution to be infused for clarity, leaks, and expiration date.
    - Prime tubing as indicated.
    - Don clean gloves before insertion.
    - Assess extremities and veins. If hair removal is needed, clip it with scissors or shave it with an electric shaver.
- Client Education
    - Identify the client and explain the procedure.
    - Place the client in a comfortable position.

Intraprocedure

- Nursing Actions
    - Use a clean tourniquet or blood pressure cuff (especially for older adults), 4 to 6 inches above the selected site to compress only venous blood flow.
    - Select vein by choosing:
        - Distal veins first on the nondominant hand
        - A site that is not painful or bruised and will not interfere with activity
        - A vein that is resilient with a soft, bouncy feeling

    - Additional methods to enhance venous access include:
        - Gravity, fist clenching, friction with alcohol, and heat
        - Percussion with gentle tapping
    - Avoid:
        - Varicosed veins that are permanently dilated and tortuous
        - Veins in the inner wrist with bifurcations, in flexion areas, near valves (appearing as bumps), in lower extremities, and in the antecubital fossa (except for emergency access)
        - Veins that are sclerosed or hard
        - Veins in an extremity with impaired sensitivity (scar tissue, paralysis), lymph nodes removed, recent infiltration, or arteriovenous fistula/graft
- Untie the tourniquet or deflate the BP cuff.
- Cleanse the area at the site using friction in a circular motion from the middle and outward with alcohol, iodine preparation, or chlorhexidine. Allow to air dry for 1 to 2 min.
- Remove cover from catheter, grasp plastic hub, and examine device for smooth edges.
- Retie the tourniquet, or reinflate the BP cuff.
- Anchor the vein below the site of insertion.
- Pull skin taut and hold it.
- Warn the client of a sharp, quick stick.
- Insert the catheter into the skin with bevel up at an angle of 10° to 30° using steady, smooth motion.
- Advance the catheter through the skin and into the vein, maintaining a 10 to 30° angle. Flashback of blood will confirm placement in vein.
- Lower the hub of the catheter close to the skin to prepare for threading into the vein, approximately ¼ in.
- Loosen the needle from the catheter and pull back slightly on the needle so that it no longer extends past the tip of the catheter.
- Use the thumb and index finger to advance the catheter into the vein until the hub rests against the insertion site.
- Stabilize the IV catheter with one hand and release the tourniquet with the other.
- Apply pressure approximately 1¼ in (3 cm) above the insertion site with the middle finger and stabilize the catheter with the index finger.
- Remove the needle and activate the safety device.
- Maintain pressure above the IV site and connect the appropriate equipment to the hub of the IV catheter.

- Apply dressing per facility protocol. The dressing is usually left in place until the catheter is removed, unless it becomes damp, loose, or soiled.
- Avoid encircling the entire extremity with tape, and taping under the sterile dressing.
- If continuous IV infusion is prescribed, regulate IV infusion rate according to the provider's order.
- Dispose of used equipment properly.
- Document in chart:
  - Date and time of insertion
  - Insertion site and appearance
  - Catheter size
  - Type of dressing
  - IV fluid and rate (if applicable)
  - Number, locations, and conditions of site-attempted cannulations
  - Client response
  - Sample documentation: 1/1/2010, 1635, #22-gauge IV catheter inserted into left wrist cephalic vein (1 attempt) with sterile occlusive dressing applied. IV D_5LR infusing at 100 mL/hr per infusion pump without redness or edema at the site. Tolerated without complications. J. Doe, RN

Postprocedure

- Nursing Actions
  - Maintaining patency of IV access
    - Do not stop a continuous infusion or allow blood to back up into the catheter for any length of time. Clots can form at the tip of the needle or catheter and can be lodged against the vein wall, blocking the flow of fluid.
    - Instruct the client not to manipulate flow rate device, change settings on IV pump, or lie on the tubing.
    - Make sure the IV insertion site dressing is not too tight.
    - Flush intermittent IV catheters with appropriate solution after every medication administration or every 8 to 12 hr when not in use.
    - Monitor site and infusion rate at least every hour.
  - Discontinuing IV therapy
    - Check order/prepare equipment.
    - Perform hand hygiene.
    - Don clean gloves.
    - Remove tape and dressing, stabilizing IV.

- Clamp IV tubing.
- Apply sterile gauze pad over the site without putting pressure on the vein. Do not use alcohol.
- Using the other hand, withdraw the catheter by pulling straight back from the site.
- Elevate and apply pressure for 2 min.
- Assess the site.
- Apply tape over gauze.
- Use pressure dressing, if needed.
- Assess the catheter for intactness.
- Document.

Complications

- Complications require notification of the provider and complete documentation. All IVs should be restarted with new tubing and catheters.

COMPLICATIONS	FINDINGS	TREATMENT	PREVENTION
Infiltration	Pallor, local swelling at the site, decreased skin temperature around the site, damp dressing, slowed infusion	• Stop the infusion and remove the catheter. • Elevate the extremity. • Encourage active range of motion. • Apply warm compresses three to four times/day. • Restart the infusion proximal to the site or in another extremity.	• Carefully select site and catheter. • Secure the catheter.
Phlebitis/ thrombophlebitis	Edema; throbbing, burning, or pain at the site; increased skin temperature; erythema; a red line up the arm with a palpable band at the vein site; slowed infusion	• Promptly discontinue the infusion and remove the catheter. • Elevate the extremity. • Apply warm compresses three to four times/day. • Restart the infusion proximal to the site or in another extremity. • Culture the site and catheter if drainage is present.	• Rotate sites at least every 72 hr. • Avoid the lower extremities. • Use hand hygiene. • Use surgical aseptic technique.

COMPLICATIONS	FINDINGS	TREATMENT	PREVENTION
Hematoma	Ecchymosis at site	• Do not apply alcohol. • Apply pressure after IV catheter removal. • Use warm compress and elevation after bleeding stops.	• Minimize tourniquet time. • Remove the tourniquet before starting IV infusion. • Maintain pressure after IV catheter removal.
Cellulitis	Pain; warmth; edema; induration; red streaking; fever, chills, and malaise	• Promptly discontinue the infusion and remove catheter. • Elevate the extremity. • Apply warm compresses three to four times/day. • Culture the site and cannula if drainage is present. • Administer: ○ Antibiotics ○ Analgesics ○ Antipyretics	• Rotate sites at least every 72 hr. • Avoid the lower extremities. • Use hand hygiene. • Use surgical aseptic technique.
Fluid overload	Distended neck veins, increased blood pressure, tachycardia, shortness of breath, crackles in the lungs, edema	• Stop infusion. • Raise the head of the bed. • Assess vital signs. • Adjust rate as prescribed. • Administer diuretics if prescribed.	• Use an infusion pump. • Monitor I&O.
Catheter embolus	Missing catheter tip when discontinued; severe pain at the site with migration, or no symptoms if no migration	• Place the tourniquet high on the extremity to limit venous flow. • Prepare for removal under x-ray or via surgery. • Save the catheter after removal to determine the cause.	• Do not reinsert the stylet into the catheter.

CHAPTER 4: INTRAVENOUS THERAPY

Application Exercises

1. When assessing the IV site for phlebitis, the nurse should look for which of the following findings? (Select all that apply.)

   ____ Red line on affected extremity
   ____ An increased rate of infusion
   ____ Palpable, hard mass or band above insertion site
   ____ Cool, pale skin
   ____ Pain at site

2. Which of the following techniques will minimize the risk of catheter embolism?

   A. Use hand hygiene before and after IV insertion.
   B. Rotate the IV sites at least every 72 hr.
   C. Administer anticoagulants.
   D. Once in the vein, never put the stylet back through the catheter.

3. The nurse checks for patency of an IV saline lock by

   A. assessing the site for redness.
   B. flushing the IV saline lock with 0.9% normal saline.
   C. asking the client if the site is painful.
   D. checking the date of insertion.

4. A nurse is caring for a client receiving dextrose 5% in water IV at 100 mL/hr. Which of the following may indicate fluid overload? (Select all that apply)

   ____ Decreased blood pressure
   ____ Bradycardia
   ____ Shortness of breath
   ____ Crackles heard in lungs
   ____ Distended neck veins.

CHAPTER 4: INTRAVENOUS THERAPY

Application Exercises Answer Key

1. When assessing the IV site for phlebitis, the nurse should look for which of the following findings? (Select all that apply.)

  __X__ **Red line on affected extremity**

  _____ An increased rate of infusion

  __X__ **Palpable, hard mass or band above insertion site**

  _____ Cool, pale skin

  __X__ **Pain at site**

A red line over the vein of the affected extremity; a palpable, hardened band above the insertion site; and pain at the site are signs and symptoms of phlebitis. The rate of the infusion slows down with phlebitis. The skin is warm and red.

NCLEX® Connection: Pharmacological and Parenteral Therapies, Parenteral/Intravenous Therapy

2. Which of the following techniques will minimize the risk of catheter embolism?

  A. Use hand hygiene before and after IV insertion.

  B. Rotate the IV sites at least every 72 hr.

  C. Administer anticoagulants.

  D. Once in the vein, never put the stylet back through the catheter.

Reinsertion of the stylet can damage the catheter, causing a small portion to break off and enter the venous system. Hand hygiene will prevent infection. Rotating IV sites will prevent phlebitis and thrombosis. A catheter embolism is not related to blood clotting.

NCLEX® Connection: Pharmacological and Parenteral Therapies, Parenteral/Intravenous Therapy

3. The nurse checks for patency of an IV saline lock by

  A. assessing the site for redness.

  B. flushing the IV saline lock with 0.9% normal saline.

  C. asking the client if the site is painful.

  D. checking the date of insertion.

Free flow of solution through the IV indicates patency. Absence of redness and reports of pain are not positive indicators of IV patency. How long an IV has been in will not determine if it is still patent.

NCLEX® Connection: Pharmacological and Parenteral Therapies, Parenteral/Intravenous Therapy

4. A nurse is caring for a client receiving dextrose 5% in water IV at 100 mL/hr. Which of the following may indicate fluid overload? (Select all that apply)

    ______ Decreased blood pressure

    ______ Bradycardia

    __X__ **Shortness of breath**

    __X__ **Crackles heard in lungs**

    __X__ **Distended neck veins.**

    Findings of fluid overload include increased blood pressure, tachycardia, shortness of breath, crackles heard in the lungs, and distended neck veins.

NCLEX® Connection: Pharmacological and Parenteral Therapies, Parenteral/Intravenous Therapy

UNIT 1 PHARMACOLOGICAL PRINCIPLES

Chapter 5 Adverse Effects, Interactions, and Contraindications

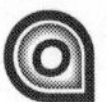

Overview

- To ensure safe medication administration and prevent errors, the nurse must know why a medication is prescribed and the intended therapeutic effect. In addition the nurse must be aware of potential side/adverse effects, interactions, contraindications, and precautions.
- Every medication has the potential to cause side effects and/or adverse effects. Side effects are usually expected when a medication is given at a therapeutic dose. Adverse effects are undesired, inadvertent, and unexpected dangerous effects of the medication. Adverse effects can occur at both therapeutic and higher than therapeutic doses.
- Medications are chemicals that affect the body. When more than one medication is given there is a potential for an interaction. In addition, medications can interact with foods.
- Contraindications and precautions of specific medications refer to client conditions that make it unsafe or potentially harmful to administer these medications.

Side/Adverse Medication Effects

- These effects may be classified according to body systems

SIDE/ADVERSE MEDICATION EFFECTS	NURSING INTERVENTIONS/CLIENT EDUCATION
Central nervous system (CNS) effects may result from either CNS stimulation (excitement) or CNS depression.	• If CNS stimulation is expected, clients may be at risk for seizures, and precautions should be taken. • If CNS depression is likely, clients should be advised not to drive or participate in other activities that can be dangerous.
Extrapyramidal symptoms (EPS) (abnormal body movements) may include involuntary fine motor tremors, rigidity, uncontrollable restlessness, and acute dystonias (spastic movements and/or muscle rigidity affecting the head, neck, eyes, facial area, and limbs). These may occur within a few hr or may take months to develop.	• Extrapyramidal symptoms are more often associated with medications affecting the CNS, such as those used to treat mental health disorders.

SIDE/ADVERSE MEDICATION EFFECTS	NURSING INTERVENTIONS/CLIENT EDUCATION
Anticholinergic effects are side effects that are a result of muscarinic receptor blockade. Most effects are seen in the eye, smooth muscle, exocrine glands, and the heart.	• Teach clients how to manage these effects. For example, dry mouth may be relieved by sipping on liquids; photophobia can be managed by use of sunglasses; and urinary retention may be reduced by urinating before taking the medication.
Cardiovascular effects may involve blood vessels and the heart.	• Antihypertensives can cause orthostatic hypotension. • Instruct clients about signs of postural hypotension (lightheadedness, dizziness). If these occur, advise the client to sit or lie down. Postural hypotension can be minimized by getting up and changing position slowly.
Gastrointestinal (GI) effects may result from local irritation of the GI tract. Stimulation of the vomiting center also results in adverse effects.	• NSAIDs may cause GI upset. Advise the client to take these medications with food.
Hematologic effects are relatively common and potentially life-threatening with some groups of medications.	• Bone marrow depression/suppression is generally associated with anticancer medications and hemorrhagic disorders with anticoagulants and thrombolytics. Educate clients taking anticoagulants about signs and symptoms of bleeding (bruising, discolored urine/stool, petechiae, bleeding gums). Tell clients to notify the provider if these effects occur.
Hepatotoxicity may occur with many medications. Because most medications are metabolized in the liver, the liver is particularly vulnerable to drug-induced injury. Damage to liver cells can impair metabolism of many medications, causing medication accumulation in the body and producing adverse effects. Many medications can alter normal values of liver function tests with no obvious clinical signs of liver dysfunction.	• When two or more medications that are hepatotoxic are combined, the risk for liver damage is increased. • Liver function tests are indicated when a client starts a medication known to be hepatotoxic and periodically thereafter.
Nephrotoxicity may occur with a number of medications, but is primarily the result of certain antimicrobial agents and NSAIDs. Damage to the kidneys may interfere with medication excretion leading to medication accumulation and adverse effects.	• Aminoglycosides may cause renal damage. Monitor serum creatinine and BUN levels of clients taking an aminoglycoside.

SIDE/ADVERSE MEDICATION EFFECTS	NURSING INTERVENTIONS/CLIENT EDUCATION
Toxicity is an adverse medication effect that is considered severe and may be life-threatening. It may be caused by an excessive dose, but can also occur at therapeutic dose levels.	• Liver damage will occur with an acetaminophen (Tylenol) overdose. There is a greater risk of liver damage with chronic alcohol use. The antidote acetylcysteine (Mucomyst) may be used to minimize liver damage.
Allergic reaction occurs when an individual develops an immune response to a medication. The individual has been previously exposed to the medication and has developed antibodies.	• Allergic reactions range from minor to serious. Mild rashes and hives can be treated with diphenhydramine (Benadryl). • Before administering any medications, take a complete medication history.
Anaphylactic reaction is a life-threatening, immediate allergic reaction that causes respiratory distress, severe bronchospasm, and cardiovascular collapse.	• Treat with epinephrine, bronchodilators, and antihistamines. Provide respiratory support and inform the provider.
Immunosuppression is decreased or absent immune response.	• Glucocorticoids depress the immune response and increase the risk for infection. • Monitor clients taking a glucocorticoid for signs and symptoms of infection.

Drug-Drug Interactions

	CONSEQUENCES OF DRUG-DRUG INTERACTIONS
TYPE OF INTERACTION	NURSING IMPLICATIONS/INTERVENTIONS
Increase therapeutic effects	• Some medications may be given together to increase therapeutic effects. Clients with asthma are instructed to use albuterol (Proventil), a $beta_2$-adrenergic agonist inhaler, 5 min prior to using triamcinolone acetonide (Azmacort), a glucocorticoid inhaler, to increase the absorption of triamcinolone acetonide.
Increase side/adverse effects	• Clients may take two medications that have the same side/adverse effect. Taking these two medications together increases the risk of these effects. Diazepam (Valium) and hydrocodone bitartrate 5 mg/acetaminophen 500 mg (Vicodin) both have CNS depressant effects. When these medications are used together, the client has an increased risk for CNS depression.
Decrease therapeutic effects	• One medication can increase the metabolism of a second medication and therefore decrease the serum level and effectiveness of the second medication. For example: phenytoin (Dilantin) increases hepatic medication-metabolizing enzymes that affect warfarin (Coumadin) and thereby decreases the serum level and the effect of warfarin.

CONSEQUENCES OF DRUG-DRUG INTERACTIONS	
TYPE OF INTERACTION	NURSING IMPLICATIONS/INTERVENTIONS
Decrease side/ adverse effects	• One medication can be given to counteract the side/adverse effects of another medication. Ondansetron hydrochloride (Zofran), an antiemetic, may be administered to counteract the side effects of nausea and vomiting for a client receiving chemotherapy.
Increase serum levels, leading to toxicity	• One medication can decrease the metabolism of a second medication and therefore increase the serum level of the second medication. This may lead to toxicity. Fluconazole (Diflucan) inhibits hepatic medication-metabolizing enzymes that affect aripiprazole (Abilify) and thereby increases serum levels of this medication.

<table>
<tr><th colspan="2">OVER-THE-COUNTER (OTC) MEDICATIONS</th></tr>
<tr><th>INTERACTIONS</th><th>NURSING IMPLICATIONS/INTERVENTIONS</th></tr>
<tr><td>Ingredients in OTC medications may interact with other OTC or prescription medications.</td><td rowspan="3">• Obtain a complete medication history.
• Instruct clients to follow the manufacturer's recommendation for dosage.</td></tr>
<tr><td>Inactive ingredients such as dyes, alcohol, or preservatives may cause adverse reactions.</td></tr>
<tr><td>Potential for overdose exists because of the use of several preparations (including prescription medications) with similar ingredients.</td></tr>
<tr><td>Interactions of certain prescription and OTC medications can interfere with therapeutic effects.</td><td>• Clients are advised to use caution and to check with their provider before using any OTC preparations such as antacids, laxatives, decongestants, or cough syrups. For example, antacids can interfere with the absorption of ranitidine (Zantac) and other medications. Advise clients to take antacids 1 hr apart from other medications.</td></tr>
</table>

Medication-Food Interactions

- Food may alter medication absorption and/or may contain substances that react with certain medications.
- Examples include:

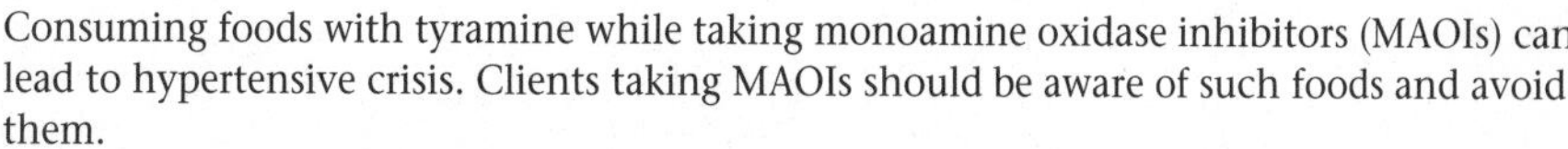

  - Consuming foods with tyramine while taking monoamine oxidase inhibitors (MAOIs) can lead to hypertensive crisis. Clients taking MAOIs should be aware of such foods and avoid them.
  - Vitamin K can decrease the therapeutic effects of warfarin (Coumadin) and place clients at risk for developing blood clots. Clients taking warfarin should include a consistent amount of vitamin K in their diet.

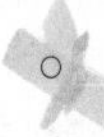

- Tetracycline can interact with a chelating agent such as milk, and form an insoluble, unabsorbable compound. Instruct clients not to take tetracycline within 2 hr of consuming any dairy products.
- Grapefruit juice seems to act by inhibiting presystemic medication metabolism in the small bowel, thus increasing absorption of certain oral medications. This either increases effects or adverse reactions. Clients should be instructed not to drink grapefruit juice if they are taking such a medication.

Contraindications and Precautions

- A specific medication may be contraindicated for a client based on the client's condition. For example, penicillins are contraindicated for clients who have an allergy to this medication.
- Precautions should be taken for a client who is more likely to have an adverse reaction than another client. Morphine sulfate (Duramorph) depresses respiratory function, so it should be used with caution for clients who have asthma or impaired respiratory function.
- The US Food and Drug Administration places medications in categories based on risk to a fetus.
    - Category A: There is no evidence of risk to fetus during pregnancy based on adequate and well-controlled studies.
    - Category B: There is no evidence of risk to animal fetus based on studies but there are no adequate and well-controlled studies in pregnant women.
    - Category C: Adverse effects have been demonstrated on animal fetuses. There are no adequate and well-controlled studies in pregnant women but use of the medication during pregnancy may be warranted based on the potential benefits.
    - Category D: Adverse effects have been demonstrated on human fetuses based on data from investigational or marketing experience, but use of the medication during pregnancy may be warranted based on the potential benefits.
    - Category X: Adverse effects have been demonstrated on animal and human fetuses based on studies and data from investigational or marketing experience. The use of the medication is contraindicated during pregnancy because the risks outweigh the potential benefits.

CHAPTER 5: ADVERSE EFFECTS, INTERACTIONS, AND CONTRAINDICATIONS

 Application Exercises

1. Which of the following statements by a client receiving warfarin (Coumadin) indicates a need for further teaching?

   A. "I take a laxative about once a week."

   B. "I apply sunscreen before I go outside."

   C. "I need an antacid after a spicy meal."

   D. "I use aspirin when I have a headache."

2. A nurse is ready to administer the first dose of a new oral penicillin prescription to a client. The client states she took penicillin 3 years ago and developed a rash. Based on this information, the nurse should

   A. give the medication as prescribed and observe for a reaction.

   B. administer the medication intravenously to bypass gastric absorption.

   C. withhold the medication and inform the provider of the client's previous reaction.

   D. combine the medication with an antihistamine to decrease the possibility of a reaction.

3. A nursing responsibility for a client receiving an antihypertensive medication is to

   A. increase the dose if the client experiences tachycardia.

   B. teach the client to change positions slowly to avoid dizziness or fainting.

   C. instruct the client to check his blood pressure every 8 hr.

   D. discontinue the client's medication if blood pressure decreases.

4. Do drug-drug interactions produce increased or decreased medication effects? Explain.

CHAPTER 5: ADVERSE EFFECTS, INTERACTIONS, AND CONTRAINDICATIONS

Application Exercises Answer Key

1. Which of the following statements by a client receiving warfarin (Coumadin) indicates a need for further teaching?

   A. "I take a laxative about once a week."

   B. "I apply sunscreen before I go outside."

   C. "I need an antacid after a spicy meal."

   D. "I use aspirin when I have a headache."

   Aspirin decreases platelet aggregation. Warfarin suppresses coagulation. Concurrent use increases the risk for bleeding. If used concurrently, dosage adjustments will be necessary. Taking a laxative once a week, using sunscreen when outside and needing an antacid after a spicy meal does not require further teaching.

NCLEX® Connection: Pharmacological and Parenteral Therapies, Adverse Effects/ Contraindications/Side Effects/Interactions

2. A nurse is ready to administer the first dose of a new oral penicillin prescription to a client. The client states she took penicillin 3 years ago and developed a rash. Based on this information, the nurse should

   A. give the medication as prescribed and observe for a reaction.

   B. administer the medication intravenously to bypass gastric absorption.

   C. withhold the medication and inform the provider of the client's previous reaction.

   D. combine the medication with an antihistamine to decrease the possibility of a reaction.

   The client was exposed to penicillin 3 years ago and is now sensitized to the medication. Re-exposure to this medication can cause an allergic reaction, ranging from mild to life threatening. Therefore, it is important for the provider to be informed of the client's prior sensitization. The provider may choose to use a different medication.

NCLEX® Connection: Pharmacological and Parenteral Therapies, Adverse Effects/ Contraindications/Side Effects/Interactions

3. A nursing responsibility for a client receiving an antihypertensive medication is to

   A. increase the dose if the client experiences tachycardia.

   B. teach the client to change positions slowly to avoid dizziness or fainting.

   C. instruct the client to check his blood pressure every 8 hr.

   D. discontinue the client's medication if blood pressure decreases.

   Orthostatic hypotension is a common side effect of antihypertensives. Changing positions slowly allows the body to adjust to the change and prevents dizziness or fainting. It is not within the scope of practice for the nurse to change the dose, it is not necessary for the client to check his blood pressure every 8 hr, and it is not within the scope of practice for the nurse to discontinue the client's medication.

NCLEX® Connection: Pharmacological and Parenteral Therapies, Medication Administration

4. Do drug-drug interactions produce increased or decreased medication effects? Explain.

   Drug-drug interactions may produce increased or decreased medication effects. These effects can be beneficial or detrimental to the client.

NCLEX® Connection: Pharmacological and Parenteral Therapies, Adverse Effects/Contraindications/Side Effects/Interactions

UNIT 1 PHARMACOLOGICAL PRINCIPLES

Chapter 6 Individual Considerations of Medication Administration

Individual Considerations of Medication Administration

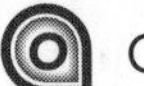

Overview

- Various factors may affect how clients respond to medications. It is important for nurses to recognize these factors in order to individualize nursing care when administering medications.

Factors Affecting Medication Dosages and Responses

- Body weight – Because medications are absorbed and distributed in body tissue, individuals with a greater body mass may require larger doses.

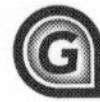

- Age – Young children with immature liver and kidney function, and older adults, often with reduced liver and kidney function, may require proportionately smaller medication doses.
- Gender – Females may respond differently to medications than males due to a higher proportion of body fat and the effects of female hormones.
- Genetics – Genetic factors such as missing enzymes can alter the metabolism of certain medications, thus enhancing or reducing medication action.
- Biorhythmic cycles – Responses to certain medications vary with the biologic rhythms of the body. For example, hypnotic medications work better when given at the usual sleep time than at other times.
- Tolerance – Reduced responsiveness to a medication may be either congenital (genetic factors) or acquired (stimulation of liver enzymes or other physiologic variations). Cross-tolerance may occur with other chemically similar medications.
- Accumulation – Medication concentration in the body can be increased by the inability to metabolize or excrete a medication rapidly enough, resulting in a toxic medication effect. For older adults, decreased renal function is the major cause of medication accumulation leading to toxicity.
- Psychological factors – Emotional state and expectations can influence the effects of a medication. A term used to describe positive medication effects influenced by psychological factors is the placebo effect.
- Medical Conditions
    - Inadequate gastric acid inhibits the absorption of medications that require an acid medium to dissolve.

- Diarrhea causes oral medications to pass too quickly through the GI tract to be absorbed.
- Vascular insufficiency prevents distribution of a medication to affected tissue.
- Liver disease/failure impairs medication metabolism, which may cause toxicity.
- Kidney disease/failure prevents or delays medication excretion, which may cause toxicity.

Pharmacology and Children

- While most medications administered to adults are useful for children, the dosages are different. Pediatric dosages are based on body weight or body surface area (BSA). Neonates (< 1 month old) and infants (1 month to 1 year old) have immature liver and kidney function, alkaline gastric juices, and an immature blood-brain barrier. Certain medication dosages are based on age due to greater risk for decreased skeletal bone growth, acute cardiopulmonary failure, or hepatic toxicity.
- Additional pharmacokinetic factors specific to children include:
    - Decreased gastric acid production and slower gastric emptying time
    - Decreased first-pass medication metabolism
    - Increased absorption of topical medications (greater body surface area and thinner skin)
    - Lower blood pressure (more blood flow to the liver and brain and less blood flow to the kidneys)
    - Higher body water content (dilutes water-soluble medications)
    - Decreased serum protein-binding sites (until age 1). There may be an increase in serum medication level of protein-binding medications
- Be particularly alert when administering medications to children due to the risk for medication errors.
    - Dosages are usually based on weight or body surface area (BSA).
    - Most medications are not tested on children.
    - Adult medication forms and concentrations may require dilution, calculation, preparation, and administration of very small doses.
    - Limited sites exist for IV medication administration.

Pharmacology and Older Adults (65+ Years)

- Physiologic changes associated with aging that impact pharmacokinetics include:
    - Increased gastric pH (alkaline)
    - Decreased GI motility and gastric emptying time
    - Decreased blood flow through cardiovascular system, liver, and kidneys

  - Decreased hepatic enzyme function
  - Decreased kidney function and glomerular filtration rate
  - Decreased protein-binding sites
  - Decreased body water, increased body fat, and decreased lean body mass
- Other factors affecting medication therapy for older adults may include:
  - Impaired memory or altered mental state
  - Changes in vision and hearing
  - Decreased mobility and dexterity
  - Poor adherence
  - Reduced financial resources
  - Polypharmacy
    - The practice of taking several medications simultaneously (prescribed and/or over-the-counter [OTC]) together with diminished bodily functions and certain medical conditions can contribute to the potential for medication toxicity.
- Nursing interventions for older adults:
  - Decreasing the risk of adverse medication effects
    - Obtain a complete medication history and include all OTC medications.
    - Make sure medication therapy starts at the lowest possible dose.
    - Assess/monitor for therapeutic and adverse effects.
    - Assess/monitor for drug-drug and drug-food interactions.
    - Document findings.
    - Notify the provider of adverse effects.
  - Promoting adherence
    - Give clear and concise instructions, verbally and in writing.
    - Ensure that the dosage form is appropriate. Administer liquid forms to clients who have difficulty swallowing.
    - Provide clearly marked containers that are easy to open.
    - Assist the client to set up a daily calendar with the use of pill containers.
    - Suggest that the client obtain assistance from a friend, neighbor, or relative.

Pharmacology and Pregnancy and Lactation

- Pregnancy – any medication ingested by a woman who is pregnant will be distributed to the fetus, as well.
    - Medications are classified according to potential harm to the fetus. In general, most medications should be considered potentially harmful to the fetus; therefore, benefits of maternal medication administration must be weighed against possible fetal risk.
    - Medications are most commonly used during pregnancy as nutritional supplements (iron, vitamins, minerals) and for the treatment of nausea, vomiting, gastric acidity, and mild discomforts.
    - Chronic medical conditions such as diabetes or hypertension must be managed with careful maternal-fetal monitoring. Live virus vaccines (e.g., measles, mumps, polio, rubella, yellow fever) are contraindicated due to possible teratogenic effects.
- Lactation – most medications taken by lactating women are secreted in breast milk. Medications that have an extended half-life or medications that are known to be harmful to infants should be avoided. For medications that are safe, give the medication immediately after breastfeeding to minimize medication concentration in the next feeding.

CHAPTER 6: INDIVIDUAL CONSIDERATIONS OF MEDICATION ADMINISTRATION

Application Exercises

1. When giving a medication that is highly protein-bound to an infant, will there be more or less free medication available? Will medication effects be increased or decreased? Explain.

2. A woman who is breastfeeding is to begin taking an antimicrobial medication. She tells the nurse she doesn't want to take the medication because it may harm her baby. Which of the following is an appropriate response by the nurse?

   A. "You should tell your doctor that you do not want to take this medication."

   B. "Taking the medication immediately after breastfeeding will minimize effects on your baby."

   C. "You can bottle feed your baby while taking this medication."

   D. "The medication cannot pass through your breast milk to your baby."

3. An older adult client who is hospitalized reports an inability to sleep at night. The client is given a hypnotic medication at 2200. The next morning the client is drowsy and wants to sleep instead of eating breakfast. The nurse is aware that this effect is most likely due to

   A. reduced cardiac function.

   B. first-pass effect.

   C. reduced hepatic function.

   D. delayed toxic effect.

CHAPTER 6: INDIVIDUAL CONSIDERATIONS OF MEDICATION ADMINISTRATION

Application Exercises Answer Key

1. When giving a medication that is highly protein-bound to an infant, will there be more or less free medication available? Will medication effects be increased or decreased? Explain.

   More free medication will be available due to fewer protein-binding sites. Medication effects will be increased with greater potential for toxicity.

NCLEX® Connection: Pharmacological and Parenteral Therapies, Expected Actions/ Outcomes

2. A woman who is breastfeeding is to begin taking an antimicrobial medication. She tells the nurse she doesn't want to take the medication because it may harm her baby. Which of the following is an appropriate response by the nurse?

   A. "You should tell your doctor that you do not want to take this medication."

   B. "Taking the medication immediately after breastfeeding will minimize effects on your baby."

   C. "You can bottle feed your baby while taking this medication."

   D. "The medication cannot pass through your breast milk to your baby."

   Taking any medication right after breastfeeding will decrease the concentration of the medication in the next feeding. Instructing the client to talk to the doctor is a nontherapeutic response because it does not address the client's concern. There is no indication that the client should stop breastfeeding and give the baby formula. Some of the medication may pass through the breast milk.

NCLEX® Connection: Pharmacological and Parenteral Therapies, Adverse Effects/ Contraindications/Side Effects/Interactions

3. An older adult client who is hospitalized reports an inability to sleep at night. The client is given a hypnotic medication at 2200. The next morning the client is drowsy and wants to sleep instead of eating breakfast. The nurse is aware that this effect is most likely due to

   A. reduced cardiac function.

   B. first-pass effect.

   C. reduced hepatic function.

   D. delayed toxic effect.

   Reduced hepatic function may prolong the half-life of a medication and increase the length of response of a medication. This effect is not due to reduced cardiac function, first-pass effect, or delayed toxic effect.

NCLEX® Connection: Pharmacological and Parenteral Therapies, Expected Actions/ Outcomes

UNIT 2: MEDICATIONS AFFECTING THE NERVOUS SYSTEM

- Anxiety Disorders
- Depression
- Bipolar Disorders
- Psychoses
- Behavioral Disorders
- Substance Abuse
- Chronic Neurologic Disorders
- Eye and Ear Disorders
- Miscellaneous Central Nervous System Medications
- Sedative-Hypnotics

NCLEX® CONNECTIONS

When reviewing the chapters in this unit, keep in mind the relevant sections of the NCLEX® outline, in particular:

CLIENT NEEDS: PHARMACOLOGICAL AND PARENTERAL THERAPIES

Relevant topics/tasks include:

- Adverse Effects/Contraindications/Side Effects/Interactions
  - Assess the client for actual or potential side effects and adverse effects of medications.
- Expected Actions/Outcomes
  - Obtain information about prescribed medication for the client.
- Medication Administration
  - Educate the client about medications.

UNIT 2 MEDICATIONS AFFECTING THE NERVOUS SYSTEM

Chapter 7 Anxiety Disorders

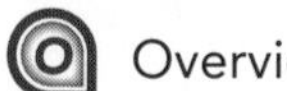

Overview

- The major medications used to treat anxiety disorders include:
    - Benzodiazepine sedative hypnotic anxiolytics such as diazepam (Valium)
    - Atypical anxiolytic/nonbarbiturate anxiolytics such as buspirone (BuSpar)
    - Selective Serotonin Reuptake Inhibitors (SSRI antidepressants) such as paroxetine (Paxil)
- Other classifications that may be used include:
    - Antidepressants, such as
        - Amitriptyline (Elavil), a tricyclic antidepressant (TCA)
        - Phenelzine (Nardil), a monoamine oxidase inhibitor (MAOI)
        - Venlafaxine (Effexor), a serotonin-norepinephrine reuptake inhibitor
        - Sertraline (Zoloft), a selective serotonin reuptake inhibitor
    - CNS stimulants, such as methylphenidate (Ritalin, Concerta)
    - Antihistamines, such as hydroxyzine (Vistaril)
    - Beta blockers, such as propranolol (Inderal)
    - Anticonvulsants, such as gabapentin (Neurontin)

MEDICATION CLASSIFICATION: SEDATIVE HYPNOTIC ANXIOLYTIC – BENZODIAZEPINE

- Select Prototype Medication: diazepam (Valium)
- Other Medications:
    - Alprazolam (Xanax)
    - Lorazepam (Ativan)
    - Chlordiazepoxide (Librium)
    - Clorazepate (Tranxene)
    - Oxazepam (Serax)
    - Clonazepam (Klonopin)

Purpose

- Expected Pharmacological Action
  - Diazepam enhances the inhibitory effects of gamma-aminobutyric acid (GABA) in the central nervous system (CNS). Relief from anxiety occurs rapidly following administration.
- Therapeutic Uses
  - Generalized anxiety disorder (GAD) and panic disorder
  - Other uses for benzodiazepines include:
    - Seizure disorders
    - Insomnia
    - Muscle spasm
    - Alcohol withdrawal (for prevention and treatment of acute symptoms)
    - Induction of anesthesia

Complications

SIDE/ADVERSE EFFECTS	NURSING INTERVENTIONS/CLIENT EDUCATION
CNS depression, (sedation, light-headedness, ataxia, decreased cognitive function)	• Advise clients to observe for symptoms. Instruct the client to notify the provider if symptoms occur. • Advise clients to avoid hazardous activities (driving, operating heavy equipment/machinery).
Anterograde amnesia (difficulty recalling events that occur after dosing)	• Advise clients to observe for symptoms. Instruct clients to notify the provider if symptoms occur.
Acute toxicity • Oral toxicity (drowsiness, lethargy, confusion) • IV toxicity (may lead to respiratory depression, severe hypotension, or cardiac/respiratory arrest)	• For oral toxicity, gastric lavage can be used, followed by the administration of activated charcoal or saline cathartics. • For IV toxicity, administer flumazenil (Romazicon) to counteract sedation and reverse side effects. • Monitor the client's vital signs, maintain patent airway, and provide fluids to maintain blood pressure. • Have resuscitation equipment available.
Paradoxical response (insomnia, excitation, euphoria, anxiety, rage)	• Advise clients to watch for manifestations of overdose. Notify the provider if these occur. • Advise clients to observe for symptoms. Instruct the client to notify the provider and stop the medication if symptoms occur.
Withdrawal symptoms, which occur infrequently with short-term use(anxiety, insomnia, diaphoresis, tremors, light-headedness)	• Advise clients who have been taking diazepam regularly and in high doses to taper the dose over several weeks.

Contraindications/Precautions

- Diazepam is a Pregnancy Risk Category D medication.
- Benzodiazepines are classified under Schedule IV of the Controlled Substances Act.
- Diazepam is contraindicated in clients with sleep apnea and/or respiratory depression.
- Use diazepam cautiously in clients with substance abuse and liver disease.

Interactions

MEDICATION/FOOD INTERACTIONS	NURSING INTERVENTIONS/CLIENT EDUCATION
CNS depressants (alcohol, barbiturates, opioids) may result in respiratory depression.	• Advise clients to observe for symptoms and notify the provider if symptoms occur. • Advise clients to avoid hazardous activities (driving, operating heavy equipment/ machinery).

Nursing Administration

- Advise clients to take the medication as prescribed and to avoid abrupt discontinuation of treatment to prevent withdrawal symptoms.
- When discontinuing benzodiazepines that have been taken regularly for long periods and in higher doses, taper the dose over several weeks.
- Administer the medication with meals or snacks if GI upset occurs.
- Advise clients to swallow sustained-release tablets and to avoid chewing or crushing the tablets.
- Inform clients about the possible development of dependency during and after treatment and to notify the provider if symptoms occur.

MEDICATION CLASSIFICATION: ATYPICAL ANXIOLYTIC/NONBARBITURATE ANXIOLYTIC

- Select Prototype Medication: buspirone (BuSpar)

Purpose

- Expected Pharmacological Action
  - The exact antianxiety mechanism of this medication is unknown. This medication binds to serotonin and dopamine receptors. Abuse is much less likely than with other anxiolytics, and use of buspirone does not result in sedation or potentiate the effects of other CNS depressants.
- Therapeutic Uses
  - Panic disorder, obsessive-compulsive disorder, social anxiety disorder, and post-traumatic stress disorder

Complications

SIDE/ADVERSE EFFECTS	NURSING INTERVENTIONS/CLIENT EDUCATION
Dizziness, nausea, headache, light-headedness, agitation	• Advise the client to take with food to decrease nausea. • Instruct client that most side effects are self-limiting.

Contraindications/Precautions

- Buspirone is Pregnancy Risk Category B.
- Buspirone is not recommended for use by nursing mothers.

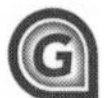

- Use buspirone cautiously in older adult clients and clients with liver and/or renal dysfunction.
- Buspirone is contraindicated for concurrent use with MAOI antidepressants or for 14 days after MAOIs are discontinued. Hypertensive crisis may result.

Interactions

MEDICATION/FOOD INTERACTIONS	NURSING INTERVENTIONS/CLIENT EDUCATION
Erythromycin, ketoconazole, and grapefruit juice may increase the effects of buspirone.	• Advise clients to avoid the use of these antimicrobial agents. • Advise clients to avoid drinking grapefruit juice.

Nursing Administration

- Advise clients to take the medication with meals to prevent gastric irritation.
- Advise clients that effects do not occur immediately. It may take a week to notice the first therapeutic effects and several more weeks for the full benefit. Medication should be taken on a regular basis and not PRN.
- Instruct clients that tolerance, dependence, or withdrawal symptoms are not an issue with this medication.

MEDICATION CLASSIFICATION: SELECTIVE SEROTONIN REUPTAKE INHIBITORS (SSRI ANTIDEPRESSANTS)

- Select Prototype Medication: Paroxetine
- Other Medications:
    - Sertraline
    - Escitalopram (Lexapro)
    - Fluoxetine (Prozac)
    - Fluvoxamine (Luvox)

Purpose

- Expected Pharmacological Action
    - Paroxetine selectively inhibits serotonin reuptake, allowing more serotonin to stay at the junction of the neurons.
    - It does not block uptake of dopamine or norepinephrine.
    - Paroxetine produces CNS stimulation, which can cause insomnia.
    - The medication has a long effective half-life. A timeframe of about 4 weeks is necessary to produce therapeutic medication levels.
- Therapeutic Uses
    - Paroxetine
        - GAD
        - Panic disorder
            - Decreases both the frequency and intensity of panic attacks and also prevents anticipatory anxiety about attacks
        - Obsessive-compulsive disorder (OCD)
            - Reduces symptoms by increasing serotonin
        - Social anxiety disorder
        - Posttraumatic stress disorder (PTSD)
        - Depressive disorders
    - Sertraline is indicated for panic disorder, OCD, social anxiety disorder, and PTSD.
    - Escitalopram is indicated for GAD and OCD.
    - Fluoxetine is used for panic disorder and OCD.
    - Fluvoxamine is used for OCD and social anxiety disorder.

Complications

SIDE/ADVERSE EFFECTS	NURSING INTERVENTIONS/CLIENT EDUCATION
Early adverse effects (first few days/weeks): nausea, diaphoresis, tremor, fatigue, drowsiness	• Advise clients that these effects should soon subside. • Instruct clients to report symptoms to the provider. • Instruct clients to take the medication as prescribed.
Later adverse effects (after 5 to 6 weeks of therapy): sexual dysfunction (impotence, delayed or absent orgasm, delayed or absent ejaculation, decreased sexual interest)	• Instruct clients to report problems with sexual function (may be managed with dose reduction, medication holiday, changing medications).
Weight gain	• Advise clients to follow a well-balanced diet and exercise regularly.
GI bleeding	• Use caution in clients with a history of GI bleed or ulcers and in clients taking other medications that affect blood coagulation. • Advise clients to report signs of bleeding such as dark stool or coffee ground emesis.
Hyponatremia (more likely in older adult clients taking diuretics)	• Obtain baseline serum sodium, and monitor level periodically throughout treatment.
Serotonin syndrome • Agitation, confusion, disorientation, difficulty concentrating, anxiety, hallucinations, hyperreflexia, incoordination, tremors, fever, diaphoresis • Usually begins 2 to 72 hr after initiation of treatment • Resolves when the medication is discontinued	• Watch for and advise clients to report any of these symptoms, which could indicate a lethal problem.
Bruxism: grinding and clenching of teeth, usually during sleep	• Bruxism should be reported to the provider, who may: ○ Switch the client to another class of medication ○ Treat bruxism with low-dose buspirone ○ Advise the client to use a mouth guard during sleep
Withdrawal syndrome • Nausea, sensory disturbances, anxiety, tremor, malaise, unease • Minimized by tapering the medication slowly	• Advise clients that, after a long period of use, the medication will be tapered slowly to avoid withdrawal symptoms. • Advise clients not to discontinue use abruptly.

 Contraindications/Precautions

- Paroxetine is a Pregnancy Risk Category D medication.
- Paroxetine is contraindicated in clients taking MAOIs or a TCA.
- Clients taking paroxetine should avoid alcohol.
- Use paroxetine cautiously in clients with liver and renal dysfunction, seizure disorders, or a history of GI bleeding.

Interactions

MEDICATION/FOOD INTERACTIONS	NURSING INTERVENTIONS/CLIENT EDUCATION
Use of MAOI antidepressants or TCAs can cause serotonin syndrome.	Educate the client about this combination.

Nursing Administration

- Advise clients that medications may be taken with food. Sleep disturbances may be minimized by taking medication in the morning.
- Instruct clients to take the medication on a daily basis to establish therapeutic plasma levels.
- Assist with medication regimen adherence by informing clients that therapeutic effects may not be experienced for 1 to 3 weeks.

Nursing Evaluation of Medication Effectiveness

- Depending on therapeutic intent, effectiveness may be evidenced by:
    - Maintaining normal sleep pattern
    - Verbalizing feeling less anxious and more relaxed
    - Greater ability to participate in social and occupational interactions

CHAPTER 7: ANXIETY DISORDERS

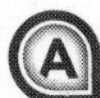 Application Exercises

1. Which of the following is an antidote for benzodiazepine overdose or toxicity?

   A. Buspirone (BuSpar)
   B. Hydroxyzine (Vistaril)
   C. Flumazenil (Romazicon)
   D. Naloxone (Narcan)

2. A nurse knows that teaching has been effective if a client who is taking a benzodiazepine for long-term treatment of anxiety makes which of the following statements?

   A. "I will only take the medication at bedtime."
   B. "I cannot take this drug if I am using a pain medication."
   C. "I will not stop taking the drug abruptly."
   D. "I will need to take this medication the rest of my life."

3. Buspirone is different from other antianxiety medications in which of the following ways?

   A. Buspirone has anticonvulsant effects.
   B. Buspirone has muscle relaxant effects.
   C. Buspirone will depress the central nervous system.
   D. Buspirone does not cause physical or psychological dependence.

4. A client has been taking buspirone for 3 days for an anxiety disorder. He calls the community mental health facility and tells the nurse that the medication has not helped him to sleep at all and that he is still feeling anxious. How should the nurse reply?

5. A client has been taking paroxetine (Paxil) to treat an anxiety disorder for several weeks. The client calls the nurse to say that he has been grinding his teeth during the night, which causes pain in his mouth and insomnia for his spouse. Which of the following measures may be used to manage bruxism (teeth grinding)? (Select all that apply.)

   _____ Concurrent administration of buspirone
   _____ Administration of a different SSRI
   _____ Use of a mouth guard
   _____ Changing to a different class of antianxiety medication
   _____ Increasing the dose of paroxetine

CHAPTER 7: ANXIETY DISORDERS

Application Exercises Answer Key

1. Which of the following is an antidote for benzodiazepine overdose or toxicity?

    A. Buspirone (BuSpar)

    B. Hydroxyzine (Vistaril)

    C. Flumazenil (Romazicon)

    D. Naloxone (Narcan)

    Flumazenil is a benzodiazepine receptor antagonist, which specifically reverses an overdose of benzodiazepines. Buspirone is a nonbarbiturate anxiolytic, and hydroxyzine is an antihistamine used for anxiety disorders. Naloxone is an opioid antagonist used to reverse an overdose of opioids, such as morphine sulfate.

NCLEX® Connection: Pharmacological and Parenteral Therapies: Expected Actions/Outcomes

2. A nurse knows that teaching has been effective if a client who is taking a benzodiazepine for long-term treatment of anxiety makes which of the following statements?

    A. "I will only take the medication at bedtime."

    B. "I cannot take this drug if I am using a pain medication."

    C. "I will not stop taking the drug abruptly."

    D. "I will need to take this medication the rest of my life."

    Abrupt discontinuation of a benzodiazepine that the client has been taking for some time may cause withdrawal symptoms. The medication may need to be tapered for several weeks before discontinuing. The other statements indicate a need for further teaching about benzodiazepine therapy.

NCLEX® Connection: Pharmacological and Parenteral Therapies: Medication Administration

3. Buspirone is different from other antianxiety medications in which of the following ways?

    A. Buspirone has anticonvulsant effects.

    B. Buspirone has muscle relaxant effects.

    C. Buspirone will depress the central nervous system.

    D. Buspirone does not cause physical or psychological dependence.

    Buspirone does not affect the CNS in the same way as do benzodiazepines. It does not cause dependence or tolerance, does not have anticonvulsant or muscle relaxant effects, and does not promote drowsiness.

NCLEX® Connection: Pharmacological and Parenteral Therapies: Adverse Effects/ Contraindications/Side Effects/Interactions

4. A client has been taking buspirone for 3 days for an anxiety disorder. He calls the community mental health facility and tells the nurse that the medication has not helped him to sleep at all and that he is still feeling anxious. How should the nurse reply?

   The initial response to buspirone takes 1 week, but it may take several weeks to reach its therapeutic peak. The medication has no hypnotic effect, so it does not promote sleep. Try nonmedication measures to promote sleep (warm bath, soothing music, avoiding caffeine and alcohol before bedtime).

NCLEX® Connection: Pharmacological and Parenteral Therapies: Expected Actions/ Outcomes

5. A client has been taking paroxetine (Paxil) to treat an anxiety disorder for several weeks. The client calls the nurse to say that he has been grinding his teeth during the night, which causes pain in his mouth and insomnia for his spouse. Which of the following measures may be used to manage bruxism (teeth grinding)? (Select all that apply.)

   __X__ **Concurrent administration of buspirone**
   _____ Administration of a different SSRI
   __X__ **Use of a mouth guard**
   __X__ **Changing to a different class of antianxiety medication**
   _____ Increasing the dose of paroxetine

   Concurrent administration of buspirone, use of a mouth guard, or changing to a different class of antianxiety medication are all ways to manage bruxism. Any SSRI may cause bruxism, so changing to another SSRI will not be effective. Increasing the dose of paroxetine would also not stop the problem.

NCLEX® Connection: Pharmacological and Parenteral Therapies: Adverse Effects/ Contraindications/Side Effects/Interactions

UNIT 2 MEDICATIONS AFFECTING THE NERVOUS SYSTEM

Chapter 8 Depression

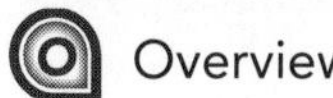

Overview

- Depression is a mood (affective) disorder and is a widespread problem, ranking high among causes of disability.
- Clients starting antidepressant medication therapy for depression need to be advised that symptom relief can take 1 to 3 weeks and possibly 2 to 3 months for full benefits to be achieved. Encourage continued adherence.
- Clients with major depression may require hospitalization with close observation and suicide precautions until the antidepressant medications reach their peak effect.
- Antidepressant mediations are classified into four main groups:
  - Tricyclic antidepressants
  - Selective serotonin reuptake inhibitors (SSRIs)
  - Monoamine oxidase inhibitors (MAOIs)
  - Atypical antidepressants

MEDICATION CLASSIFICATION: TRICYCLIC ANTIDEPRESSANTS (TCAs)

- Select Prototype Medication: Amitriptyline (Elavil)
- Other Medications
  - Imipramine (Tofranil)
  - Doxepin (Sinequan)
  - Nortriptyline (Aventyl)
  - Amoxapine (Asendin)
  - Trimipramine (Surmontil)

Purpose

- Expected Pharmacological Action
  - These medications block reuptake of norepinephrine and serotonin in the synaptic space, thereby intensifying the effects of these neurotransmitters.

- Therapeutic Uses
  - Depression
  - Depressive episodes of bipolar disorders
  - Other Uses
    - Chronic pain
    - Enuresis

Complications

SIDE/ADVERSE EFFECTS	NURSING INTERVENTIONS/CLIENT EDUCATION
Orthostatic hypotension	• Instruct clients about the signs of postural hypotension (lightheadedness, dizziness). If these occur, advise the client to sit or lie down. Orthostatic hypotension can be minimized by getting up or changing positions slowly. • Monitor blood pressure and heart rate for clients in the hospital for orthostatic changes before administration and 1 hr after. If a significant decrease in blood pressure and/or increase in heart rate is noted, do not administer the medication, and notify the provider.
Anticholinergic effects • Dry mouth • Blurred vision • Photophobia • Urinary hesitancy or retention • Constipation • Tachycardia	• Instruct clients on ways to minimize anticholinergic effects. These include: ○ Chewing sugarless gum ○ Sipping on water ○ Wearing sunglasses when outdoors ○ Eating foods high in fiber ○ Participating in regular exercise ○ Increasing fluid intake to at least 2 to 3 L/day from beverages and food sources ○ Voiding just before taking medication • Advise the client to notify the provider if symptoms persist.
Sedation	• This effect usually diminishes over time. • Advise clients to avoid hazardous activities such as driving if sedation is excessive. • Advise clients to take medication at bedtime to minimize daytime sleepiness and to promote sleep.

SIDE/ADVERSE EFFECTS	NURSING INTERVENTIONS/CLIENT EDUCATION
Toxicity resulting in cholinergic blockade and cardiac toxicity evidenced by dysrhythmias, mental confusion, and agitation, followed by seizures, coma, and possible death	• Give a 1-week supply of medication to clients who are acutely ill. • Obtain the client's baseline ECG. • Monitor vital signs frequently. • Monitor clients for signs of toxicity. • Notify the provider if signs of toxicity occur.
Decreased seizure threshold	• Monitor clients who have seizure disorders.
Excessive sweating	• Inform clients of side effect. Assist clients with frequent linen changes.

Contraindications/Precautions

- TCAs are Pregnancy Risk Category C.
- These medications are contraindicated in clients who have seizure disorders
- Use cautiously in clients who have coronary artery disease; diabetes, liver, kidney and respiratory disorders; urinary retention and obstruction; angle-closure glaucoma; benign prostatic hypertrophy; and hyperthyroidism.

Interactions

MEDICATION/FOOD INTERACTIONS	NURSING INTERVENTIONS/CLIENT EDUCATION
Concurrent use of MAOIs and St. John's wort may lead to serotonin syndrome.	• Avoid concurrent use.
Antihistamines and other anticholinergic agents have additive anticholinergic effects.	
Increased effects of epinephrine, dopamine (direct-acting sympathomimetics) occur because uptake into the nerve terminals is blocked by TCAs and they remain for a longer amount of time in the synaptic space.	
TCAs decrease the effects of ephedrine, amphetamine (indirect-acting sympathomimetics), because uptake into the nerve terminals is blocked and they are unable to reach their site of action.	
Alcohol, benzodiazepines, opioids, and antihistamines cause additive CNS depression when used concurrently.	• Advise clients to avoid other CNS depressants.

MEDICATION CLASSIFICATION: SELECTIVE SEROTONIN REUPTAKE INHIBITORS (SSRIs)

- Select Prototype Medication: Fluoxetine (Prozac)
- Other Medications
  - Citalopram (Celexa)
  - Escitalopram oxalate (Lexapro)
  - Paroxetine (Paxil)
  - Sertraline (Zoloft)

Purpose

- Expected pharmacological action
  - SSRIs selectively block reuptake of the monoamine neurotransmitter serotonin in the synaptic space, thereby intensifying the effects of serotonin.
- Therapeutic Uses
  - Major depression
  - Obsessive compulsive disorders (OCD)
  - Bulimia nervosa
  - Premenstrual dysphoric disorders
  - Panic disorders
  - Posttraumatic disorder (PTSD)

Complications

SIDE/ADVERSE EFFECTS	NURSING INTERVENTIONS/CLIENT EDUCATION
Sexual dysfunction (no orgasm, impotence, decreased libido)	• Warn clients of possible side effects and to notify the provider if intolerable. • Instruct client on ways to manage sexual dysfunction, which may include lowering dosage, discontinuing medication temporarily (medication holiday), and using adjunct medications to improve sexual function (e.g., sildenafil [Viagra] and buspirone [BuSpar]). • Inform clients that an atypical antidepressant with fewer sexual dysfunction side effects (bupropion [Wellbutrin] and nefazodone [Serzone]) may be indicated.

SIDE/ADVERSE EFFECTS	NURSING INTERVENTIONS/CLIENT EDUCATION
CNS stimulation (inability to sleep, agitation, anxiety)	• Advise clients to notify the provider. Dose may need to be lowered. • Advise clients to take dose in the morning. • Advise clients to avoid caffeinated beverages. • Teach relaxation techniques to promote sleep.
Weight loss early in therapy, may be followed by weight gain with long-term treatment	• Monitor the client's weight. • Encourage clients to participate in regular exercise and to follow a healthy, well-balanced diet.
Serotonin syndrome may begin 2 to 72 hr after starting treatment and may be lethal. Manifestations include: • Mental confusion, difficulty concentrating • Fever • Agitation • Anxiety • Hallucinations • Incoordination, hyperreflexia • Diaphoresis • Tremors	• Advise clients to observe for symptoms. If symptoms occur, instruct the client to notify the provider and stop the medication.
Withdrawal syndrome resulting in headache, nausea, visual disturbances, anxiety, dizziness, and tremors	• Instruct clients to taper dose gradually.
Hyponatremia (more likely in older adult clients taking diuretics)	• Obtain baseline serum sodium, and monitor level periodically throughout treatment.
Rash	• Advise clients that a rash can be treated with an antihistamine or withdrawal of medication.
Sleepiness, faintness, lightheadedness	• Advise clients that these side effects are not common, but can occur. • Advise clients to avoid driving if these side effects occur.
GI bleeding	• Use caution in clients with history of GI bleed and ulcers, and those taking other medications that affect blood coagulation.
Bruxism	• Advise clients to report to the provider. Advise clients to use a mouth guard. Changing to a different classification of antidepressants or adding a low dose of buspirone may be indicated.

 Contraindications/Precautions

- These medications are Pregnancy Risk Category C.
  - Fluoxetine and paroxetine may increase the risk of birth defects. Other SSRIs should be used. Late in pregnancy, use of SSRIs may increase the risk of withdrawal symptoms or pulmonary hypertension in the newborn.
- SSRIs are contraindicated in clients taking MAOIs or TCAs.
- Use cautiously in clients with liver and renal dysfunction, cardiac disease, seizure disorders, diabetes, ulcers, and a history of GI bleeding.

Interactions

MEDICATION/FOOD INTERACTIONS	NURSING INTERVENTIONS/CLIENT EDUCATION
MAOIs, TCAs, and St. John's wort increase the risk of serotonin syndrome.	• MAOIs should be discontinued for 14 days prior to starting an SSRI. If already taking fluoxetine, the client should wait 5 weeks before starting an MAOI. • Avoid concurrent use of TCAs and St. John's wort.
Fluoxetine can displace warfarin (Coumadin) from bound protein and result in increased warfarin levels.	• Monitor the client's prothrombin time (PT) and INR levels. • Assess clients for signs of bleeding and the need for dosage adjustment.
Fluoxetine can increase the levels of tricyclic antidepressants and lithium.	• Avoid concurrent use.
Fluoxetine suppresses platelet aggregation and thus increases the risk of bleeding when used concurrently with NSAIDs and anticoagulants.	• Advise clients to monitor for signs of bleeding (bruising, hematuria) and to notify the provider if they occur.

MEDICATION CLASSIFICATION: MONOAMINE OXIDASE INHIBITORS (MAOIs)

- Select Prototype Medication: phenelzine (Nardil)
- Other Medications:
  - Isocarboxazid (Marplan)
  - Tranylcypromine (Parnate)
  - Selegiline (Emsam) – transdermal MAOI

Purpose

- Expected Pharmacological Action
  - These medications block MAO-A in the brain, thereby increasing the amount of norepinephrine (NE), dopamine, and serotonin available for transmission of impulses. An increased amount of these neurotransmitters at nerve endings intensifies responses and relieves depression.
- Therapeutic Uses
  - Atypical depression
  - Bulimia nervosa
  - Obsessive compulsive disorders (OCD)

Complications

SIDE/ADVERSE EFFECTS	NURSING INTERVENTIONS/CLIENT EDUCATION
CNS stimulation (anxiety, agitation, mania, or hypomania)	• Advise clients to observe for symptoms and notify the provider if they occur.
Orthostatic hypotension	• Monitor the client's BP and HR for orthostatic changes. Hold medication and notify the provider for significant changes. Instruct the client to change positions slowly.
Hypertensive crisis resulting from intake of dietary tyramine • Severe hypertension occurs as a result of intensive vasoconstriction and stimulation of the heart • Clients will most likely experience headache, nausea, increased heart rate and blood pressure	• Administer phentolamine (Regitine) IV, a rapid-acting alpha-adrenergic blocker or nifedipine (Procardia) SL. • Provide continuous cardiac monitoring and respiratory support as indicated.
Local rash may occur with transdermal preparation.	• Choose a clean, dry area for each application. • Apply a topical glucocorticoid on the affected area.

Contraindications/Precautions

- MAOIs are Pregnancy Risk Category C.
- These medications are contraindicated in clients taking SSRIs and in those with pheochromocytoma, heart failure, cardiovascular and cerebral vascular disease, and severe renal insufficiency.
- Use cautiously in clients with diabetes and seizure disorders or those taking TCAs.
- Transdermal selegiline is contraindicated for clients taking carbamazepine (Tegretol) or oxcarbazepine (Trileptal), which may increase blood levels of the MAOI.

Interactions

MEDICATION/FOOD INTERACTIONS	NURSING INTERVENTIONS/CLIENT EDUCATION
Indirect-acting sympathomimetic medications (ephedrine, amphetamine) promote the release of norepinephrine and can lead to hypertensive crisis	• Instruct the client that OTC decongestants and cold remedies frequently contain medications with sympathomimetic action and should be avoided.
Use of tricyclic antidepressants can lead to hypertensive crisis.	• Use MAOIs and TCAs cautiously.
Use of selective serotonin reuptake inhibitors (SSRIs) can lead to serotonin syndrome.	• Avoid concurrent use.
Antihypertensives have an additive hypotensive effect.	• Monitor the client's blood pressure. • Notify the provider if there is a significant drop in the client's blood pressure. A reduced dosage of antihypertensive may be indicated.
Use of meperidine (Demerol) can lead to hyperpyrexia	• Use an alternative analgesic.
Tyramine-rich foods can lead to hypertensive crisis. Clients will most likely experience headache, nausea, increased heart rate and increased blood pressure.	• Assess the client for ability to follow strict adherence to dietary restrictions. • Inform the client of symptoms and to notify the provider if they occur. • Provide clients with written instructions regarding foods and beverages to be avoided. • Tyramine-rich foods include aged cheese, pepperoni, salami, avocados, figs, bananas, smoked fish, protein dietary supplements, soups, soy sauce, some beers, and red wine. • Advise clients to avoid taking any medications without approval of the provider.
Concurrent use of vasopressors (phenylethylamine, caffeine) may result in hypertension	• Advise clients to avoid foods that contain these agents (caffeinated beverages, chocolate, fava beans, ginseng).

MEDICATION CLASSIFICATION: ATYPICAL ANTIDEPRESSANTS

- Select Prototype Medication: bupropion HCL (Wellbutrin)

Purpose

- Expected Pharmacological Action
  - This medication acts by inhibiting dopamine uptake.
- Therapeutic Uses
  - Treatment of depression
  - Alternative to SSRIs for clients unable to tolerate sexual dysfunction side effects of SSRIs
  - Aid to quit smoking
  - Prevention of SAD (seasonal affective disorder)

Complications

SIDE/ADVERSE EFFECTS	NURSING INTERVENTIONS/CLIENT EDUCATION
Headache, dry mouth, GI distress, constipation, increased heart rate, nausea, restlessness, and insomnia	• Advise clients to observe for symptoms and to notify the provider if intolerable. • Treat headache with mild analgesic. • Advise clients to sip on fluids to treat dry mouth and to increase dietary fiber to prevent constipation.
Suppresses appetite and often causes weight loss	• Monitor client's weight and food intake.
Seizures	• Avoid administering to clients at risk for seizures, such as a client who has a head injury. • Monitor clients for seizures and treat accordingly.

Contraindications/Precautions

- Bupropion is a Pregnancy Risk Category B.
- This medication is contraindicated in clients taking MAOIs.
- Use cautiously in clients who have seizure disorders.

Interactions

MEDICATION/FOOD INTERACTIONS	NURSING INTERVENTIONS/CLIENT EDUCATION
MAOIs such as phenelzine (Nardil) increase the risk of toxicity.	• MAOIs should be discontinued 2 weeks prior to beginning treatment with bupropion.

OTHER ATYPICAL ANTIDEPRESSANTS

AGENT	PHARMACOLOGICAL ACTION	NURSING IMPLICATIONS
Venlafaxine (Effexor), duloxetine (Cymbalta)	These agents inhibit serotonin and norepinephrine reuptake thereby increasing the amount of these neurotransmitters available in the brain for impulse transmission. There is also a minimal amount of dopamine blockade.	• Side effects include headache, nausea, agitation, anxiety and sleep disturbances. • Monitor for hyponatremia, especially in older adult clients. • Monitor for weight loss. • Monitor for increase in diastolic pressure. • Discuss ways to manage interference with sexual functioning. • Advise clients not to stop medication abruptly.
Mirtazapine (Remeron)	This agent increases the release of serotonin and norepinephrine and thereby increases the amount of neurotransmitters available for impulse transmission.	• Therapeutic effects may occur sooner with less sexual dysfunction than with SSRIs. • Mirtazapine is generally well tolerated. Clients may experience sleepiness that can be exacerbated by other CNS depressants (alcohol, benzodiazepines), weight gain, and elevated cholesterol.
Reboxetine (Edronax)	This agent selectively inhibits the reuptake of norepinephrine, thereby increasing the amount of neurotransmitters available for impulse transmission.	• This medication has similar results as with SSRIs. • Reboxetine is generally well tolerated but clients may experience dry mouth, decreased blood pressure, constipation, sexual dysfunction, and urinary hesitancy or retention. • Weight gain and sleepiness do not occur. • This medication should not be combined with an MAOI.
Trazodone (Desyrel)	This agent has moderate selective blockade of serotonin receptors, which allows more serotonin to be available for impulse transmission.	• This agent is usually used with another antidepressant agent. Sedation may be a problem or this medication may be indicated for a client with insomnia caused by an SSRI. • Priapism may be an adverse effect and clients should be instructed to seek medical attention immediately if this occurs.

Nursing Administration

- Instruct clients to take these medications as prescribed on a daily basis to establish therapeutic plasma levels.
- Assist with medication regimen adherence by informing clients that therapeutic effects may not be experienced for 1 to 3 weeks. Full therapeutic effects may take 2 to 3 months.
- Instruct clients to continue therapy after improvement in symptoms. Sudden discontinuation of medication can result in relapse.
- Advise the client that therapy usually continues for 6 months after resolution of symptoms and may continue for a year or longer.

- Suicide prevention can be facilitated by prescribing only a week's worth of medication for an acutely ill client, and then only prescribing 1 month's worth of medication at a time, especially with TCAs.
- For SSRIs:
    - Advise clients to take medication in the morning to minimize sleep disturbances
    - Advise clients to take medications with food to minimize GI disturbances.

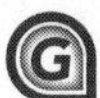

    - Obtain baseline sodium levels for older adult clients taking diuretics and monitor periodically.
- For MAOIs:
    - Give clients a list of tyramine-rich food so hypertensive crises can be avoided.
    - Advise the client to avoid taking any other prescription or nonprescription medications unless approved by the provider.
- For bupropion HCL:
    - Advise clients with SAD to take medication beginning in the autumn each year and gradually taper dose and discontinue by spring.

Nursing Evaluation of Medication Effectiveness

- Depending on therapeutic intent, effectiveness may be evidenced by:
    - Verbalizing improvement in mood
    - Ability to perform ADLs
    - Improved sleeping and eating habits
    - Increased interaction with peers

CHAPTER 8: DEPRESSION

 Application Exercises

1. A client starting phenelzine (Nardil) for treatment of depression should be monitored for which of the following effects?

   A. Orthostatic hypotension
   B. Respiratory depression
   C. GI bleeding
   D. Rash

2. A nurse is providing teaching to a client who is starting amitriptyline (Elavil) for treatment of depression. Which of the following should be included? (Select all that apply.)

   _____ Therapeutic effects should be experienced immediately.
   _____ Stop taking the medication after a week of improved mood.
   _____ Change positions slowly to minimize dizziness.
   _____ Decrease dietary fiber intake to control diarrhea.
   _____ Chew sugarless gum to prevent dry mouth.

3. Which of the following foods should be avoided by a client who is taking an MAOI?

   A. Fresh vegetables
   B. Cheese
   C. Apples
   D. Grilled steak

4. A nurse is caring for a group of clients who take antidepressants. The nurse should educate the client who takes which of the following medications about the possible occurrence of sexual dysfunction as an adverse effect?

   A. Fluoxetine (Prozac)
   B. Phenelzine (Nardil)
   C. Bupropion HCl (Wellbutrin)
   D. Amitriptyline (Elavil)

5. A nurse is caring for a client who has been taking an SSRI antidepressant for the past two days. Which of the following assessment findings should alert the nurse to the possibility that the client is developing serotonin syndrome?

   A. Bruising
   B. Fever
   C. Abdominal pain
   D. Urinary retention

CHAPTER 8: DEPRESSION

Application Exercises Answer Key

1. A client starting phenelzine (Nardil) for treatment of depression should be monitored for which of the following effects?

 A. Orthostatic hypotension

 B. Respiratory depression

 C. GI bleeding

 D. Rash

 Orthostatic hypotension is a side effect of MAOIs. Clients experience CNS stimulation, not depression. GI bleeding is a side effect of aspirin and NSAIDs. Rash is a side effect of fluoxetine (Prozac).

NCLEX® Connection: Pharmacological and Parenteral Therapies, Adverse Effects/Contraindications/Side Effects/Interactions

2. A nurse is providing teaching to a client who is starting amitriptyline (Elavil) for treatment of depression. Which of the following should be included? (Select all that apply.)

 ______ Therapeutic effects should be experienced immediately.

 ______ Stop taking the medication after a week of improved mood.

 __X__ Change positions slowly to minimize dizziness.

 ______ Decrease dietary fiber intake to control diarrhea.

 __X__ Chew sugarless gum to prevent dry mouth.

 Orthostatic hypotension, experienced as dizziness and lightheadedness, is a side effect of amitriptyline and can be minimized by changing positions slowly. Dry mouth is a side effect of amitriptyline and can be minimized by chewing sugarless gum. Therapeutic effects may take several weeks to be achieved. Medication should not be stopped abruptly and therapy will most likely last 6 to 12 months to prevent relapse. Clients should increase dietary fiber to prevent constipation.

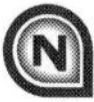

NCLEX® Connection: Pharmacological and Parenteral Therapies, Medication Administration

3. Which of the following foods should be avoided by a client who is taking an MAOI?

 A. Fresh vegetables

 B. Cheese

 C. Apples

 D. Grilled steak

 Cheese contains dietary tyramine that can interact with MAOIs to precipitate hypertensive crisis. Tyramine is not contained in fresh vegetables, apples, or grilled steak.

NCLEX® Connection: Pharmacological and Parenteral Therapies, Medication Administration

4. A nurse is caring for a group of clients who take antidepressants. The nurse should educate the client who takes which of the following medications about the possible occurrence of sexual dysfunction as an adverse effect?

   A. Fluoxetine (Prozac)

   B. Phenelzine (Nardil)

   C. Bupropion HCl (Wellbutrin)

   D. Amitriptyline (Elavil)

   Clients with prescriptions for SSRI antidepressants, such as fluoxetine (Prozac) are at risk for problems with sexual dysfunction. Phenelzine (an MAOI antidepressant), bupropion HCl (an atypical antidepressant, and amitriptyline (a TCA) do not cause sexual dysfunction.

NCLEX® Connection: Pharmacological and Parenteral Therapies, Adverse Effects/ Contraindications/Side Effects/Interactions

5. A nurse is caring for a client who has been taking an SSRI antidepressant for the past two days. Which of the following assessment findings should alert the nurse to the possibility that the client is developing serotonin syndrome?

   A. Bruising

   B. Fever

   C. Abdominal pain

   D. Urinary retention

   Fever, along with changes in mental status, tremors, and hyperreflexia, is a sign of serotonin syndrome. Bruising, abdominal pain, and urinary retention are not expected findings.

NCLEX® Connection: Pharmacological and Parenteral Therapies, Adverse Effects/ Contraindications/Side Effects/Interactions

UNIT 2 MEDICATIONS AFFECTING THE NERVOUS SYSTEM

Chapter 9 Bipolar Disorders

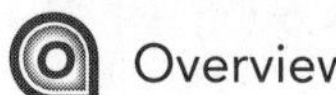

Overview

- Bipolar disorders are primarily managed with mood stabilizing medications such as lithium carbonate (Lithane, Eskalith, Lithobid).
- Other medications used to treat bipolar disorders include antiepileptic medications such as:
    - Valproic acid (Depakote)
    - Carbamazepine (Tegretol)
    - Lamotrigine (Lamictal)
  - Atypical antipsychotics – These can be useful in early treatment to promote sleep and to decrease anxiety and agitation. These medications also demonstrate mood-stabilizing properties.
  - Anxiolytics – Clonazepam (Klonopin) and lorazepam (Ativan) can be useful in treating acute mania and managing the psychomotor agitation often seen in mania.

MEDICATION CLASSIFICATION: MOOD STABILIZER

- Select Prototype Medication: lithium carbonate

Purpose

- Expected Pharmacological Action
  - Lithium produces neurochemical changes in the brain, including serotonin receptor blockade.
  - There is evidence that the use of lithium can show a decrease in neuronal atrophy and/or an increase in neuronal growth..
- Therapeutic Uses
  - Lithium is used in the treatment of bipolar disorders. Lithium controls episodes of acute mania, helps prevent the return of mania or depression, and decreases the incidence of suicide.
  - Other uses:
    - Alcoholism
    - Bulimia
    - Schizophrenia

Complications

- Effects with therapeutic lithium levels (some effects will resolve within a few weeks)

SIDE/ADVERSE EFFECTS	NURSING INTERVENTIONS/CLIENT EDUCATION
Gastrointestinal distress (nausea, diarrhea, abdominal pain)	• Advise clients that symptoms are usually transient. • Administer medication with meals or milk.
Fine hand tremors that can interfere with purposeful motor skills and can be exacerbated by factors such as stress and caffeine	• Administer beta-adrenergic blocking agents such as propranolol (Inderal). • Adjust to lowest possible dosage, give in divided doses, or use long-acting formulations. • Advise clients to report an increase in tremors.
Polyuria, mild thirst	• Use a potassium-sparing diuretic, such as spironolactone (Aldactone). • Instruct clients to maintain adequate fluid intake by consuming at least 2,000 to 3,000 mL of fluid from beverages and food sources.
Weight gain	• Assist clients to follow a healthy diet and regular exercise regimen.
Renal toxicity	• Monitor the client's I&O. • Adjust dosage and keep dose low. • Assess baseline kidney function and monitor kidney function periodically.
Goiter and hypothyroidism with long-term treatment	• Obtain the client's baseline T_3, T_4, and TSH levels prior to starting treatment, and then annually. • Advise clients to monitor for signs of hypothyroidism (cold, dry skin; decreased heart rate, weight gain). • Administer levothyroxine (Synthroid) to manage hypothyroid symptoms.
Bradydysrhythmia, hypotension, and electrolyte imbalances	• Encourage clients to maintain adequate fluid intake.

- Signs and symptoms of toxicity

SIGNS AND SYMPTOMS OF TOXICITY			
Early signs	Less than 1.5 mEq/L	Diarrhea, nausea, vomiting, thirst, polyuria, muscle weakness and slurred speech	• Advise clients to discontinue medication and notify the provider. • Administer new dosage based on serum lithium levels.
Advanced signs	1.5 to 2.0 mEq/L	Ongoing gastrointestinal distress including nausea, vomiting, and diarrhea, mental confusion, and poor coordination and coarse tremors	• Advise clients to discontinue medication and notify the provider. • Administer new dosage based on serum lithium levels. • If symptoms are severe, it may be necessary to promote excretion.
Severe toxicity	Greater than 2.0 to 2.5 mEq/L	Extreme polyuria of dilute urine, tinnitus, blurred vision, ataxia, seizures, severe hypotension leading to coma and possibly death from respiratory complications	• Give alert clients an emetic. • Perform gastric lavage or administer urea, mannitol, or aminophylline to increase the rate of excretion.
	Greater than 2.5 mEq/L	Rapid progression of symptoms leading to coma and death	Hemodialysis

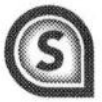

Contraindications/Precautions

- Lithium is Pregnancy Risk Category D. This medication is teratogenic, especially during the first trimester.
- Discourage clients from breastfeeding if lithium therapy is necessary.
- Use cautiously in clients with renal dysfunction, heart disease, sodium depletion, and dehydration.

Interactions

MEDICATION/FOOD INTERACTIONS	NURSING INTERVENTIONS/CLIENT EDUCATION
Sodium is excreted with the use of diuretics. Reduced serum sodium decreases lithium excretion, which can lead to toxicity.	• Monitor clients for signs of toxicity. • Advise clients to observe for symptoms and to notify the provider. • Encourage clients to maintain a diet adequate in sodium, and to drink 2,000 mL to 3,000 mL of water each day from food and beverage sources.
Concurrent use of NSAIDs (ibuprofen [Motrin] and celecoxib [Celebrex]) will increase renal reabsorption of lithium, leading to toxicity.	• Avoid use of NSAIDs. • Use aspirin as a mild analgesic.
Anticholinergics (antihistamines, tricyclic antidepressants) can induce urinary retention and polyuria, leading to abdominal discomfort.	• Advise clients to avoid medications with anticholinergic effects.

Nursing Administration

- Monitor plasma lithium levels while undergoing treatment. At initiation of treatment, monitor levels every 2 to 3 days and then every 1 to 3 months. Lithium blood levels should be obtained in the morning, usually 12 hr after the last dose.
    - During initial treatment of a manic episode, levels should be between 0.8 to 1.4 mEq/L.
    - Maintenance level range is between 0.4 to 1.0 mEq/L.
    - Plasma levels > 1.5 mEq/L can result in toxicity.
- Care for clients who have a toxic plasma lithium level in an inpatient setting and provide supportive measures. Hemodialysis may be indicated.
- Advise clients that effects begin within 7 to 14 days.
- Advise clients to take lithium as prescribed. Lithium must be administered in 2 to 3 doses daily due to a short half life. Taking lithium with food will help decrease GI distress.
- Encourage clients to adhere to laboratory appointments needed to monitor lithium effectiveness and adverse effects. Emphasize the high risk of toxicity due to the narrow therapeutic range.
- Provide nutritional counseling. Stress the importance of adequate fluid and sodium intake.
- Instruct clients to monitor for signs of toxicity and when to contact the provider. Clients should stop taking medication and seek medical attention if experiencing diarrhea, vomiting, or excessive sweating.

MEDICATION CLASSIFICATION: MOOD-STABILIZING ANTIEPILEPTIC DRUGS (AEDs)

- Select Prototype Medications:
  - Carbamazepine (Tegretol)
  - Valproic acid (Depakote)
  - Lamotrigine (Lamictal)

Purpose

- Expected Pharmacological Action
  - AEDs help treat and manage bipolar disorders by various mechanisms, which include:
    - Slowing the entrance of sodium and calcium back into the neuron and, thus extending the time it takes for the nerve to return to its active state
    - Potentiating the inhibitory effects of gamma butyric acid (GABA)
    - Inhibiting glutamic acid (glutamate) which in turn suppresses CNS excitation
- Therapeutic Uses
  - Treatment of manic and depressive episodes, prevention of relapse of mania and depressive episodes. Especially useful for clients with mixed mania and rapid cycling bipolar disorders.

Complications

SIDE/ADVERSE EFFECTS	NURSING INTERVENTIONS/CLIENT EDUCATION
Carbamazepine	
Cognitive function is minimally affected, but CNS effects may include nystagmus, double vision, vertigo, staggering gait, headache.	• Administer low doses initially, then gradually increase dosage. • Advise clients that symptoms should subside within a few weeks. • Administer dose at bedtime.
Blood dyscrasias (leukopenia, anemia, thrombocytopenia)	• Obtain the client's baseline CBC and platelets and perform ongoing monitoring. • Observe the client for signs of bruising and bleeding of gums.
Teratogenesis	• Advise clients to avoid use in pregnancy.
Hypo-osmolarity (Promotes secretion of ADH, which inhibits water excretion by the kidneys and places clients with heart failure at risk for fluid overload)	• Monitor serum sodium. • Monitor the client for edema, decrease in urine output, and hypertension.
Skin disorders (Dermatitis, rash, Stevens-Johnson syndrome)	• Treat mild reactions with anti-inflammatory or antihistamine medications. • Advise clients to wear sunscreen • Instruct clients to notify the provider if Stevens-Johnson syndrome rash occurs and to discontinue medication.

SIDE/ADVERSE EFFECTS	NURSING INTERVENTIONS/CLIENT EDUCATION
Valproic acid	
Gastrointestinal effects (nausea vomiting, indigestion)	• Advise clients that symptoms are usually self-limiting. • Advise clients to take medication with food or switch to enteric-coated pills.
Hepatotoxicity as evidenced by anorexia, nausea, vomiting, fatigue abdominal pain, jaundice	• Assess baseline liver function and monitor liver function regularly. • Advise clients to observe for signs and symptoms and to notify the provider if they occur. • Avoid using in children younger than 2 years old. • Administer lowest effective dose.
Pancreatitis as evidenced by nausea, vomiting, and abdominal pain	• Advise clients to observe for signs and symptoms and to notify the provider immediately if they occur. • Monitor amylase levels. • Discontinue medication if pancreatitis develops.
Thrombocytopenia	• Advise clients to observe for signs and symptoms such as bruising, and to notify the provider if these occur. • Monitor the client's platelet counts.
Teratogenesis	• Advise the client to avoid use in pregnancy.
Lamotrigine	
Common effects include double or blurred vision, dizziness, headache, nausea and vomiting.	• Caution clients about performing activities requiring concentration.
Serious skin rashes including Stevens-Johnson syndrome	• Instruct client to notify provider if rash occurs. Medication should be discontinued

Contraindications/Precautions

- These medications are in Pregnancy Risk Category D and can result in birth defects.
- Carbamazepine is contraindicated in clients with bone marrow suppression or with bleeding disorders.
- Valproic acid is contraindicated in clients who have liver disorders.

Interactions

MEDICATION/FOOD INTERACTIONS	NURSING INTERVENTIONS/CLIENT EDUCATION
Carbamazepine	
• Concurrent use of carbamazepine causes a decrease in the effects of Oral contraceptives and warfarin (Coumadin) because of stimulation of hepatic drug-metabolizing enzymes.	• Advise clients to use an alternate form of birth control. • Monitor for therapeutic effects of warfarin. • Dosages may need to be adjusted.
• Grapefruit juice inhibits metabolism, thus increasing carbamazepine levels.	• Advise clients to avoid intake of grapefruit juice.
• Phenytoin and phenobarbital decrease the effects of carbamazepine by stimulating metabolism.	• Monitor phenytoin and phenobarbital levels. • Adjust dosage of medications as prescribed.
Valproic acid	
• Concurrent use of valproic acid increases the levels of phenytoin and phenobarbital.	• Monitor phenytoin and phenobarbital levels. • Adjust dosage of medications as prescribed.
Lamotrigine	
• Carbamazepine, phenytoin, and phenobarbital promote liver drug-metabolizing enzymes, thereby decreasing the effect of lamotrigine.	• Monitor for therapeutic effects. • Adjust dosage of medications as prescribed.
• Valproic acid inhibits medication-metabolizing enzymes and thus increases the half-life of lamotrigine.	• Monitor for adverse effects. • Adjust dosage of medications as prescribed.

Nursing Evaluation of Medication Effectiveness

- Depending on therapeutic intent, effectiveness may be evidenced by:
  - Relief of acute manic symptoms (flight of ideas, obsessive talking, agitation) or depressive symptoms (fatigue, poor appetite, psychomotor retardation)
  - Verbalizing improvement in mood
  - Ability to perform ADLs
  - Improved sleeping and eating habits
  - Greater interaction with peers

CHAPTER 9: BIPOLAR DISORDERS

Application Exercises

1. A client's plasma lithium level is 0.2 mEq/L. The nurse can expect to implement which of the following nursing interventions?

   A. Administer an additional oral dose of lithium.

   B. Prepare to give emergency resuscitation.

   C. Infuse 1 L of 0.9% sodium chloride over 4 hr.

   D. Prepare the client immediately for another laboratory draw.

2. The nurse is caring for a client with a new prescription for lithium carbonate. When teaching the client about ways to prevent lithium toxicity, the nurse should advise the client to do which of the following?

   A. Avoid the use of acetaminophen for headaches.

   B. Restrict intake of foods rich in sodium.

   C. Decrease fluid intake to less than 1,500 mL daily

   D. Limit aerobic activity in hot weather.

3. Which of the following is an adverse effect for which a nurse should assess a client who is taking lithium carbonate?

   A. Alopecia

   B. Tremors

   C. Constipation

   D. Urinary retention

4. A client has a prescription for valproic acid (Depakote). Which of the following laboratory values should the nurse anticipate monitoring for a client taking this medication? (Select all that apply)

   _____ Thrombocyte count

   _____ White Blood Count (WBC)

   _____ Amylase level

   _____ Liver function tests

   _____ Potassium level

CHAPTER 9: BIPOLAR DISORDERS

Application Exercises Answer Key

1. A client's plasma lithium level is 0.2 mEq/L. The nurse can expect to implement which of the following nursing interventions?

    A. Administer an additional oral dose of lithium.

    B. Prepare to give emergency resuscitation.

    C. Infuse 1 L of 0.9% sodium chloride over 4 hr.

    D. Prepare the client immediately for another laboratory draw.

    This plasma level is subtherapeutic and the client should be given an additional dose. Emergency resuscitation may be indicated if the client's laboratory value indicates toxicity. There is no indication that the client needs supplemental fluids. There is no reason to question the laboratory result.

NCLEX® Connection: Pharmacological and Parenteral Therapies: Expected Actions/Outcomes

2. The nurse is caring for a client with a new prescription for lithium carbonate. When teaching the client about ways to prevent lithium toxicity, the nurse should advise the client to do which of the following?

    A. Avoid the use of acetaminophen for headaches.

    B. Restrict intake of foods rich in sodium.

    C. Decrease fluid intake to less than 1,500 mL daily

    D. Limit aerobic activity in hot weather.

    Activities that could cause sodium/water depletion should be avoided in order to prevent lithium carbonate toxicity. Acetaminophen, rather than NSAIDs such as ibuprofen, should be used for headaches because NSAIDs interact with lithium and could cause increased blood levels of lithium. The client should make sure to take in enough sodium and increase, rather than decrease, fluid intake to prevent toxicity.

NCLEX® Connection: Pharmacological and Parenteral Therapies: Adverse Effects/Contraindications/Side Effects/Interactions

3. Which of the following is an adverse effect for which a nurse should assess a client who is taking lithium carbonate?

    A. Alopecia

    B. Tremors

    C. Constipation

    D. Urinary retention

    Fine hand tremors are a common adverse effect in clients who take lithium. Alopecia is not an adverse effect of lithium. Diarrhea and polyuria are side effects of lithium.

NCLEX® Connection: Pharmacological and Parenteral Therapies: Adverse Effects/Contraindications/Side Effects/Interactions

4. A client has a prescription for valproic acid (Depakote). Which of the following laboratory values should the nurse anticipate monitoring for a client taking this medication? (Select all that apply)

   __X__ **Thrombocyte count**
   _____ White Blood Count (WBC)
   __X__ **Amylase level**
   __X__ **Liver function tests**
   _____ Potassium level

   Valproic acid may lead to thrombocytopenia, pancreatitis or liver disease. The nurse should plan to monitor the thrombocyte count, amylase level, and liver function tests. Monitoring the WBC and potassium level would not give information regarding an adverse effect of this medication.

NCLEX® Connection: Pharmacological and Parenteral Therapies: Adverse Effects/ Contraindications/Side Effects/Interactions

UNIT 2 MEDICATIONS AFFECTING THE NERVOUS SYSTEM

Chapter 10 Psychoses

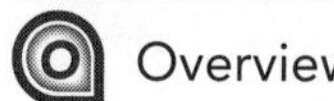

Overview

- Schizophrenia is the primary reason for the administration of antipsychotic medications.
  - The clinical course of schizophrenia usually involves acute exacerbations with intervals of semiremission.
  - Medications are used to treat:
    - Positive symptoms related to behavior, thought, and speech (agitation, delusions, hallucinations, tangential speech patterns)
    - Negative symptoms (social withdrawal, lack of emotion, lack of energy [anergia], flattened affect, decreased motivation, decreased pleasure in activities)
  - The goals of psychopharmacological treatment for schizophrenia include:
    - Suppressing acute episodes
    - Preventing acute recurrence
    - Maintaining the highest possible level of functioning
- Conventional antipsychotic medications control mainly the positive symptoms, such as hallucinations, delusions, and bizarre behavior of psychosis. These medications are reserved for clients who are:
  - Using them successfully and can tolerate the side effects
  - Violent or particularly aggressive
- Atypical antipsychotic agents are medications of choice for clients receiving initial treatment and for treating breakthrough episodes in clients on conventional medication therapy, because they are more effective with fewer adverse effects.
  - Advantages of atypical antipsychotic agents include:
    - Relief of both the positive and negative symptoms of the disease
    - Decrease in affective symptoms (depression, anxiety) and suicidal behaviors
    - Improvement of neurocognitive defects, such as poor memory
    - Fewer or no extrapyramidal symptoms (EPS), including tardive dyskinesia, because of less dopamine blockade
    - Fewer anticholinergic adverse effects because most atypical antipsychotics, with the exception of clozapine (Clozaril), cause little or no blockade of cholinergic receptors
    - Less relapse

MEDICATION CLASSIFICATION: ANTIPSYCHOTICS – CONVENTIONAL

- Select Prototype Medication: chlorpromazine (Thorazine) – low potency
- Other Medications:
  - Haloperidol (Haldol) – high potency
  - Fluphenazine (Prolixin) – high potency
  - Thiothixene (Navane) – high potency

Purpose

- Expected Pharmacological Action
  - The conventional antipsychotic medications block dopamine (D_2), acetylcholine, histamine, and norepinephrine (NE) receptors in the brain and periphery.
  - Inhibition of psychotic symptoms is believed to be a result of D_2 blockade in the brain.
- Therapeutic Uses
  - Treatment of acute and chronic psychosis
  - Schizophrenia
  - Bipolar disorders (primarily the manic phase)
  - Tourette's syndrome
  - Delusional and schizoaffective disorders
  - Dementia
  - Prevention of nausea/vomiting through blocking of dopamine in the chemoreceptor trigger zone of the medulla

Complications

SIDE/ADVERSE EFFECTS	NURSING INTERVENTIONS/CLIENT EDUCATION
Acute dystonia • The client experiences severe spasms of tongue, neck, face, or back. This is a crisis situation, which requires rapid treatment.	• Begin to monitor for side effects anywhere between 5 hr to 5 days after administration of the first dose. • Treat with anticholinergic agents, such as benztropine (Cogentin) or diphenhydramine (Benadryl). Use oral doses for less acute effects and IM or IV doses for serious effects.
Parkinsonism • Signs and symptoms include bradykinesia, rigidity, shuffling gait, drooling and tremors.	• Observe for signs and symptoms within 1 month of initiation of therapy. • Treat with benztropine, diphenhydramine, or amantadine (Symmetrel). Discontinue these medications to determine if they are still needed. If symptoms return, administer atypical antipsychotic as prescribed.
Akathisia • The client is unable to stand still or sit, and is continually pacing and agitated.	• Observe for signs and symptoms within 2 months of the initiation of treatment. • Manage symptoms with beta-blocker, benzodiazepine, or anticholinergic medication.
Late extrapyramidal symptoms (EPS), tardive dyskinesia (TD) • Manifestations include involuntary movements of the tongue and face, such as lip-smacking, which cause speech and/or eating disturbances. • TD may also include involuntary movements of arms, legs, or trunk.	• Manifestations may occur months to years after the start of therapy, and may improve following medication change or may be permanent. • Administer the lowest dosage possible to control symptoms. • Evaluate the client after 12 months of therapy and then every 3 months. If signs of TD appear, dosage should be lowered or the client should be switched to an atypical agent. • Use the AIMS test to screen for the presence of EPS.
Neuroleptic malignant syndrome • Symptoms include sudden high-grade fever, blood pressure fluctuations, dysrhythmias, muscle rigidity, and change in level of consciousness developing into coma.	• Stop antipsychotic medication. • Monitor the client's vital signs. • Apply cooling blankets. • Administer antipyretics (aspirin, acetaminophen). • Increase the client's fluid intake. • Administer diazepam (Valium) to control anxiety. • Administer dantrolene (Dantrium) to induce muscle relaxation. • Wait 2 weeks before resuming therapy. Consider switching to an atypical agent.

SIDE/ADVERSE EFFECTS	NURSING INTERVENTIONS/CLIENT EDUCATION
Anticholinergic effects • Dry mouth • Blurred vision • Photophobia • Urinary hesitancy/ retention • Constipation • Tachycardia	• Suggest these strategies to decrease anticholinergic effects: ○ Chewing sugarless gum ○ Sipping water ○ Avoiding hazardous activities ○ Wearing sunglasses when outdoors ○ Eating foods high in fiber ○ Participating in regular exercise ○ Maintaining fluid intake of 2 to 3 L of water each day from food and beverage sources ○ Voiding just before taking medication
Orthostatic hypotension	• Clients should develop tolerance in 2 to 3 months. • In the hospital setting, monitor the client's blood pressure and heart rate for orthostatic changes. If a significant decrease in blood pressure and/or increase in heart rate is noted, do not administer the medication, and notify the provider. • Instruct clients about the signs of postural hypotension (lightheadedness, dizziness). If these occur, advise the client to sit or lie down. Orthostatic hypotension can be minimized by getting up or changing positions slowly.
Sedation	• Inform clients that effects should diminish within a few weeks. • Clients may take this medication at bedtime to avoid daytime sleepiness. • Advise clients not to drive until sedation has subsided.
Neuroendocrine effects • Effects include gynecomastia (breast enlargement), galactorrhea, and menstrual irregularities	• Advise clients to observe for manifestations and to notify the provider if these occur.
Seizures • The greatest risk for developing seizures is in clients with existing seizure disorders.	• Advise clients to report seizure activity to the provider. • An increase in antiseizure medication may be necessary.
Sexual dysfunction (common in both males and females)	• Advise clients of possible side effects. • Encourage clients to report side effects to the provider. • The client may need a lower dosage or to be switched to a high-potency agent.

SIDE/ADVERSE EFFECTS	NURSING INTERVENTIONS/CLIENT EDUCATION
Skin effects • Effects include photosensitivity resulting in severe sunburn, and contact dermatitis from handling medications.	• Advise clients to avoid excessive exposure to sunlight, to use sunscreen, and to wear protective clothing. • Advise clients to avoid direct contact with medication.
Agranulocytosis	• Advise clients to observe for signs of infection (fever, sore throat), and to notify the provider if these occur. • If signs of infection appear, obtain the client's baseline WBC. Medication should be discontinued if laboratory tests indicate the presence of infection.
Severe dysrhythmias with some of the conventional antipsychotic agents	• Obtain the client's baseline ECG and potassium level prior to treatment and periodically throughout the treatment period. • Avoid concurrent use with other medications that prolong QT interval.

Contraindications/Precautions

- These medications are contraindicated in clients in a coma, and clients who have severe depression, Parkinson's disease, prolactin-dependent cancer of the breast, and severe hypotension

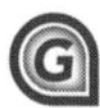

- Use of conventional antipsychotic medications is contraindicated in older clients with dementia.
- Use cautiously in clients with glaucoma, paralytic ileus, prostate enlargement, heart disorders, liver or kidney disease, and seizure disorders.

Interactions

MEDICATION/FOOD INTERACTIONS	NURSING INTERVENTIONS/CLIENT EDUCATION
Concurrent use of anticholinergic agents with other anticholinergic medications will increase anticholinergic effects.	• Advise clients to avoid over-the-counter medications that contain anticholinergic agents, such as sleep aids.
Alcohol, opioids, and antihistamines have additive CNS depressant effects.	• Advise clients to avoid alcohol and other medications that cause CNS depression. • Advise clients to avoid hazardous activities, such as driving.
By activating dopamine receptors, levodopa counteracts the effects of antipsychotic agents.	• Avoid concurrent use of levodopa and other direct dopamine receptor agonists.

Nursing Administration

- Assess clients to differentiate between EPS and worsening of psychotic disorder.
- Administer anticholinergics, beta-blockers, and benzodiazepines to control early EPS. If symptoms are intolerable, a client can be switched to a low-potency or an atypical antipsychotic agent.
- Advise clients that antipsychotic medications do not cause addiction.
- Advise clients to take medication as prescribed and to take it on a regular schedule.
- Advise clients that some therapeutic effects may be noticeable within a few days, but significant improvement may take 2 to 4 weeks, and possibly several months for full effects.
- Consider depot preparations administered IM once every 2 to 4 weeks for clients with difficulty maintaining medication regimen. Inform the client that lower doses can be used with depot preparations, which will decrease the risk of adverse effects and the development of tardive dyskinesia.
- Start administration with BID dosing, then switch to daily dosing at bedtime to decrease daytime drowsiness and promote sleep.

MEDICATION CLASSIFICATION: ANTIPSYCHOTICS – ATYPICAL

- Select Prototype Medication: risperidone (Risperdal)
- Other Medications:
  - Olanzapine (Zyprexa)
  - Quetiapine (Seroquel)
  - Aripiprazole (Abilify)
  - Ziprasidone (Geodon)
  - Clozapine (Clozaril)

Purpose

- Expected Pharmacological Action
  - These antipsychotic agents work mainly by blocking serotonin, and to a lesser degree, dopamine receptors. These medications also block receptors for norepinephrine, histamine, and acetylcholine.
- Therapeutic Uses
  - Schizophrenia (negative and positive symptoms)
  - Psychosis induced by levodopa therapy
  - Relief of psychotic symptoms in other disorders such as bipolar disorders

Complications

SIDE/ADVERSE EFFECTS	NURSING INTERVENTIONS/CLIENT EDUCATION
New onset of diabetes mellitus or loss of glucose control in clients who have diabetes	• Obtain the client's baseline fasting blood glucose and monitor throughout treatment. • Instruct the client to report signs and symptoms (increased thirst, urination, and appetite).
Weight gain	• Advise the client to follow a healthy, low-caloric diet, engage in regular exercise, and monitor weight gain.
Hypercholesterolemia with increased risk for hypertension and other cardiovascular disease	• Monitor cholesterol, triglycerides, and blood glucose if weight gain is > 14 kg (30 lb).
Orthostatic hypotension	• Monitor the client's blood pressure and heart rate for orthostatic changes. Instruct clients to change positions slowly.
Anticholinergic effects such as urinary hesitancy or retention, dry mouth	• Monitor for these effects and report their occurrence to the provider. • Educate clients about measures to relieve dry mouth, such as sipping fluids.
Agitation, dizziness, sedation, and sleep disruption	• Monitor for these effects and report to the provider if they occur. • Administer alternative medication if prescribed.
May cause mild EPS, such as tremor	• Monitor for and teach clients to recognize EPS. • Use AIMS test to screen for EPS.

Contraindications/Precautions

- Risperidone is Pregnancy Risk Category C.
- Use is contraindicated for clients with dementia. Use of all atypical antipsychotic medications may cause death related to cerebrovascular accident or infection.
- Clients should avoid the use of alcohol.
- Use cautiously in clients who have cardiovascular or cerebrovascular disease, seizures, or diabetes mellitus. Obtain a fasting blood glucose for clients who have diabetes mellitus, and monitor blood glucose carefully.

- Other atypical antipsychotic agents

MEDICATION	FORMULATIONS	COMPLICATIONS
Olanzapine	• Tablets • Oral solution • Short-acting injectable	• Olanzapine has a low risk of EPS. • Olanzapine has a high risk for diabetes, weight gain and dyslipidemia. • Other adverse effects include sedation, orthostatic hypotension and anticholinergic effects.
Quetiapine	Tablets	• Quetiapine has a low risk of EPS. • Quetiapine has a moderate risk for diabetes, weight gain, and dyslipidemia. • Other effects include cataracts, sedation, orthostatic hypotension, and anticholinergic effects. • Clients should have screening eye exam and then every 6 months.
Aripiprazole	• Tablets • Oral solution	• Aripiprazole has low or no risk of EPS, diabetes, weight gain, dyslipidemia, hypotension, and anticholinergic effects. • Other adverse effects include headache, anxiety, insomnia, sedation, and GI upset.
Ziprasidone • Affects both dopamine and serotonin; can be used for clients with concurrent depression	• Capsules • Short-acting injectable	• Ziprasidone has a low risk of EPS, diabetes, weight gain, and dyslipidemia. • Other effects include sedation, orthostatic hypotension, anticholinergic effects and rash • ECG changes and QT prolongation, which may lead to torsades de pointes.
Clozapine • The first atypical antipsychotic developed; no longer considered a first-line medication for schizophrenia because of its adverse effects	Tablets	• Clozapine has a low risk of EPS. • High risk of weight gain, diabetes and dyslipidemia. • Agranulocytosis may occur. Obtain the client's baseline WBC and then monitor weekly. • Monitor the client for signs of infection (fever, sore throat, lesions in mouth), and notify the provider if symptoms occur. • Other adverse effects include sedation, orthostatic hypotension, and anticholinergic effects.

Interactions

MEDICATION/FOOD INTERACTIONS	NURSING INTERVENTIONS/CLIENT EDUCATION
Immunosuppressive medications, such as anticancer medications, can further suppress immune function in clients taking clozapine.	• Avoid use in clients taking clozapine.
Alcohol, opioids, and antihistamines have additive CNS depressant effects.	• Advise clients to avoid alcohol and other medications that cause CNS depression. • Advise clients to avoid hazardous activities, such as driving.
By activating dopamine receptors, levodopa counteracts the effects of antipsychotic agents.	• Avoid concurrent use of levodopa and other direct dopamine receptor agonists.
Tricyclic antidepressants, amiodarone (Cordarone), and clarithromycin (Biaxin) prolong QT interval and thus increase the risk of cardiac dysrhythmias in clients taking ziprasidone.	• Use is contraindicated with ziprasidone.
Barbiturates and phenytoin (Dilantin) stimulate hepatic medication-metabolizing enzymes and thereby decrease drug levels of aripiprazole, quetiapine, and ziprasidone.	• Monitor medication effectiveness.
Fluconazole (Diflucan) inhibits hepatic medication-metabolizing enzymes and thereby increases levels of aripiprazole, quetiapine, and ziprasidone	• Monitor medication effectiveness

Nursing Administration

- Administer by oral or IM route. Risperidone is also available as a depot injection administered IM once every 2 weeks. Use for clients with difficulty adhering to medication regimen. Therapeutic effect occurs 4 to 6 weeks after the first depot injection.
- Advise clients that low doses of medication are given initially and are then gradually increased.
- Use oral disintegrating tablets for clients who may attempt to "cheek" (or pocket) tablets or have difficulty swallowing them.

Nursing Evaluation of Medication Effectiveness

- Depending on therapeutic intent, effectiveness may be evidenced by:
  - Improvement of symptoms (prevention of acute psychotic symptoms, absence of hallucinations, delusions, anxiety, and hostility)
  - Improvement in ability to perform ADLs
  - Improvement in ability to interact socially with peers
  - Improvement of sleeping and eating habits

CHAPTER 10: PSYCHOSES

 Application Exercises

1. A nurse is caring for a client who takes chlorpromazine (Thorazine) for schizophrenia. For which of the following symptoms should the nurse expect to see improvement? (Select all that apply)

   _____ Poverty of speech
   _____ Bizarre behavior
   _____ Impaired social interactions
   _____ Hallucinations
   _____ Decreased motivation

2. A nurse is teaching a client with schizophrenia ways to cope with anticholinergic effects of Fluphenazine (Prolixin). Which of the following strategies should the nurse suggest to the client to minimize anticholinergic effects?

   A. Avoid foods that can cause diarrhea.
   B. Chew sugarless gum to moisten the mouth.
   C. Use cooling measures to decrease fever.
   D. Take an antacid to relieve nausea.

3. Several hours after administering a typical antipsychotic medication, a nurse should watch for which of the following adverse effects?

   A. Shuffling gait
   B. Neck spasms
   C. Lip smacking
   D. Continuous pacing

4. A nurse is caring for a client who has a new prescription for clozapine (Clozaril) Which of the following laboratory values should the nurse plan to monitor weekly during the first few months this client is taking clozapine?

   A. Serum creatinine
   B. Serum sodium
   C. Triglycerides and cholesterol
   D. White blood cell count

CHAPTER 10: PSYCHOSES

Application Exercises Answer Key

1. A nurse is caring for a client who takes chlorpromazine (Thorazine) for schizophrenia. For which of the following symptoms should the nurse expect to see improvement? (Select all that apply)

   __X__ **Poverty of speech**

   __X__ **Bizarre behavior**

   _____ Impaired social interactions

   __X__ **Hallucinations**

   _____ Decreased motivation

   A client taking a conventional antipsychotic medication, such as chlorpromazine, should see improvement in positive symptoms such as poverty of speech, bizarre behavior, and hallucinations. Chlorpromazine is not very effective for negative symptoms such as impaired social interactions and decreased motivation.

NCLEX® Connection: Pharmacological and Parenteral Therapies: Expected Actions/ Outcomes

2. A nurse is teaching a client with schizophrenia ways to cope with anticholinergic effects of Fluphenazine (Prolixin). Which of the following strategies should the nurse suggest to the client to minimize anticholinergic effects?

   A. Avoid foods that can cause diarrhea.

   B. Chew sugarless gum to moisten the mouth.

   C. Use cooling measures to decrease fever.

   D. Take an antacid to relieve nausea.

   Chewing gum, sucking hard candies, or sipping liquids can help the client cope with dry mouth, which occurs as an anticholinergic effect of some antipsychotic medications. Constipation is an anticholinergic side effect. Fever may indicate neuroleptic malignant syndrome and should be reported to the provider. Nausea is not an anticholinergic effect.

NCLEX® Connection: Pharmacological and Parenteral Therapies: Adverse Effects/ Contraindications/Side Effects/Interactions

3. Several hours after administering a typical antipsychotic medication, a nurse should watch for which of the following adverse effects?

    A. Shuffling gait

    B. Neck spasms

    C. Lip smacking

    D. Continuous pacing

    Neck spasms are a sign of acute dystonia, a side effect that can occur anywhere between 5 hr to 5 days after administration of a typical antipsychotic medication. Shuffling gait is a sign of parkinsonism, which usually does not occur for at least one month after administration. Continuous pacing is a sign of akathisia and usually develops within 2 months of the initiation of treatment. Lip smacking is a sign of tardive dyskinesia and is an adverse effect that occurs after long-term use of at least a year.

NCLEX® Connection: Pharmacological and Parenteral Therapies: Adverse Effects/ Contraindications/Side Effects/Interactions

4. A nurse is caring for a client who has a new prescription for clozapine (Clozaril) Which of the following laboratory values should the nurse plan to monitor weekly during the first few months this client is taking clozapine?

    A. Serum creatinine

    B. Serum sodium

    C. Triglycerides and cholesterol

    D. White blood cell count

    The WBC should be monitored carefully during the first few months of treatment due to the risk for agranulocytosis. Although triglycerides and cholesterol should be monitored for clients taking clozapine, they do not require weekly monitoring. Serum sodium and creatinine are not routinely monitored for clients taking clozapine.

NCLEX® Connection: Pharmacological and Parenteral Therapies: Adverse Effects/ Contraindications/Side Effects/Interactions

UNIT 2 MEDICATIONS AFFECTING THE NERVOUS SYSTEM

Chapter 11 Behavioral Disorders

 Overview

- Various medications may be used to manage behavioral disorders in children and adolescents. Parents should understand that pharmacological management should be accompanied by behavioral modification techniques.
- Medications include selective serotonin reuptake inhibitors, tricyclic antidepressants, antipsychotics, nonbarbiturate anxiolytics, CNS stimulants, and norepinephrine selective reuptake inhibitors.

MEDICATION CLASSIFICATION: SELECTIVE SEROTONIN REUPTAKE INHIBITORS (SSRIs)

- Select Prototype Medication: fluoxetine (Prozac)
- Other Medications:
  - Citalopram (Celexa)
  - Escitalopram oxalate (Lexapro)
  - Paroxetine (Paxil)
  - Sertraline (Zoloft)

Purpose

- Expected Pharmacological Action
  - SSRIs selectively block reuptake of the monoamine neurotransmitter serotonin in the synaptic space, thereby intensifying the effects that can be produced.
- Therapeutic Uses
  - Major depression
  - Bulimia nervosa
  - Panic, school phobia, separation anxiety disorder
  - Posttraumatic stress disorder (PTSD)
  - Obsessive compulsive disorder (OCD)
  - Attention-deficit hyperactivity disorder (ADHD) in children (and adults)

Complications

SIDE/ADVERSE EFFECTS	NURSING INTERVENTIONS/CLIENT EDUCATION
CNS stimulation (inability to sleep, agitation, anxiety)	• Advise clients to notify provider. Dose may need to be lowered. • Advise clients to take dose in the morning. • Advise clients to avoid chocolate and caffeinated beverages. • Teach relaxation techniques to promote sleep.
Weight loss early in therapy, may be followed by weight gain with long-term treatment	• Monitor client weight. • Encourage clients to participate in regular exercise and to follow a healthy, well-balanced diet.
Serotonin syndrome may begin 2 to 72 hr after starting treatment and it can be lethal. Symptoms include: • Mental confusion, difficulty concentrating • Agitation • Anxiety • Hallucinations • Incoordination, hyperreflexia • Tremors • Fever • Diaphoresis	• Advise clients to observe for symptoms and to notify the provider and stop the medication if symptoms occur.
Withdrawal syndrome (headache, nausea, visual disturbances, anxiety)	• Instruct clients to taper the dose gradually.
Rash	• Advise clients that a rash can be treated with an antihistamine or withdrawal of medication.
Sleepiness, faintness, lightheadedness	• Advise clients that these side effects are not common, but can occur. • Advise clients to avoid driving if these side effects occur.
GI bleeding	• Use caution in clients with history of GI bleed and ulcers and in clients taking other medications that affect blood coagulation.
Bruxism	• Advise clients to report to the provider. • Advise clients to use mouth guard, and that changing to a different classification of antidepressants or adding a low dose of buspirone (BuSpar) may be indicated.

Contraindications/Precautions

- Contraindicated in clients taking MAOIs and tricyclic antidepressants
- Use cautiously in clients with liver and renal dysfunction, cardiac disease, seizure disorders, diabetes, ulcers, and a history of GI bleeding.

Interactions

MEDICATION/FOOD INTERACTIONS	NURSING INTERVENTIONS/CLIENT EDUCATION
MAOIs and tricyclic antidepressants increase the risk of serotonin syndrome.	• MAOIs should be discontinued for 14 days prior to starting an SSRI. If already taking fluoxetine, clients should wait 5 weeks before starting an MAOI. • Concurrent use with tricyclic antidepressants is not recommended.
Fluoxetine can displace warfarin (Coumadin) from bound protein and result in increased warfarin levels.	• Monitor the client's prothrombin time (PT) and INR levels. • Assess clients for signs of bleeding. • A dosage adjustment may be required.
Fluoxetine can increase the levels of tricyclic antidepressants and lithium.	• Avoid concurrent use.
Fluoxetine suppresses platelet aggregation and thus increases the risk of bleeding when used concurrently with NSAIDs and anticoagulants.	• Advise clients to monitor for signs of bleeding (bruising, hematuria) and to notify the provider if they occur.

Nursing Administration

- Assess use of alcohol and other CNS depressants, especially with adolescents.
- Medications may be taken with food. Sleep disturbances may be minimized by taking medication in the morning.
- Instruct clients to take the medication on a daily basis to establish therapeutic plasma levels.
- Suggest weekly dosing for clients with difficulty adhering to the medication regimen.
- Assist clients with adherence by informing them that therapeutic effects may not be experienced for 1 to 3 weeks.
- Instruct clients to continue therapy after improvement in symptoms. Sudden discontinuation of medication can result in relapse.

Nursing Evaluation of Medication Effectiveness

- Depending on therapeutic intent, effectiveness may be evidenced by the following:
  - For depression:
    - Verbalizing improvement in mood
    - Improved sleeping and eating habits
    - Increased interaction with peers
  - For ADHD:
    - Less hyperactivity
    - Greater ability to pay attention

MEDICATION CLASSIFICATION: TRICYCLIC ANTIDEPRESSANTS (TCAs)

- Select Prototype Medication: amitriptyline (Elavil)
- Other Medications:
  - Imipramine (Tofranil)
  - Clomipramine (Anafranil)
  - Nortriptyline (Aventyl)

Purpose

- Expected Pharmacological Action
  - These medications block reuptake of the monoamine neurotransmitters norepinephrine and serotonin in the synaptic space, thereby intensifying the effects that these neurotransmitters produce.
- Therapeutic Uses
  - Depression
  - Depressive episodes of bipolar disorders
  - Autistic disorder
  - ADHD
  - Panic, school phobia, separation anxiety disorder
  - PTSD
  - OCD

Complications

SIDE/ADVERSE EFFECTS	NURSING INTERVENTIONS/CLIENT EDUCATION
Orthostatic hypotension	○ Monitor blood pressure with first dose. Instruct client to change positions slowly.
Anticholinergic effects • Dry mouth • Blurred vision • Photophobia • Urinary hesitancy or retention • Constipation • Tachycardia	• Instruct clients about ways to minimize anticholinergic effects. These include: ○ Chewing sugarless gum ○ Sipping on water ○ Avoiding hazardous activities ○ Wearing sunglasses when outdoors ○ Eating foods high in fiber ○ Participating in regular exercise ○ Increasing fluid intake to at least 2 to 3 L/day from beverages or food sources ○ Voiding just before taking medication • Advise clients to notify the provider if symptoms are intolerable
Weight gain	• Monitor client weight. • Encourage clients to participate in regular exercise and to follow a healthy, low-caloric diet.
Sedation	• Advise clients that this side effect usually diminishes over time. • Advise clients to avoid hazardous activities such as driving if sedation is excessive. • Advise clients to take medication at bedtime to minimize daytime sleepiness and to promote sleep.
Toxicity resulting in cholinergic blockade and cardiac toxicity evidenced by dysrhythmias mental confusion, and agitation, followed by seizures and coma	• Give clients who are acutely ill a 1-week supply of medication. • Obtain the client's baseline ECG. • Monitor vital signs frequently. • Monitor clients for signs of toxicity and notify the provider if signs of toxicity occur.
Decreased seizure threshold	• Monitor clients who have seizure disorders.
Excessive sweating	• Inform clients of this side effect and assist with frequent linen changes.

Contraindications/Precautions

- Use cautiously in clients who have seizure disorders; diabetes; liver, kidney and respiratory disorders; and hyperthyroidism.

Interactions

MEDICATION/FOOD INTERACTIONS	NURSING INTERVENTIONS/CLIENT EDUCATION
Concurrent use of monoamine oxidase inhibitors (MAOIs) causes hypertension.	Avoid concurrent use with TCAs.
Antihistamines and other anticholinergic agents have additive anticholinergic effects.	Avoid concurrent use with TCAs.
TCAs block uptake of epinephrine, NE (direct-acting sympathomimetics) in the synaptic space, leading to decreased intensity of their effects.	Avoid concurrent use with TCAs.
TCAs inhibit uptake of ephedrine, amphetamine (indirect-acting sympathomimetics) and reduce their ability to get to the site of action in the nerve terminal, leading to decreased responses to these medications.	Avoid concurrent use with TCAs.
Alcohol, benzodiazepines, opioids, and antihistamines cause additive CNS depression when used concurrently.	Advise clients to avoid other CNS depressants.

Nursing Administration

- Instruct clients to take this medication as prescribed on a daily basis to establish therapeutic plasma levels.
- Assist with medication regimen compliance by informing clients that therapeutic effects may not be experienced for 1 to 3 weeks. Full therapeutic effects may take 2 to 3 months.
- Instruct clients to continue therapy after improvement in symptoms. Sudden discontinuation of the medication can result in relapse.

- Give only a week's worth of medication at a time for an acutely ill client.

Nursing Evaluation of Medication Effectiveness

- Depending on therapeutic intent, effectiveness may be evidenced by the following:
    - For depression:
        - Verbalizing improvement in mood
        - Improved sleeping and eating habits
        - Increased interaction with peers
    - For autistic disorder: Decreased anger and compulsive behavior
    - For ADHD: less hyperactivity, greater ability to pay attention

MEDICATION CLASSIFICATION: ATYPICAL ANXIOLYTIC: NONBARBITURATE ANXIOLYTIC

- Select Prototype Medication: buspirone (BuSpar)

Purpose

- Expected Pharmacological Action
  - The exact antianxiety mechanism of this medication is unknown. Buspirone binds to serotonin and dopamine receptors. There is no potential for abuse, and use of buspirone does not result in sedation or potentiate the effects of other CNS depressants.
- Therapeutic Uses
  - Panic disorder, obsessive-compulsive disorder, social anxiety disorder, and post-traumatic stress disorder

Complications

SIDE/ADVERSE EFFECTS	NURSING INTERVENTIONS/CLIENT EDUCATION
CNS effects (dizziness, nausea, headache, light-headedness, agitation)	• Advise clients to take with food to decrease nausea. • Instruct clients that most side effects are self-limiting.

Contraindications/Precautions

- Buspirone is contraindicated for concurrent use with MAOI antidepressants or for 14 days after MAOIs are discontinued. Hypertensive crisis may result.

Interactions

MEDICATION/FOOD INTERACTIONS	NURSING INTERVENTIONS/CLIENT EDUCATION
Erythromycin, ketoconazole, and grapefruit juice increase the effects of buspirone.	• Take complete medication history. • Advise clients to avoid drinking grapefruit juice.

Nursing Administration

- Advise clients to take the medication with meals to prevent gastric irritation.
- Advise clients that effects do not occur rapidly and may take a week to start, and several more for the full benefit to be felt.
- Advise clients to take the medication on a regular basis and not PRN.

Nursing Evaluation of Medication Effectiveness

- Depending on therapeutic intent, effectiveness may be evidenced by the following:
  - For depression:
    - Verbalizing improvement in mood
    - Improved sleeping and eating habits
    - Increased interaction with peers
  - For anxiety disorders:
    - Decrease in anxiety symptoms
    - Improvement in functioning

MEDICATION CLASSIFICATION: CNS STIMULANTS

- Select Prototypes and Other Medications

MEDICATION	SHORT – ACTING	INTERMEDIATE ACTING	LONG-ACTING
Methylphenidate	Ritalin, Methylin	Ritalin SR, Methylin ER	Ritalin LA, Concerta, Daytrana (transdermal)
Dexmethylphenidate	Focalin		
Dextroamphetamine	Dexedrine		Dexedrine Spansule
Amphetamine mixture	Adderall		Adderall-XR

Purpose

- Expected Pharmacological Action
  - These medications raise the levels of norepinephrine, serotonin, and dopamine into the CNS.
- Therapeutic Uses
  - ADHD
  - Conduct disorder

Complications

SIDE/ADVERSE EFFECTS	NURSING INTERVENTIONS/CLIENT EDUCATION
CNS stimulation (insomnia, restlessness)	• Advise clients to observe for symptoms and notify the provider if they occur. • Administer the last dose before 4 p.m.
Weight loss	• Monitor the client's weight and compare to baseline height and weight. • Administer medication immediately before or after meals. • Promote good nutrition in children. • Encourage children to eat at regular meal times and avoid unhealthy foods for snacks.
Cardiovascular effects (dysrhythmias, chest pain, high blood pressure) • These medications may increase the risk of sudden death in clients with heart abnormalities.	• Monitor the client's vital signs and ECG. • Advise clients to observe for symptoms and to notify the primary care provider if they occur.
Development of psychotic symptoms such as hallucinations, paranoia	• Instruct clients to report symptoms immediately and to discontinue the medication if they occur.
Withdrawal reaction	• Advise clients to not stop taking medication suddenly. Doing so may lead to depression and severe fatigue.
Hypersensitivity skin reaction to transdermal methylphenidate (hives, papules)	• Remove the patch and notify the provider.

Contraindications/Precautions

- These medications are contraindicated in clients who have a history of drug abuse, cardiovascular disorders, severe anxiety, and psychosis.

Interactions

MEDICATION/FOOD INTERACTIONS	NURSING INTERVENTIONS/CLIENT EDUCATION
Concurrent use of MAOIs may cause hypertensive crisis.	• Avoid concurrent use.
Concurrent use of caffeine may increase CNS stimulant effects.	• Instruct clients to avoid foods that contain caffeine.
Methylphenidate inhibits metabolism of phenytoin (Dilantin), warfarin (Coumadin), and phenobarbital, leading to increased serum levels.	• Monitor clients for adverse effects (CNS depression, signs of bleeding). • Concurrent use of these medications should be used cautiously.
OTC cold and decongestant medications with sympathomimetic action can increase CNS stimulant effects.	• Instruct clients to avoid use of OTC medications.

Nursing Administration

- Advise clients to swallow sustained-release tablets whole and to not chew or crush the tablets.
- Teach clients the importance of administering the medication on a regular schedule.
- Teach clients who use transdermal medication (Daytrana) to place the patch on one hip daily in the morning and leave it in place no longer than 9 hr. Alternate hips daily.
- Instruct parents and clients that ADHD is not cured by medication and should be managed with an overall treatment plan that may include family therapy and cognitive therapy.
- Instruct parents that these medications have special handling procedures controlled by federal law. Handwritten prescriptions are required for medication refills.
- Instruct parents in safety and storage of medications.
- Advise parents that these medications have a high potential for abuse.

Nursing Evaluation of Medication Effectiveness

- Depending on therapeutic intent, effectiveness may be evidenced by:
    - Improvement of symptoms of ADHD, such as increased ability to focus and complete tasks, interact with peers, and manage impulsivity
    - Improved ability to stay awake

MEDICATION CLASSIFICATION: NOREPINEPHRINE SELECTIVE REUPTAKE INHIBITOR

- Select Prototype Medication: atomoxetine (Strattera)

Purpose

- Expected Pharmacological Action
    - Blocks reuptake of norepinephrine at synapses in the CNS. Atomoxetine is not a stimulant medication.
- Therapeutic Uses
    - ADHD

Complications

- Atomoxetine is usually tolerated well with minimal side effects.

SIDE/ADVERSE EFFECTS	NURSING INTERVENTIONS/CLIENT EDUCATION
Appetite suppression, weight loss, growth suppression	• Monitor the client's weight and compare to baseline height and weight. • Administer medication right before meals. • Encourage children to eat at regular meal times and avoid unhealthy foods for snacks.
GI effects (nausea and vomiting)	• Advise client to take with food if these occur.
Suicidal ideation (in children and adolescents)	• Clients should be monitored for signs of depression. • Advise clients to report change in mood, excessive sleeping, agitation, and irritability.
Hepatotoxicity	• Advise client to report signs of liver damage (flu-like symptoms, yellowing skin, abdominal pain).

Contraindications/Precautions

- Use cautiously in clients with cardiovascular disorders.

Interactions

MEDICATION/FOOD INTERACTIONS	NURSING INTERVENTIONS
• Concurrent use of MAOIs may cause hypertensive crisis.	• Avoid concurrent use.
• Paroxetine (Paxil), fluoxetine (Prozac), or quinidine gluconate (Quinidine Duratabs) inhibit hepatic metabolizing enzymes, thereby increasing levels of atomoxetine.	• Teach clients to watch for and report increased adverse reactions of atomoxetine. • Dosage of atomoxetine may need to be reduced if used concurrently with these medications.

Nursing Administration

- Note any changes in the child's behavior related to dosing and timing of medications.
- Administer the medication in a daily dose in the morning, or in two divided doses, morning and afternoon, with or without food.
- Instruct clients that effects may take at least one week to fully develop.

Nursing Evaluation of Medication Effectiveness

- Depending on therapeutic intent, effectiveness may be evidenced by:
  - Improvement of symptoms of ADHD such as increase in ability to focus and complete tasks, interact with peers, and manage impulsivity.

MEDICATION CLASSIFICATION: ANTIPSYCHOTICS – ATYPICAL

- Select Prototype Medication: risperidone (Risperdal)
- Other Medications:
  - Olanzapine (Zyprexa)
  - Quetiapine (Seroquel)

Purpose

- Expected Pharmacological Action
  - These antipsychotic agents work mainly by blocking serotonin, and to a lesser degree, dopamine receptors. These medications also block receptors for norepinephrine, histamine, and acetylcholine.
- Therapeutic Uses
  - Pervasive development disorders (PDD) including autistic disorder
  - Conduct disorder
  - Post-Traumatic Stress Disorder (PTSD)
  - Relief of psychotic symptoms

Complications

SIDE/ADVERSE EFFECTS	NURSING INTERVENTIONS/CLIENT EDUCATION
New onset of diabetes or loss of glucose control in clients with diabetes	• Obtain the client's baseline fasting blood glucose and monitor periodically throughout treatment. • Instruct clients to report signs and symptoms such as increased thirst, urination, and appetite.
Weight gain	• Advise clients to follow a healthy, low-caloric diet, engage in regular exercise, and monitor weight gain.
Hypercholesterolemia with increased risk for hypertension and other cardiovascular disease	• Monitor cholesterol, triglycerides, and blood glucose if weight gain is more than 14 kg (30 lb).
Orthostatic hypotension	• Monitor blood pressure with first dose. Instruct client to change positions slowly.
Anticholinergic effects (urinary hesitancy or retention, dry mouth)	• Monitor for these adverse effects and report their occurrence to the provider. • Encourage client to use measures to relieve dry mouth such as sipping fluids throughout the day.
Agitation, dizziness, sedation, and sleep disruption	• Monitor for these adverse effects and report their occurrence to the provider. • Administer an alternative medication if prescribed.
May cause mild extrapyramidal side effects, such as tremor	• Monitor for and teach clients to recognize extrapyramidal side effects. These are usually dose related.

Contraindications/Precautions

- Clients should avoid the use of alcohol.
- Use cautiously in clients with cardiovascular disease, seizures, or diabetes mellitus. Obtain a baseline fasting glucose for clients with diabetes mellitus and monitor carefully.

Interactions

MEDICATION/FOOD INTERACTIONS	NURSING INTERVENTIONS/CLIENT EDUCATION
• Alcohol, opioids, and antihistamines cause additive CNS depressant effects.	• Advise clients to avoid alcohol and other medications that cause CNS depression. • Advise clients to avoid hazardous activities, such as driving.
• By activating dopamine receptors, levodopa counteracts effects of antipsychotic agents.	• Avoid concurrent use of levodopa and other direct dopamine receptor agonists.
• Tricyclic antidepressants, amiodarone (Cordarone), and clarithromycin (Biaxin) prolong QT interval and thus increase the risk of cardiac dysrhythmias.	• Avoid concurrent use.
• Barbiturates and phenytoin (Dilantin) promote hepatic drug-metabolizing enzymes, thereby decreasing drug levels of quetiapine.	• Monitor medication effectiveness.
• Medications that inhibit CYP3A4, such as fluconazole (Diflucan), inhibit hepatic drug-metabolizing enzymes, thereby increasing drug levels of aripiprazole, quetiapine, and ziprasidone.	• Monitor for adverse effects.

Nursing Administration

- Administer by oral or IM route.
- Advise clients that low doses of medication are given initially and are then gradually increased.

Nursing Evaluation of Medication Effectiveness

- Depending on therapeutic intent, effectiveness may be evidenced by the following:
  - For PDD: Reduction of hyperactivity and improvement in mood
  - For conduct disorder: decrease in aggressiveness
  - For PTSD:
    - Decrease in aggressiveness and reduction of flashbacks
    - Improvement of psychotic symptoms (prevention of acute psychotic symptoms and absence of hallucinations, delusions, anxiety, and hostility)
    - Improvement in ability to perform ADLs
    - Improvement in ability to interact socially with peers
    - Improvement of sleeping and eating habits

CHAPTER 11: BEHAVIORAL DISORDERS

Application Exercises

1. A nurse is teaching the parents of a child who has a new prescription for fluoxetine (Prozac) about possible reactions during the first three days of treatment. For which of the following manifestations should the nurse teach the family to stop the medication and notify the provider immediately?

    A. Diaphoresis

    B. Fever

    C. Nausea

    D. Headache

2. An adolescent client has just begun taking amitriptyline (Elavil) for depression. Which of the following nursing interventions should the nurse teach the client in order to minimize an adverse effect of his medication?

    A. Wear sunglasses when outdoors.

    B. Check temperature daily while taking this medication.

    C. Take medication first thing in the morning before eating.

    D. Add extra calories to the diet as between-meal snacks.

3. A nurse is caring for a school-age child who recently began a prescription for atomoxetine (Strattera). For which of the following possible complications should the nurse monitor the child?

    A. Renal toxicity

    B. Liver damage

    C. Seizure activity

    D. Adrenal insufficiency

4. A nurse is caring for a school-age child who has just been prescribed methylphenidate (Concerta) to treat ADHD. Which of the following should the nurse teach the client and family about this medication?

    A. Apply the patch once daily at bedtime.

    B. Take oral medication once daily in the morning.

    C. Take oral medication early in the morning and again at bedtime.

    D. Apply the patch on awakening and remove at bedtime.

CHAPTER 11: BEHAVIORAL DISORDERS

Application Exercises Answer Key

1. A nurse is teaching the parents of a child who has a new prescription for fluoxetine (Prozac) about possible reactions during the first three days of treatment. For which of the following manifestations should the nurse teach the family to stop the medication and notify the provider immediately?

   A. Diaphoresis

   B. Fever

   C. Nausea

   D. Headache

   Fever, tremors, hyperreflexia, agitation, and hallucinations are some of the manifestations of serotonin syndrome, which may occur between 2 and 72 hours after beginning treatment with fluoxetine and other SSRI medications. The family should stop the medication and notify the provider if these symptoms occur. Diaphoresis is a side effect the client may be taught to expect; however, it will not warrant stopping the medication and notifying the provider. Nausea and headache are signs of abrupt withdrawal from SSRI medications and are not manifestations to watch for during the first three days of therapy.

NCLEX® Connection: Pharmacological and Parenteral Therapies: Adverse Effects/ Contraindications/Side Effects/Interactions

2. An adolescent client has just begun taking amitriptyline (Elavil) for depression. Which of the following nursing interventions should the nurse teach the client in order to minimize an adverse effect of his medication?

   A. Wear sunglasses when outdoors.

   B. Check temperature daily while taking this medication.

   C. Take medication first thing in the morning before eating.

   D. Add extra calories to the diet as between-meal snacks.

   Wearing sunglasses when outdoors will decrease photophobia, an anticholinergic effect that may be experienced when taking a tricyclic antidepressant medication such as amitriptyline. Checking the temperature daily while taking a TCA is not necessary. Taking the medication at bedtime rather than in the morning will prevent daytime sleepiness. Following a low-calorie diet plan rather than adding extra calories as snacks will help prevent weight gain, a common adverse effect.

NCLEX® Connection: Pharmacological and Parenteral Therapies: Adverse Effects/ Contraindications/Side Effects/Interactions

3. A nurse is caring for a school-age child who recently began a prescription for atomoxetine (Strattera). For which of the following possible complications should the nurse monitor the child?

   A. Renal toxicity

   B. Liver damage

   C. Seizure activity

   D. Adrenal insufficiency

   Liver damage may occur while taking atomoxetine. The nurse should monitor for signs such as jaundice, upper abdominal tenderness, darkening of urine, and elevated liver enzymes. Renal toxicity, seizure activity, and adrenal insufficiency are not complications expected when taking atomoxetine.

NCLEX® Connection: Pharmacological and Parenteral Therapies: Adverse Effects/Contraindications/Side Effects/Interactions

4. A nurse is caring for a school-age child who has just been prescribed methylphenidate (Concerta) to treat ADHD. Which of the following should the nurse teach the client and family about this medication?

   A. Apply the patch once daily at bedtime.

   B. Take oral medication once daily in the morning.

   C. Take oral medication early in the morning and again at bedtime.

   D. Apply the patch on awakening and remove at bedtime.

   Concerta is a long-acting formulation of methylphenidate that should be taken once daily in the morning. A long-acting methylphenidate (Daytrana) transdermal patch is available, which should be put on in the morning and removed after no more than 9 hours each day. Short-acting methylphenidate (Ritalin) is taken orally 2 or 3 times daily. The last dose is taken no later than late afternoon or early evening so as not to interfere with the child's sleep.

NCLEX® Connection: Pharmacological and Parenteral Therapies: Medication Administration

UNIT 2 MEDICATIONS AFFECTING THE NERVOUS SYSTEM

Chapter 12 Substance Abuse

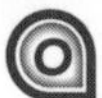

Overview

- Abstinence syndrome occurs when a client abruptly withdraws from a drug on which he is physically dependent.
- Withdrawing from a substance that has the potential to cause addiction can cause an abstinence syndrome. Symptoms of abstinence syndrome can be distressing and may lead to coma and death.
- Major Drugs of Abuse

SUBSTANCE	WITHDRAWAL SYMPTOMS
Alcohol	• Effects usually start within 4 to 12 hr of the last intake of alcohol, peak after 24 to 48 hr, and subside within 5 to 7 days, unless alcohol withdrawal delirium occurs. • Symptoms include nausea; vomiting; tremors; restlessness and inability to sleep; depressed mood or irritability; increased heart rate, blood pressure, respiratory rate, and temperature; and tonic-clonic seizures. Illusions are also common. • Alcohol withdrawal delirium may occur 2 to 3 days after cessation of alcohol, and may last 2 to 3 days, and is considered a medical emergency. Findings include severe disorientation, psychotic symptoms (hallucinations), severe hypertension, and cardiac dysrhythmias that may progress to death.
Opioids, including heroin and prescription medications	• Characteristic withdrawal syndrome occurs within 1 hr to several days of cessation of drug use. • Symptoms include agitation, insomnia, flu-like symptoms, rhinorrhea, yawning, sweating, and diarrhea. • Symptoms are non-life-threatening, although suicidal ideation may occur.
Nicotine	• Abstinence syndrome is evidenced by irritability, nervousness, restlessness, insomnia, and difficulty concentrating.

MEDICATIONS TO SUPPORT WITHDRAWAL/ABSTINENCE FROM ALCOHOL

Detoxification

INTENDED EFFECTS	NURSING INTERVENTIONS/CLIENT EDUCATION
Benzodiazepines: chlordiazepoxide (Librium), diazepam (Valium), lorazepam (Ativan)	
• Maintenance of the client's vital signs within normal limits • Decrease in the risk of seizures • Decrease in the intensity of symptoms	• Administer around the clock or PRN. • Use chlordiazepoxide only if the client is able to tolerate oral intake. Otherwise, use IV route for diazepam and lorazepam. The client may continue with diazepam and lorazepam orally. • Obtain the client's baseline vital signs. • Monitor the client's vital signs and neurological status on an ongoing basis. • Provide for seizure precautions (padded side rails, suction equipment at bedside).
Adjunct medications: carbamazepine (Tegretol), clonidine (Catapres), propranolol (Inderal)	
• Decrease in seizures ○ Carbamazepine • Depression of autonomic response (decrease in blood pressure, heart rate, diaphoresis) ○ Clonidine and propranolol • Decrease in cravings ○ Propranolol	• Provide for seizure precautions (padded side rails and suction equipment at bedside). • Obtain the client's baseline vital signs and continue to monitor on a regular basis.

Abstinence Maintenance (Following Detoxification)

INTENDED EFFECTS	NURSING INTERVENTIONS/CLIENT EDUCATION
Disulfiram (Antabuse)	
• Disulfiram is a daily oral medication that is a type of aversion (behavioral) therapy. • Disulfiram used concurrently with alcohol will cause acetaldehyde syndrome to occur. • Effects include nausea, vomiting, weakness, sweating, palpitations, and hypotension. • Acetaldehyde syndrome can progress to respiratory depression, cardiovascular suppression, seizures, and death.	• Inform clients of the potential dangers of drinking any alcohol. • Advise clients to avoid any products that contain alcohol (cough syrups, aftershave lotion). • Encourage clients to wear a medical alert bracelet. • Encourage clients to participate in a 12-step self-help program. • Advise clients that medication effects (potential for acetaldehyde syndrome with alcohol ingestion) persist for 2 weeks following discontinuation of disulfiram.

INTENDED EFFECTS	NURSING INTERVENTIONS/CLIENT EDUCATION
Naltrexone (ReVia)	
Naltrexone is a pure opioid antagonist that suppresses the craving and pleasurable effects of alcohol (also used for opioid withdrawal).	• Take an accurate history to determine if clients are also dependent on opioids. Use of naltrexone will initiate withdrawal syndrome. • Advise clients to take the medication with meals to decrease gastrointestinal distress. • Suggest monthly IM injects for clients with difficulty adhering to regimen.
Acamprosate (Campral)	
Acamprosate decreases unpleasant effects resulting from abstinence (anxiety, restlessness).	• Inform clients that diarrhea may result. • Advise clients to maintain adequate fluid intake and to receive adequate rest. • Advise clients to avoid use in pregnancy

MEDICATIONS TO SUPPORT WITHDRAWAL/ABSTINENCE FROM OPIOIDS

INTENDED EFFECTS	NURSING INTERVENTIONS/CLIENT EDUCATION
Methadone (Dolophine) substitution	
• Methadone substitution is an oral opioid agonist that replaces the opioid to which the client is addicted. • This will prevent abstinence syndrome from occurring and remove the need for the client to obtain illegal drugs. • It is used for withdrawal and long-term maintenance. • Dependence will be transferred from the illegal opioid to methadone.	• Inform clients that the methadone dose must be slowly tapered to produce detoxification. • Encourage clients to participate in a 12-step self-help program. • Inform clients that medication must be administered from a an approved treatment center.
Clonidine (Catapres)	
• Clonidine assists with withdrawal of symptoms related to autonomic hyperactivity (diarrhea, nausea, vomiting). • Clonidine therapy does not reduce the craving for opioids.	• Obtain baseline vital signs. • Advise clients to avoid activities that require mental alertness until drowsiness subsides. • Encourage clients to chew gum or suck on hard candy and to sip small amounts of water or suck on ice chips to treat dry mouth.
Buprenorphine (Subutex), buprenorphine combined with naloxone (Suboxone)	
• These medications are agonist-antagonist opioids used for detoxification and maintenance. • These medications decrease feelings of craving and may be effective in maintaining adherence.	• Inform clients that medication must be administered from an approved treatment center. • Administer sublingually.

MEDICATIONS TO SUPPORT WITHDRAWAL/ABSTINENCE FROM NICOTINE

INTENDED EFFECTS	NURSING INTERVENTIONS/CLIENT EDUCATION
Bupropion (Zyban)	
Bupropion decreases nicotine craving and symptoms of withdrawal.	• To treat dry mouth, encourage clients to chew gum or suck on hard candy and to sip small amounts of water or suck on ice chips. • Advise clients to avoid caffeine and other CNS stimulants to control insomnia.
Nicotine replacement therapy (nicotine gum [Nicorette] and nicotine patch [Nicotrol])	
These nicotine replacements are pharmaceutical product substitutes for the nicotine in cigarettes or chewing tobacco.	• Clients should avoid using any nicotine products while pregnant or breastfeeding. • Nicotine gum: ○ Use of chewing gum is not recommended for longer than 6 months. ○ Advise clients to chew gum slowly and intermittently over 30 min. ○ Advise clients to avoid eating or drinking 15 min prior to and while chewing the gum. • Nicotine patch: ○ Clients should apply a nicotine patch to an area of clean, dry skin each day. ○ Advise clients to avoid using any nicotine products while the patch is on. ○ Follow product directions for dosage times. ○ Advise clients to stop using patches and to notify the provider if local skin reactions occur. ○ Remove the patch prior to MRI scan and replace when the scan is completed.

Nursing Evaluation of Medication Effectiveness

- Depending on therapeutic intent, effectiveness may be evidenced by:
    - Absence of injury
    - Abstinence from substance
    - Regular attendance at self-help group

CHAPTER 12: SUBSTANCE ABUSE

Application Exercises

1. A nurse is caring for a client who is withdrawing from alcohol. Which of the following medications should the nurse expect to administer to decrease craving?

   A. Carbamazepine (Tegretol)
   B. Methadone (Dolophine)
   C. Propranolol (Inderal)
   D. Clonidine (Catapres)

2. Which of the following medications may be used to for short-term management of alcohol detoxification? (Select all that apply.)

   _____ Lorazepam (Ativan)
   _____ Diazepam (Valium)
   _____ Disulfiram (Antabuse)
   _____ Naltrexone (ReVia)
   _____ Acamprosate (Campral)

3. A nurse is providing teaching to a client who is prescribed clonidine (Catapres) to assist with maintenance of abstinence from opioids. The nurse should instruct the client to watch for which of the following side effects?

   A. Diarrhea
   B. Dry mouth
   C. Agitation
   D. Headaches

4. Match the treatment goal with the appropriate medication

_____ Alcohol withdrawal	A. Methadone (Dolophine)
_____ Heroin withdrawal	B. Naloxone (Narcan)
_____ Nicotine withdrawal	C. Bupropion (Zyban)
_____ Alcohol abstinence	D. Chlordiazepoxide (Librium)
_____ Morphine overdose	E. Disulfiram (Antabuse)

CHAPTER 12: SUBSTANCE ABUSE

Application Exercises Answer Key

1. A nurse is caring for a client who is withdrawing from alcohol. Which of the following medications should the nurse expect to administer to decrease craving?

   A. Carbamazepine (Tegretol)

   B. Methadone (Dolophine)

   C. Propranolol (Inderal)

   D. Clonidine (Catapres)

   Propranolol is administered to decrease craving and control autonomic responses such as elevated heart rate and blood pressure. Clonidine provides relief for somatic symptoms of withdrawal. Carbamazepine is an antiepileptic agent administered to prevent seizures. Methadone is used for opioid withdrawal.

NCLEX® Connection: Pharmacological and Parenteral Therapies: Expected Actions/Outcomes

2. Which of the following medications may be used to for short-term management of alcohol detoxification? (Select all that apply.)

   __X__ **Lorazepam (Ativan)**

   __X__ **Diazepam (Valium)**

   ______ Disulfiram (Antabuse)

   ______ Naltrexone (ReVia)

   ______ Acamprosate (Campral)

   Lorazepam and diazepam are both benzodiazepines used short-term for detoxification. They decrease anxiety and prevent seizures. Disulfiram is administered to assist the client maintain abstinence from alcohol. Clients who drink alcohol while taking disulfiram may experience a mild reaction such as nausea and vomiting or a more severe reaction that can lead to respiratory depression and death. Naltrexone is a pure opioid antagonist that suppresses the craving and pleasurable effects of alcohol. Acamprosate decreases unpleasant effects resulting from abstinence (anxiety, restlessness).

NCLEX® Connection: Pharmacological and Parenteral Therapies: Expected Actions/Outcomes

3. A nurse is providing teaching to a client who is prescribed clonidine (Catapres) to assist with maintenance of abstinence from opioids. The nurse should instruct the client to watch for which of the following side effects?

   A. Diarrhea

   B. Dry mouth

   C. Agitation

   D. Headaches

   Dry mouth is a common side effect of clonidine and can be managed by chewing gum or sipping water throughout the day. Clonidine may cause constipation and drowsiness and is used to decrease the autonomic symptoms of diarrhea and agitation. Headaches are not associated with clonidine use.

NCLEX® Connection: Pharmacological and Parenteral Therapies, Adverse Effects/Contraindications/Side Effects/Interactions

4. Match the treatment goal with the appropriate medication

Answer	Treatment goal	Medication
D	Alcohol withdrawal	A. Methadone (Dolophine)
A	Heroin withdrawal	B. Naloxone (Narcan)
C	Nicotine withdrawal	C. Bupropion (Zyban)
E	Alcohol abstinence	D. Chlordiazepoxide (Librium)
B	Morphine overdose	E. Disulfiram (Antabuse)

NCLEX® Connection: Pharmacological and Parenteral Therapies, Adverse Effects/Contraindications/Side Effects/Interactions

UNIT 2 MEDICATIONS AFFECTING THE NERVOUS SYSTEM

Chapter 13 Chronic Neurologic Disorders

Overview

- Medications administered for chronic neurologic disorders are used to manage symptoms and improve quality of life.
- Chronic neurologic disorders include myasthenia gravis, Parkinson's disease, and seizure disorder.

MEDICATION CLASSIFICATION: CHOLINESTERASE INHIBITORS

- Select Prototype Medication: neostigmine (Prostigmin)
- Other Medications:
  - Ambenonium (Mytelase)
  - Pyridostigmine (Mestinon)
  - Edrophonium (Tensilon)

Purpose

- Expected Pharmacological Action
  - Cholinesterase inhibitors prevent the enzyme cholinesterase (ChE) from inactivating acetylcholine (ACh), thereby increasing the amount of ACh available at receptor sites. Transmission of nerve impulses is increased at all sites responding to ACh as a transmitter.
- Therapeutic Uses

	NEOSTIGMINE	AMBENOMIUM	PYRIDOSTIGMINE	EDROPHONIUM
Treatment of myasthenia gravis	X	X	X	
Diagnosis of myasthenia gravis				X
Reversal of nondepolarizing neuromuscular blocking agents	X		X	X

Complications

SIDE/ADVERSE EFFECTS	NURSING INTERVENTIONS/CLIENT EDUCATION
Excessive muscarine stimulation as evidenced by increased GI motility, increased GI secretions, bradycardia, and urinary urgency	• Advise the client of potential side effects. If effects become intolerable, instruct the client to notify the provider. • Side effects may be treated with atropine.
Cholinergic crisis (excessive muscarinic stimulation and respiratory depression from neuromuscular blockade)	• Muscarinic effects can be treated with atropine. • Provide respiratory support through mechanical ventilation and oxygen.

Contraindications/Precautions

- Cholinesterase inhibitors are Pregnancy Risk Category C.
- These medications are contraindicated in clients with obstruction of GI and GU system
- Use cautiously in clients with seizure disorders, hyperthyroidism, peptic ulcer disease, asthma, bradycardia, and hypotension.

Interactions

MEDICATION/FOOD INTERACTIONS	NURSING INTERVENTIONS/CLIENT EDUCATION
Atropine counteracts the effects of neostigmine.	• Atropine is used to treat neostigmine toxicity. • Monitor the client closely and provide mechanical ventilation until the client has regained full muscle function.
Neostigmine reverses neuromuscular blockade caused by neuromuscular blocking agents after surgical procedures and overdose.	• Monitor the client for return of respiratory function. Support respiratory function as necessary. If used to treat overdose, provide mechanical ventilation until the client has regained full muscle function.
Succinylcholine increases neuromuscular blockade.	• Avoid concurrent use.

Nursing Administration

- Neostigmine may be given PO, IM, IV, or subcutaneously.
- Instruct clients to take medications as prescribed.
- Advise clients that dosage is very individualized, starts at very low doses, and is titrated until desired muscle function is achieved.

- Encourage clients to participate in self-dosage adjustments. This can be accomplished by having the client:
  - Keep records of medication administration and effects
  - Recognize signs of inadequate dosing, such as difficulty swallowing and signs of overmedication, such as urinary urgency
  - Modify dosage based on response
- Advise clients to wear a medical alert bracelet.

Nursing Evaluation of Medication Effectiveness

- Depending on therapeutic intent, effectiveness may be evidenced by:
  - Fewer episodes of fatigue
  - Improvement in strength as demonstrated by chewing, swallowing, and performing activities of daily living (ADLs) such as bathing, walking, eating, and dressing

MEDICATION CLASSIFICATION: ANTI-PARKINSON'S MEDICATIONS

- Select Prototype Medications:
  - Dopaminergics: levodopa (Dopar, Larodopa) or levodopa plus carbidopa (Sinemet)
  - Dopamine agonists: pramipexole (Mirapex)
  - Centrally acting anticholinergics: benztropine (Cogentin)
  - Dopamine releaser (Antiviral): amantadine (Symmetrel)
- Other Medications:
  - Dopamine agonists: ropinirole (Requip), bromocriptine (Parlodel)
  - Centrally acting anticholinergics: trihexyphenidyl (Artane)

Purpose

- Expected Pharmacological Action
  - These medications do not halt the progression of Parkinson's disease (PD). However, they do offer symptomatic relief from dyskinesias (bradykinesia, resting tremors, and muscle rigidity) and an increase in the ability to perform ADLs by maintaining the balance between dopamine and acetylcholine in the extrapyramidal nervous system.

CLASSIFICATIONS	EXPECTED PHARMACOLOGICAL ACTION
Dopaminergics	• Levodopa crosses the blood-brain barrier and is taken up by dopaminergic nerve terminals and converted to dopamine (DA). This newly synthesized DA is released into the synaptic space and causes stimulation of DA receptors. • Carbidopa is used to augment levodopa by decreasing the amount of levodopa that is converted to DA in the intestine and periphery. This results in greater amounts of levodopa reaching the CNS.
Dopamine agonists	• These agents act directly on DA receptors.
Centrally acting anticholinergics	• These agents block acetylcholine at muscarinic receptors, which assists in maintaining balance between dopamine and acetylcholine in the brain.
Antiviral	• Antivirals stimulate DA release, prevent dopamine reuptake, and may block cholinergic and glutamate receptors.

- Therapeutic Uses
    - Levodopa may be used as a first-line medication for PD treatment.
    - Pramipexole is used as monotherapy in early-stage PD and used in conjunction with levodopa in late-stage PD. It is used more often in younger clients who are better able to tolerate daytime drowsiness and postural hypotension.

Complications

SIDE/ADVERSE EFFECTS	NURSING INTERVENTIONS/CLIENT EDUCATION
Dopaminergics: levodopa (Usually dose dependent)	
Nausea and vomiting, drowsiness	• Administer with food, and in small doses and at the start of treatment.
Dyskinesias (head bobbing, tics, grimacing, tremors)	• Decrease the dosage. The decrease may result in resumption of PD symptoms.
Orthostatic hypotension	• Monitor the client's blood pressure. • Instruct clients about signs of postural hypotension (lightheadedness, dizziness). If these occur, advise the client to sit or lie down. Postural hypotension can be minimized by getting up slowly and avoiding sudden changes of position.
Cardiovascular effects from $beta_1$ stimulation (tachycardia, palpitations, irregular heartbeat)	• Monitor the client's vital signs. • Monitor ECG. • Notify the provider if symptoms occur. • Use cautiously in clients who have cardiovascular disorders.
Psychosis (visual hallucinations, nightmares)	• Administer antipsychotic medications as prescribed.
Discoloration of sweat and urine	• Advise clients that this is a harmless side effect.
Activation of malignant melanoma	• Avoid use of medication in clients who have skin lesions that have not been diagnosed.

SIDE/ADVERSE EFFECTS	NURSING INTERVENTIONS/CLIENT EDUCATION
Dopamine agonists: pramipexole	
Sudden inability to stay awake	• Advise clients to notify the provider immediately if this occurs.
Daytime sleepiness	• Advise clients of the potential for drowsiness and to avoid hazardous activities. • Advise clients to avoid other CNS depressants such as alcohol.
Orthostatic hypotension	• Instruct clients about the signs of postural hypotension (lightheadedness, dizziness). If these occur, advise clients to sit or lie down. Postural hypotension can be minimized by getting up slowly. Advise clients to avoid sudden changes of position.
Psychosis (visual hallucinations, nightmares)	• Administer antipsychotic medications, such as clozapine (Clozaril), if symptoms occur.
Dyskinesias (head bobbing, tics, grimacing, tremors)	• Decrease dosage of medication.
Nausea	• Advise clients to take medication with food.
Centrally acting anticholinergics: benztropine	
Nausea, vomiting	• Advise clients to take medication with food but to avoid high-protein snacks.
Atropine-like effects (dry mouth, blurred vision, mydriasis, urinary retention, constipation)	• Advise clients to observe for symptoms and notify the provider if they occur. • Monitor I&O and assess clients for urinary retention. • Advise clients to chew sugarless gum, eat foods high in fiber, and increase fluid intake to 2 to 3 L/day from beverage and food sources.
Antihistamine effects (sedation, drowsiness)	• Advise clients to avoid hazardous activities while taking the medication.
Antiviral: amantadine	
CNS effects (confusion, dizziness, restlessness)	• Advise clients to avoid hazardous activities while taking the medication.
Atropine-like effects (dry mouth, blurred vision, mydriasis, urinary hesitancy or retention, constipation)	• Advise clients to observe for symptoms and notify the provider. • Monitor I&O, and assess clients for hesitancy or urinary retention. • Advise clients to chew sugarless gum, eat high-fiber foods, and increase fluid intake to 2 to 3 L/day from beverage and food.
Discoloration of skin, also called livido reticularis	• Advise clients that discoloration of the skin will subside when the medication is discontinued.
Levodopa plus carbidopa	
Abnormal movements, psychiatric disorders	• Advise clients of potential side effects and to notify the provider if they occur.

Contraindications/Precautions

- Levodopa
  - This medication is Pregnancy Risk Category C.
  - Contraindicated in clients with malignant melanoma
  - Do not use within 2 weeks of MAOI use.
  - Use cautiously in clients who have heart disease, clients who have psychiatric disorders, and older adult clients.

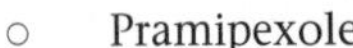

- Pramipexole
  - This medication is Pregnancy Risk Category C.
  - Use cautiously in clients with liver and kidney impairment.
- Benztropine
  - Contraindicated in clients with narrow-angle glaucoma

  - Use cautiously in older adults, the very young, and in clients who have enlarged prostate glands and a history of urinary retention.

Interactions

MEDICATION/FOOD INTERACTIONS	NURSING INTERVENTIONS/CLIENT EDUCATION
Dopaminergics: levodopa	
Proteins interfere with levodopa absorption and transport across the blood-brain barrier. High-protein meals decrease therapeutic effects.	• Proteins trigger an "off episode." • Advise clients to eat protein in several portions during the day.
Conventional-antipsychotic agents (chlorpromazine [Compazine], haloperidol [Haldol]) decrease therapeutic effects.	• Avoid concurrent use. • If the client experiences levodopa-induced psychosis, clozapine and quetiapine may be prescribed rather than conventional antipsychotic agents.
Pyridoxine (Vitamin B_6) decreases therapeutic effects.	• Advise clients to avoid vitamin preparations that contain pyridoxine.
Concurrent use of MAOIs may result in hypertensive crisis.	• Concurrent use is contraindicated.
Carbidopa, dopamine agonists, anticholinergics, Catechol O-methyltransferase (COMT) inhibitors, and dopamine releasers increase therapeutic effects.	• These medications can be used concurrently to increase the beneficial effects of levodopa.
Dopamine agonists: pramipexole	
Use with levodopa can decrease motor control fluctuations and allow for lower dosage of levodopa. Concurrent use can also increase the risk of orthostatic hypotension and dyskinesias.	• Monitor clients for these interactions.

MEDICATION/FOOD INTERACTIONS	NURSING INTERVENTIONS/CLIENT EDUCATION
Levodopa plus carbidopa	
Beneficial interactions include allowing for lower dosage of levodopa, reduced cardiovascular responses to dopamine in the periphery, and decreased nausea.	• Monitor clients for therapeutic effects.

Nursing Administration

- Instruct family members to assist clients with the medication at home.
- Instruct clients about the possible sudden loss of the effects of medication and to notify the provider if symptoms occur.
- Inform clients that effects may not be noticeable for several weeks to several months.
- Medication "holidays" may be indicated, but must be monitored in a hospital setting.
- Advise clients to avoid high-protein meals and snacks.

Nursing Evaluation of Medication Effectiveness

- Depending on therapeutic intent, effectiveness may be evidenced by:
  - Improvement of symptoms as demonstrated by absence of tremors, and reduction of irritability and stiffness.
  - Increase in ability to perform ADLs.

MEDICATION CLASSIFICATION: ANTIEPILEPTICS (AEDs)

- Select Prototype Medications:
  - Barbiturates:
    - Phenobarbital (Luminal)
    - Primidone (Mysoline)
  - Hydantoins: phenytoin (Dilantin)
  - Benzodiazepines:
    - Diazepam (Valium)
  - Lorazepam (Ativan)
  - Carbamazepine (Tegretol)
  - Ethosuximide (Zarontin)

    - Valproic acid (Depakote)
    - Gabapentin (Neurontin)
- Other Medications:
    - Lamotrigine (Lamictal)
    - Oxcarbazepine (Trileptal)

Purpose

- Expected Pharmacological Action
    - AEDs control seizure disorders by various mechanisms, which include:
        - Slowing the entrance of sodium and calcium back into the neuron and, thus extending the time it takes for the nerve to return to its active state
        - Suppressing neuronal firing, which decreases seizure activity and prevents propagation of seizure activity into other areas of the brain
        - Decreasing seizure activity by enhancing the inhibitory effects of gamma butyric acid (GABA)
- Therapeutic Uses

MEDICATION	THERAPEUTIC USES
Phenobarbital	• Phenobarbital is used for partial seizures and generalized tonic-clonic seizures. • This medication is not effective against absence seizures.
Phenytoin	• Phenytoin is effective against all major forms of epilepsy except absence seizures. • Use IV route for status epilepticus. • Phenytoin is an antidysrhythmic.
Carbamazepine	• Carbamazepine is used for the treatment of partial (simple and complex) seizures, tonic-clonic seizures, bipolar disorder, and trigeminal and glossopharyngeal neuralgias.
Ethosuximide	• Ethosuximide is only indicated for absence seizures.
Valproic acid	• Valproic acid is used for partial, generalized, and absence seizures; bipolar disorder; and migraine headaches.
Gabapentin	• Gabapentin is used as a single agent for control of partial seizures. • This medication is also used for neuropathic pain and the prevention of migraine headaches.
Diazepam	• Diazepam is used in status epilepticus.

Complications

SIDE/ADVERSE EFFECTS	NURSING INTERVENTIONS/CLIENT EDUCATION
Barbiturates: phenobarbital	
CNS effects in adults manifest as drowsiness, sedation, confusion, and anxiety. In children, CNS effects manifest as irritability and hyperactivity.	• Advise clients to observe for symptoms and to notify the provider if they occur. • Advise clients to avoid hazardous activities, such as driving.
Toxicity (nystagmus, ataxia, respiratory depression, coma, pinpoint pupils, hypotension, death)	• Stop medication. Administer oxygen and maintain respiratory function with ventilatory support. • Monitor the client's vital signs.
Hydantoins: phenytoin	
CNS effects (nystagmus, sedation, ataxia, double vision, cognitive impairment)	• Monitor for symptoms and notify the provider if symptoms occur.
Gingival hyperplasia (softening and overgrowth of gum tissue, tenderness, and bleeding gums)	• Advise clients to maintain good oral hygiene (dental flossing, massaging gums).
Skin rash	• Stop medication if rash develops.
Teratogenic (cleft palate, heart defects)	• Avoid use in pregnancy.
Cardiovascular effects (dysrhythmias, hypotension)	• Administer at slow IV rate and in dilute solution to prevent adverse CV effects.
Endocrine and other effects (coarsening of facial features, hirsutism, and interference with vitamin D metabolism)	• Instruct clients to report changes. • Encourage clients to consume adequate amounts of calcium and vitamin D.
Carbamazepine	
Cognitive function is minimally affected, but CNS effects (nystagmus, double vision, vertigo, staggering gait, headache) can occur.	• Administer in low doses initially and then gradually increase dosage. • Administer dose at bedtime.
Blood dyscrasias (leukopenia, anemia, thrombocytopenia)	• Obtain the client's baseline CBC and platelets. Perform ongoing monitoring of CBC and platelets. • Observe clients for signs of bruising and bleeding of gums.
Hypo-osmolarity (Carbamazepine promotes secretion of ADH, which inhibits water excretion by the kidneys and places clients who have heart failure at risk for fluid overload.	• Monitor serum sodium periodically. • Monitor the client for edema, decrease in urine output, and hypertension.
Skin disorders (dermatitis, rash, Stevens-Johnson syndrome)	• Treat mild reactions with anti-inflammatory or antihistamine medications. • Medication should be discontinued if there is a severe reaction.

SIDE/ADVERSE EFFECTS	NURSING INTERVENTIONS/CLIENT EDUCATION
Ethosuximide	
Gastrointestinal effects (nausea, vomiting)	• Administer with food.
CNS effects (sleepiness, lightheadedness, fatigue)	• Administer low initial dosage. • Advise clients to avoid hazardous activities, such as driving.
Valproic acid	
Gastrointestinal effects (nausea, vomiting, indigestion)	• Advise clients to take medication with food. Enteric-coated formulation can decrease symptoms.
Hepatotoxicity (anorexia, abdominal pain, jaundice)	• Assess baseline liver function and monitor liver function periodically. • Advise clients to observe for signs (anorexia, nausea, vomiting, abdominal pain, jaundice), and notify the provider if symptoms occur. • This medication should not be used for children younger than 3 years old. • Medication should be prescribed in lowest effective dose.
Pancreatitis as evidenced by nausea, vomiting, and abdominal pain	• Advise clients to observe for symptoms and to notify the provider immediately if these symptoms occur. • Monitor amylase levels. • Medication should be discontinued if pancreatitis develops.
Thrombocytopenia	• Advise clients to observe for symptoms such as bruising, and to notify the provider if these occur. • Monitor the client's platelet counts.
Gabapentin	
CNS effects (drowsiness, nystagmus)	• Administer low initial dosage. • Advise clients to avoid hazardous activities, such as driving.
Diazepam	
Respiratory depression	• Monitor the client's vital signs. • Have resuscitation equipment ready. • Administer oxygen.
Anterograde amnesia	• Monitor clients for memory loss. • Notify the provider if symptoms occur.

Contraindications/Precautions

- The following medications are in Pregnancy Risk Category D.
  - Barbiturates are contraindicated in clients with intermittent porphyria.
  - Phenytoin are contraindicated in clients with sinus bradycardia, sinoatrial blocks, second- and third-degree AV block, or Stokes-Adams syndrome.
  - Carbamazepine is contraindicated in clients with bone marrow suppression or with bleeding disorders.
  - Valproic acid is contraindicated in clients with liver disorders.

Interactions

MEDICATION/FOOD INTERACTIONS	NURSING INTERVENTIONS/CLIENT EDUCATION
Phenytoin	
Phenytoin causes a decrease in the effects of oral contraceptives, warfarin (Coumadin), and glucocorticoids because of the stimulation of hepatic drug-metabolizing enzymes.	• Dose of oral contraceptives may need to be adjusted or an alternative form of birth control used. • Monitor for therapeutic effects of warfarin and glucocorticoids. Dosages may need to be adjusted.
Alcohol, diazepam (Valium), cimetidine (Tagamet), and valproic acid increase phenytoin levels.	• Advise clients to avoid alcohol use. • Monitor serum levels.
Carbamazepine (Tegretol), phenobarbital, and chronic alcohol use decrease phenytoin levels.	• Encourage the client to avoid use of alcohol.
Additive CNS depressant effects can occur with concurrent use of CNS depressants (barbiturates, alcohol).	• Advise clients to avoid concurrent use of alcohol and other CNS depressants.
Carbamazepine	
Carbamazepine causes a decrease in the effects of oral contraceptives and warfarin (Coumadin) because of the stimulation of hepatic drug-metabolizing enzymes.	• Advise clients to increase dose of oral contraceptives. • Monitor for therapeutic effects of warfarin with PT and INR. • Dosages may need to be adjusted.
Grapefruit juice inhibits metabolism, and thus increases carbamazepine levels.	• Advise clients to avoid intake of grapefruit juice.
Phenytoin and phenobarbital decrease the effects of carbamazepine.	• Concurrent use is not recommended.
Valproic acid	
Concurrent use with valproic acid increases the levels of phenytoin and phenobarbital.	• Monitor phenytoin and phenobarbital levels. • Adjust dosage of medications as prescribed.

Nursing Administration

- Monitor therapeutic plasma levels. Be aware of therapeutic levels for medications prescribed. Notify the provider of results.
- Advise clients taking antiepileptic medications that treatment provides for control of seizures, not cure of disorder.
- Encourage clients to keep a seizure frequency diary to monitor effectiveness of therapy.
- Advise clients to take medications as prescribed and not to stop medications without consulting the provider. Sudden cessation of medication may trigger seizures.
- Advise clients to avoid hazardous activities (driving, operating heavy machinery) until seizures are fully controlled.
- Advise clients who are traveling to carry extra medication to avoid interruption of treatment in locations where their medication is not available.
- Advise clients of childbearing age to avoid pregnancy, because medications may cause birth defects and congenital abnormalities.
- Advise the client that phenytoin doses must be individualized. Dosing usually starts twice a day and can be switched to once a day dosing with an extended-release form when maintenance dose has been established.
- Advise clients that phenytoin has a narrow therapeutic range, and strict adherence to the medication regimen is imperative to prevent toxicity or therapeutic failure.

Nursing Evaluation of Medication Effectiveness

- Depending on therapeutic intent, effectiveness may be evidenced by:
    - Absence or decreased occurrence of seizures
    - Ability to perform ADLs
    - Absence of injury

CHAPTER 13: CHRONIC NEUROLOGIC DISORDERS

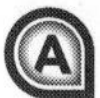

Application Exercises

1. Teaching for a client taking phenytoin (Dilantin) for a seizure disorder should include which of the following?

    A. Taking the medication with an antacid to prevent GI upset

    B. Practicing good hygiene, using a soft toothbrush, and flossing daily

    C. Using an OTC sleeping aid if difficulty sleeping

    D. Limiting daily alcohol intake to one glass of wine

2. A client has been diagnosed with absence seizures. The nurse understands that which of the following medications are used to treat this type of seizure? (Select all that apply)

    _____ Phenytoin (Dilantin)

    _____ Ethosuximide (Zarontin)

    _____ Gabapentin (Neurontin)

    _____ Carbamazepine (Tegretol)

    _____ Valproic acid (Depakote)

3. A nurse is providing teaching for a client who has just begun taking levodopa/carbidopa (Sinemet). To prevent food interactions from occurring, the client should be advised to avoid:

    A. High-protein meals

    B. Beverages containing caffeine

    C. Carbohydrate-containing snacks

    D. Foods high in fat

4. A client is taking pramipexole (Mirapex) to treat early Parkinson's disease. Which of the following should be included when teaching the client about possible adverse effects?

    A. Hallucinations

    B. Memory loss

    C. Diarrhea

    D. Discoloration of urine

CHAPTER 13: CHRONIC NEUROLOGIC DISORDERS

Application Exercises

1. Teaching for a client taking phenytoin (Dilantin) for a seizure disorder should include which of the following?

   A. taking the medication with an antacid to prevent GI upset.

   B. practicing good hygiene, using a soft toothbrush, and flossing daily.

   C. using an OTC sleeping aid if difficulty sleeping.

   D. limiting daily alcohol intake to one glass of wine.

   Gingival hyperplasia can occur with phenytoin use. Good oral hygiene can help minimize the effects. Antacids will interfere with absorption. OTC sleeping aids can have an additive CNS depressant effect. Clients taking phenytoin for seizure control should abstain from drinking any alcohol.

NCLEX® Connection: Pharmacological and Parenteral Therapies: Medication Administration

2. A client has been diagnosed with absence seizures. The nurse understands that which of the following medications are used to treat this type of seizure? (Select all that apply)

   ______ Phenytoin (Dilantin)

   __X__ **Ethosuximide (Zarontin)**

   ______ Gabapentin (Neurontin)

   ______ Carbamazepine (Tegretol)

   __X__ **Valproic acid (Depakote)**

   Ethosuximide and valproic acid are used to treat absence seizures. Phenytoin is effective against all major forms of epilepsy except absence seizures. Gabapentin is used as a single agent for control of partial seizures. Carbamazepine is used for the treatment of partial (simple and complex) seizures, tonic-clonic seizures, bipolar disorder, and trigeminal and glossopharyngeal neuralgias.

NCLEX® Connection: Pharmacological and Parenteral Therapies: Expected Actions/Outcomes

3. A nurse is providing teaching for a client who has just begun taking levodopa/carbidopa (Sinemet). To prevent food interactions from occurring, the client should be advised to avoid:

   A. High-protein meals

   B. Beverages containing caffeine

   C. Carbohydrate-containing snacks

   D. Foods high in fat

   The amino acids in protein foods interfere with levodopa absorption and can cause a decreased effect of the medication. Caffeine, carbohydrates, and fats do not interact with this medication.

NCLEX® Connection: Pharmacological and Parenteral Therapies: Adverse Effects/Contraindications/Side Effects/Interactions

4. A client is taking pramipexole (Mirapex) to treat early Parkinson's disease. Which of the following should be included when teaching the client about possible adverse effects?

    A. Hallucinations

    B. Memory loss

    C. Diarrhea

    D. Discoloration of urine

    Hallucinations may occur when taking pramipexole. Memory loss, diarrhea, and discoloration of urine are not expected adverse effects of this medication.

NCLEX® Connection: Pharmacological and Parenteral Therapies: Adverse Effects/ Contraindications/Side Effects/Interactions

UNIT 2 MEDICATIONS AFFECTING THE NERVOUS SYSTEM

Chapter 14 Eye and Ear Disorders

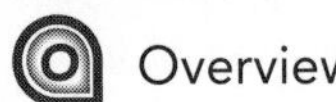

Overview

- Eye Disorders:
  - Glaucoma is the leading cause of blindness in the U.S. Damage to the optic nerve occurs when aqueous humor is not allowed to exit from the anterior chamber of the eye. This results in the buildup of aqueous humor, increased intraocular pressure (IOP), and loss of vision.
    - Types of glaucoma include:
      - Primary open-angle glaucoma (POAG)
        - POAG occurs in about 90% of people with glaucoma.
        - Peripheral vision is lost gradually, with central visual field loss occurring if damage to the optic nerve continues.
        - Symptoms usually occur only with widespread damage. IOP greater than 21 mm Hg is the highest risk factor for POAG.
        - Treatment includes medication therapy to reduce IOP. Surgical intervention is indicated if IOP cannot be reduced by medications.
      - Angle-closure glaucoma
        - This is an acute disorder with a sudden onset, resulting in irreversible blindness within 1 to 2 days without emergency treatment.
        - Symptoms include acute onset of ocular pain, seeing halos around lights, blurred vision, and photophobia. The optic nerve is damaged when the aqueous humor builds up as a result of displacement of the iris.
    - POAG is treated with the following medications:
      - Beta-adrenergic blockers
      - Alpha$_2$-adrenergic agonists
      - Prostaglandin analogs
      - Cholinergic agonists
      - Carbonic anhydrase inhibitors
      - Nonselective adrenergic agonists
    - Although several other classes of glaucoma medications may be used to treat angle-closure glaucoma, osmotic agents are first-line medications used to control symptoms until corrective surgery can be implemented.

- Ear disorders
  - Acute otitis media
    - This condition occurs most often in young children.
    - A bacterial or a viral infection causes a buildup of fluid in the middle ear (middle ear effusion).
    - The major symptom is acute onset of pain. Objective findings include erythema, bulging of the tympanic membrane, and fever.
    - Treatment for bacterial infection, especially in infants and young children, is an antibiotic. Treatment for viral infection is symptomatic.
      - Because of the increase in antibiotic-resistant bacteria, the current trend is to observe children over age 2 and prescribe antibiotics only if symptoms do not resolve or worsen over several days.
  - Otitis externa
    - This condition, also known as "swimmer's ear," is caused by a bacterial infection of the external auditory canal.
    - Any object that abrades or leaves moisture in the canal facilitates colonization of bacteria and the onset of otitis externa.
    - Treatment usually resolves infection within 10 days.
  - Medications for treating otitis media include:
    - Oral penicillins
    - Other antimicrobials, oral or parenteral
  - Otitis externa is usually treated by topical antimicrobial/anti-inflammatory combination.
    - Incidence of acute otitis media in infants and children can be reduced by yearly influenza vaccination and vaccination with pneumococcal conjugate vaccine (PCV).

MEDICATIONS FOR EYE DISORDERS

MEDICATION CLASSIFICATION: BETA ADRENERGIC BLOCKERS

- Nonselective beta blockers (which have both $beta_1$ and $beta_2$ properties):
  - Timolol (Timoptic, Betimol)
  - Carteolol (Ocupress)
  - Metipranolol (OptiPranolol)
  - Levobunolol (Betagan Liquifilm, AKBeta)
- Cardiac selective $beta_1$ blockers: betaxolol (Betoptic) and levobetaxolol (Betaxon)

Purpose

- Expected Pharmacological Action
  - Beta blockers decrease IOP by decreasing the amount of aqueous humor produced.
- Therapeutic Uses
  - Topical beta blockers are used primarily to treat POAG. They may also be prescribed in combination with other topical medications to lower IOP.
  - These medications are occasionally used to treat closed-angle glaucoma on an emergency basis.

Complications

SIDE/ADVERSE EFFECTS	NURSING INTERVENTIONS/CLIENT EDUCATION
Reports of temporary stinging discomfort in the eye immediately after drop is instilled	• Educate clients that this effect is transient.
Occasional conjunctivitis, blurred vision, photophobia, dry eyes	• Instruct clients to report symptoms to the provider.
Systemic effects of beta blockade on heart and lungs may occur.	• Warn clients that overdose could cause or increase the chance of systemic effects. • When taking $beta_1$ blockers, clients should monitor pulse rate for bradycardia. • Use $beta_1$ blockers for clients who have chronic respiratory disease.

Contraindications/Precautions

- Betaxolol and levobetaxolol are contraindicated for clients who have bradycardia and AV heart block, and should be used carefully in clients who have heart failure.

Interactions

MEDICATION/FOOD INTERACTIONS	NURSING INTERVENTIONS/CLIENT EDUCATION
Oral beta blockers or a calcium channel blocker can increase cardiovascular and respiratory effects.	• Instruct clients to inform the provider if they are taking any of these medications.
Beta blockers can interfere with some effects of insulin	• Advise clients who have diabetes to monitor their blood glucose.

Nursing Administration

- Instill one drop in the affected eye once or twice daily as prescribed.
- Review the proper method of instilling eye drops and provide instruction to a family member if indicated.

- Use sterile technique when handling the applicator portion of the container. Avoid touching any part of the applicator and keep the lid in place when not in use.
- Hold gentle pressure on the nasolacrimal duct for 30 to 60 seconds immediately after instilling the drop(s) to prevent or minimize any expected systemic effect.

- Monitor pulse rate/rhythm as indicated for beta blocker.

MEDICATION CLASSIFICATION: ALPHA$_2$ ADRENERGIC AGONISTS

- Select Prototype Medication: brimonidine (Alphagan)
- Other Medication: apraclonidine (Iopidine)

Purpose

- Expected Pharmacological Action
  - Brimonidine decreases production and may also decrease outflow of aqueous humor to lower IOP.
- Therapeutic Uses
  - Brimonidine is used as a first-line medication for long-term topical treatment of POAG.
  - Apraclonidine is a short-term therapy for POAG only and is also used preoperatively for laser eye surgeries.

Complications

SIDE/ADVERSE EFFECTS	NURSING INTERVENTIONS/CLIENT EDUCATION
Localized stinging discomfort and pruritus of conjunctiva; sensation that a foreign body is in the eye	• Advise clients not to rub their eyes.
Blurred vision, headache, dry mouth	• Instruct clients to report symptoms
Reddened sclera caused by blood-vessel engorgement	• Inform clients of the possibility of this effect.
Hypotension, drowsiness (brimonidine crosses the blood-brain barrier)	• Advise clients to use caution with driving and other tasks, and to inform the provider if dizziness and/or weakness occur.

Contraindications/Precautions

- Advise clients who wear soft contact lenses that brimonidine should be administered with lenses removed. Delay insertion of the lens at least 15 minutes after administration to prevent absorption of medication into the lens.

Interactions

MEDICATION/FOOD INTERACTIONS	NURSING INTERVENTIONS/CLIENT EDUCATION
Antihypertensive medications may intensify hypotension caused by brimonidine.	Instruct clients to inform the provider if they are taking any antihypertensive medications.

Nursing Administration

- Review proper method of administering eye drops and minimizing systemic effects
- Monitor blood pressure for hypotension as needed

MEDICATION CLASSIFICATION: PROSTAGLANDIN ANALOGS

- Select Prototype Medication: latanoprost (Xalatan)
- Other Medications:
    - Travoprost (Travatan)
    - Bimatoprost (Lumigan)
    - Unoprostone (Rescula)

Purpose

- Expected Pharmacological Action
    - Latanoprost increases aqueous humor outflow through relaxation of ciliary muscle.
- Therapeutic Uses
    - These agents are topical first-line medications for clients with POAG and ocular hypertension.

Complications

SIDE/ADVERSE EFFECTS	NURSING INTERVENTIONS/CLIENT EDUCATION
Permanent increased brown pigmentation, usually occurring in individuals with brown-colored iris (May also cause pigmentation of lids, lashes)	• Inform clients about the possibility of this effect.
Stinging, burning, reddened conjunctiva	• Instruct clients not to rub their eyes.
Blurred vision	• Instruct clients to report to the provider.
Migraine (rare adverse effect)	• Instruct clients to report to the provider.

Second-line Topical Medications for Glaucoma

CLASSIFICATION	PROTOTYPE	PURPOSE	SIDE/ADVERSE EFFECTS
Direct-acting cholinergic agonist	Pilocarpine (Isopto Carpine, Pilocar)	• Second-line treatment for POAG; lowers IOP indirectly through ciliary contraction • Also used to treat closed-angle glaucoma	• Retinal detachment • System effects, such as bradycardia • Decreased visual acuity
Carbonic anhydrase inhibitor	Dorzolamide (Trusopt) Also available in combination with Timolol (called Cosopt)	• Second-line treatment for POAG, which decreases aqueous humor production • Timolol/dorzolamide combination produces increased effect of both medications	• Localized allergic reactions in up to 15% • Blurred vision, dryness, photophobia
Adrenergic agonist	Dipivefrin (Propine)	• Converted to epinephrine after administration • Increases outflow of aqueous humor in POAG	• Local eye irritation, headache • Contraindicated for clients with closed-angle glaucoma

MEDICATION CLASSIFICATION: OSMOTIC AGENTS

- Select Prototype Medication: mannitol (Osmitrol)
- Other Medications:
  - Urea (Ureaphil)
  - Glycerin (Osmoglyn)
  - Isosorbide (Ismotic)

Purpose

- Expected Pharmacological Action
  - Osmotic agents decrease intraocular pressure rapidly by drawing fluid rapidly from the anterior chamber of the eye.
- Therapeutic Uses
  - These agents treat the rapid progression of closed-angle glaucoma to prevent blindness.

MEDICATION CLASSIFICATION: CARBONIC ANHYDRASE INHIBITOR (SYSTEMIC)

- Select Prototype Medication: acetazolamide (Diamox)
- Other Medications: methazolamide (GlaucTabs, Neptazane)

Purpose

- Expected Pharmacological Action
  - Reduces production of aqueous humor by causing diuresis through renal effects
- Therapeutic Uses
  - These medications are used to quickly lower IOP in clients for whom other medications have been ineffective.
  - Acetazolamide, a non-antimicrobial sulfonamide, can be used as an emergency medication prior to surgery for acute angle closure glaucoma and as a second-line medication for treatment of POAG.
  - Acetazolamide may also be used to treat glaucoma, acute mountain sickness, seizures, and heart failure (as a diuretic).

Complications

SIDE/ADVERSE EFFECTS	NURSING INTERVENTIONS/CLIENT EDUCATION
• Severe allergic reactions (anaphylaxis) • Possible cross-sensitivity with sulfonamides	• Educate client about signs/symptoms to report. • Ask about sulfonamide allergy.
• Rare serious blood disorders, such as bone marrow depression	• Educate clients to recognize and immediately report symptoms.
• GI side effects (nausea and diarrhea)	• Report GI symptoms and weight loss to provider.
• Electrolyte depletion (sodium and potassium), altered liver function	• Prepare clients for the need to obtain regular laboratory testing.
• Generalized flu-like symptoms (headache, fever, body aches)	• Educate client about possible reactions.
• Central nervous system disturbances (paresthesias of extremities, fatigue, sleepiness, rarely seizures)	• Educate client about possible reactions. • Medication may be discontinued.
• Glucose disturbances in clients with diabetes mellitus	• Teach clients who have diabetes to closely monitor blood glucose and watch for signs of hypo- or hyperglycemia.

 Contraindications/Precautions:

- Acetazolamide is Pregnancy Risk Category C (teratogenic).
- Use during lactation only after evaluation by the provider.

Interactions

MEDICATION/FOOD INTERACTIONS	NURSING INTERVENTIONS/CLIENT EDUCATION
Serious effects, such as metabolic acidosis, can occur in clients using high-dose aspirin.	• Question clients about aspirin use and notify the provider.
Acetazolamide may increase the risk of toxic effects of quinidine.	• Instruct clients to notify the provider of concurrent use and to watch for signs of toxicity such as decreased heart rate.
Acetazolamide may decrease blood levels of lithium.	• Teach clients taking lithium to watch for increased symptoms of mania. Lithium levels should be monitored regularly.
Acetazolamide may increase osteomalacia, an adverse effect of phenytoin.	• Teach clients taking phenytoin to watch for bone pain or weakness and report symptoms to the provider.
Sodium bicarbonate increases the risk of kidney stones.	• Question clients about the use of sodium bicarbonate and other over-the-counter antacids.

Nursing Administration

- Acetazolamide may be administered orally as a tablet or a capsule. It is also available for parenteral administration.

Nursing Evaluation of Medication Effectiveness

- Depending on therapeutic intent, effectiveness may be evidenced by:
  - Reduced IOP
  - Safe self-administration of medication
  - Prevention or minimization of systemic effects

MEDICATIONS FOR EAR DISORDERS

MEDICATION CLASSIFICATION: ANTIMICROBIALS

- Select Prototype Medication: amoxicillin (Amoxil)
- Other Medication: amoxicillin/clavulanate (Augmentin) PO
- The following antibiotics are used to treat acute otitis media in clients who have a penicillin allergy or penicillin-resistant otitis media.
  - Ceftriaxone (Rocephin) IM, IV (severe illness)
  - Cefdinir (Omnicef) PO
  - Cefuroxime (Ceftin) PO, IM, IV
  - Cefpodoxime (Vantin) PO
  - Azithromycin (Zithromax) PO, IV
  - Clindamycin (Cleocin), PO, IM, IV (a macrolide antibiotic)

Purpose

- Expected Pharmacological Action
  - Eradication of infection
- Therapeutic Uses
  - Used to treat otitis media and various other bacterial infections throughout the body

Complications

SIDE/ADVERSE EFFECTS	NURSING INTERVENTIONS/CLIENT EDUCATION
Possible allergic reaction is the most common risk when taking penicillin	• Question the client and family regarding the presence of penicillin or other antibiotic allergy. • The client may need alternative medication. • A skin test may be used to test for sensitivity.
GI upset (usually less with amoxicillin than with ampicillin)	• Educate family to inform the provider of severe diarrhea, especially in an infant or young child.
Suprainfection with other microbes, such as oral candidiasis	• Report symptoms of new infection to the provider.

Contraindications/Precautions

- Amoxicillin is contraindicated for clients with severe allergy to penicillin, cephalosporins.
- Use cautiously in infants less than 3 months of age because of immature renal system and increased risk for toxicity.

Nursing Administration

- Amoxicillin is usually prescribed 3 times daily, PO.
- Amoxicillin may be taken with meals.
- As with all antibiotics, instruct client to take full course of medication.

Nursing Evaluation of Medication Effectiveness

- Depending on therapeutic intent, effectiveness may be evidenced by:
  - No presence of infection
  - No reoccurrence of infection

MEDICATION CLASSIFICATION: FLUOROQUINOLONE ANTIBIOTIC PLUS STEROID MEDICATION

- Select Prototype Medication: ciprofloxacin plus dexamethasone (Cipro HC) otic drops
- Other Medications:
  - Acetic acid 2% solution otic drops (Vasolate)
  - Ciprofloxacin plus dexamethasone otic drops (Ciprodex)
  - Ofloxacin otic drops (Floxin)

Purpose

- Expected Pharmacological Action
  - The bactericidal effect of the ciprofloxacin and anti-inflammatory effect of the dexamethasone should decrease pain, edema, and erythema in the ear canal.
- Therapeutic Uses
  - These medications are used to treat otitis externa.

Complications

SIDE/ADVERSE EFFECTS	NURSING INTERVENTIONS/CLIENT EDUCATION
CNS effects (dizziness, lightheadedness, tremors, restlessness, convulsions)	• Instruct clients to inform the provider if any of these occur.
Rash	• Question the client/family about allergies to fluoroquinolone antibiotics or to steroids such as dexamethasone or cortisone.

Nursing Administration

- Review the method for instilling otic drops.
- Inform clients that movement of the tragus or pinna may be very painful when instilling otic drops.
- Warm the medication by gently rolling the container between hands before instilling drops. Cold drops may cause dizziness.
- Keep clients in a side-lying position for 30 to 60 seconds with the affected ear up after instilling drops.
- Instruct client/family to prevent otic medications from being placed in the eye or ingested orally.
- Teach client/family to prevent otitis externa by:
    - Keeping foreign bodies, such as cotton swabs, out of the ear canal, and avoiding the use of manual measures to remove cerumen
    - Drying the ear canal after bathing or swimming, using a towel and tilting the head to promote drainage
    - Avoiding the use of earplugs except for swimming

Nursing Evaluation of Medication Effectiveness

- Depending on therapeutic intent, effectiveness may be evidenced by:
    - Subsiding of symptoms
    - Use of measures to prevent reinfection

CHAPTER 14: EYE AND EAR DISORDERS

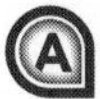

Application Exercises

1. After instilling an eye drop that has a systemic effect, the nurse should press on which of the following to prevent absorption into the circulation?

   A. The bony orbit

   B. The nasolacrimal duct

   C. The conjunctival sac

   D. The outer canthus of the eye

2. A client has a new prescription for brimonidine (Alphagan) ophthalmic, 1 drop twice daily in his right eye. He tells the nurse he also wears soft contact lenses and wants to know if he can put the drop in his eye with the lenses in place. Which of the following should the nurse tell this client?

   A. "Go ahead and put the drop in your eye with the contact lens in place."

   B. "Take the contact lens out of your eye, then instill the eye drop and immediately reinsert the contact lens."

   C. "Take the contact lens out of your eye; then instill the eye drop and wait at least 15 minutes before putting the contact lens back in place."

   D. "You will need to discontinue the use of contact lenses while using brimonidine eye drops."

3. A nurse is caring for a client who has just been diagnosed with angle-closure glaucoma. Which of the following should the nurse expect?

   A. Insidious onset of painless loss of vision

   B. Gradual reduction in peripheral vision

   C. Report of seeing halos around lights

   D. An IOP of 12 mm Hg

4. A nurse is caring for a 6-year-old child who has just been diagnosed with influenza and bilateral otitis media. The child's parent asks the nurse, "Why didn't the doctor want to give my child antibiotics for her ear infection? I think she'd get better sooner if she had them." How should the nurse reply?

CHAPTER 14: EYE AND EAR DISORDERS

Application Exercises Answer Key

1. After instilling an eye drop that has a systemic effect, the nurse should press on which of the following to prevent absorption into the circulation?

   A. The bony orbit

   B. The nasolacrimal duct

   C. The conjunctival sac

   D. The outer canthus of the eye

   The nurse should gently press the nasolacrimal duct with a gloved hand and a clean tissue for 30 to 60 seconds. This prevents movement of the medication into the circulation and thus minimizes or prevents systemic effects from taking place. Pressing any of the other structures will not prevent the medication from reaching circulation.

NCLEX® Connection: Pharmacological and Parenteral Therapies: Medication Administration

2. A client has a new prescription for brimonidine (Alphagan) ophthalmic, 1 drop twice daily in his right eye. He tells the nurse he also wears soft contact lenses and wants to know if he can put the drop in his eye with the lenses in place. Which of the following should the nurse tell this client?

   A. "Go ahead and put the drop in your eye with the contact lens in place."

   B. "Take the contact lens out of your eye, then instill the eye drop and immediately reinsert the contact lens."

   C. "Take the contact lens out of your eye; then instill the eye drop and wait at least 15 minutes before putting the contact lens back in place."

   D. "You will need to discontinue the use of contact lenses while using brimonidine eye drops."

   Brimonidine interacts with plastic contact lenses and the client needs to wait 15 minutes after instilling the eye drop before reinserting the contact lens.

NCLEX® Connection: Pharmacological and Parenteral Therapies: Medication Administration

3. A nurse is caring for a client who has just been diagnosed with angle-closure glaucoma. Which of the following should the nurse expect?

   A. Insidious onset of painless loss of vision

   B. Gradual reduction in peripheral vision

   C. Report of seeing halos around lights

   D. An IOP of 12 mm Hg

   Reports of seeing halos around lights is an expected finding in clients with angle-closure glaucoma. Onset is acute with irreversible blindness occurring within 1 to 2 days without emergency treatment. An IOP of 12 mm Hg is within the expected reference range. A client with angle-closure glaucoma will have increased IOP.

NCLEX® Connection: Pharmacological and Parenteral Therapies: Expected Effects/Outcomes

4. A nurse is caring for a 6-year-old child who has just been diagnosed with influenza and bilateral otitis media. The child's parent asks the nurse, "Why didn't the doctor want to give my child antibiotics for her ear infection? I think she'd get better sooner if she had them." How should the nurse reply?

    "Ear infections caused by a virus are not cured by antibiotics. If your child has a viral infection, giving antibiotics makes it more likely that bacteria become resistant to antibiotics, which could be a problem when your daughter develops a bacterial infection in the future." The nurse should also reinforce to the parent the need to inform the provider if symptoms do not subside or worsen in the next few days.

 **NCLEX® Connection: Pharmacological and Parenteral Therapies: Medication Administration**

UNIT 2 MEDICATIONS AFFECTING THE NERVOUS SYSTEM

Chapter 15 Miscellaneous Central Nervous System Medications

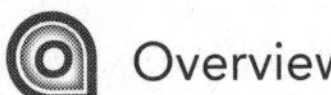

Overview

- Neuromuscular blocking agents have various uses including assisting with sedation during general anesthesia, control of seizures during electroconvulsive therapy, and suppression of gag reflex during endotracheal intubation.
  - Medications include succinylcholine (Anectine) and vecuronium (Norcuron).
- Muscle relaxants and antispasmodic agents can affect both the central and peripheral nervous systems.
  - These agents are used with spasticity related to muscle injury, cerebral palsy, spinal cord injury, and multiple sclerosis.
  - Agents include diazepam (Valium), baclofen (Lioresal), and dantrolene (Dantrium).
  - Bethanechol (Urecholine), a muscarinic agonist, is used for urinary retention.
  - Oxybutynin (Ditropan), a muscarinic antagonist, is used for neurogenic bladder.

MEDICATION CLASSIFICATION: NEUROMUSCULAR BLOCKING AGENTS

- Select Prototype Medication:
  - Depolarizing neuromuscular blocker: succinylcholine (Anectine)
  - Nondepolarizing neuromuscular blockers: pancuronium (Pavulon)
- Other Medications:
  - Nondepolarizing neuromuscular blockers: atracurium (Tracrium), Vecuronium (Norcuron)

Purpose

- Expected Pharmacological Action
  - Neuromuscular blocking agents block acetylcholine (ACh) at the neuromuscular junction, resulting in muscle relaxation and hypotension. They do not cross the blood-brain barrier, so complete paralysis can be achieved without loss of consciousness or decreased pain sensation.

MEDICATION	ACTION
Succinylcholine	• Succinylcholine mimics ACh by binding with cholinergic receptors at the neuromuscular junction. This agent fills the cholinergic receptors, preventing ACh from binding with them, and causes sustained depolarization of the muscle, resulting in muscle paralysis. • Reversal agent: Pseudocholinesterase enzyme
Pancuronium, atracurium, vecuronium	• These agents block ACh from binding with cholinergic receptors at the motor end plate. Muscle paralysis occurs because of inhibited nerve depolarization and skeletal muscle contraction. • Reversal agent: Neostigmine (Prostigmin)

- Therapeutic Uses
  - Neuromuscular blocking agents are used as adjuncts to general anesthesia to promote muscle relaxation.
  - These agents are used to control spontaneous respiratory movements in clients receiving mechanical ventilation.
  - These agents are used as seizure control during electroconvulsive therapy.
  - Neuromuscular blocking agents are used during endotracheal intubation and endoscopy.

Complications

SIDE/ADVERSE EFFECTS	NURSING INTERVENTIONS/CLIENT EDUCATION
Respiratory arrest from paralyzed respiratory muscles	• Maintain continuous cardiac and respiratory monitoring. • Have equipment ready for resuscitation and mechanical ventilation. • Monitor clients for return of respiratory function when medication is discontinued.
Hypotension	• Monitor for decreased blood pressure. Administer antihistamine if indicated.
Succinylcholine	
Low pseudocholinesterase activity can lead to prolonged apnea.	• Test the client's blood, or administer a small test dose for clients suspected of having low levels of pseudocholinesterase. • Withhold medication if pseudocholinesterase activity is low.
Signs of malignant hyperthermia include muscle rigidity accompanied by increased temperature, reaching levels as high as 43° C (109.4° F).	• Monitor the client's vital signs. • Stop succinylcholine and other anesthetics. • Ice or infusion of iced saline can be used to cool the client. • Administer dantrolene to decrease metabolic activity of skeletal muscle.
After 12 to 24 hr postoperative, clients may experience muscle pain in the upper body and back.	• Advise clients that this response is not unusual and eventually will subside. • Notify the provider to consider short-term use of muscle relaxant.
Hyperkalemia	• Monitor potassium levels.

Contraindications/Precautions

- These medications are Pregnancy Risk Category C.
- Succinylcholine is contraindicated in clients with risk of hyperkalemia (clients with major trauma, severe burns).
- Use cautiously in clients who have myasthenia gravis, respiratory dysfunction, and fluid and electrolyte imbalances.

Interactions

MEDICATION/FOOD INTERACTIONS	NURSING INTERVENTIONS/CLIENT EDUCATION
General anesthetics are often used concurrently in surgery.	• Dosage of tubocurarine should be reduced to prevent extreme neuromuscular blockade.
Aminoglycosides and tetracyclines can increase the effects of neuromuscular blockade.	• Take complete medication history of clients who are to receive neuromuscular blockade.
Neostigmine and other cholinesterase inhibitors increase the effects of depolarizing neuromuscular blockers, such as succinylcholine.	• Monitor clients during neuromuscular blockade reversal after surgery.

Nursing Administration

- Clients must receive continuous cardiac and respiratory monitoring during therapy.
- Monitor clients for respiratory depression and have life support equipment available.
- Carefully monitor clients for return of respiratory function.

Nursing Evaluation of Medication Effectiveness

- Depending on therapeutic intent, effectiveness may be evidenced by:
  - Muscle relaxation during surgery
  - No spontaneous respiratory movements in clients receiving mechanical ventilation
  - Absence of seizures in clients receiving electroconvulsive therapy
  - Successful endotracheal intubation

MEDICATION CLASSIFICATION: MUSCLE RELAXANTS AND ANTISPASMODICS

- Select Prototype Medication:
  - Centrally acting muscle relaxants: diazepam (Valium)
  - Peripherally acting muscle relaxants: dantrolene (Dantrium)
- Other Medications:
  - Centrally acting muscle relaxants:
    - Baclofen (Lioresal)
    - Cyclobenzaprine (Flexeril)
    - Metaxalone (Skelaxin)
    - Tizanidine (Zanaflex)

Purpose

EXPECTED PHARMACOLOGICAL ACTION	THERAPEUTIC USES
Diazepam	
Diazepam acts in the CNS to enhance GABA and produce sedative effects and depress spasticity of muscles.	• Relief of: ○ Muscle spasm related to muscle injury and spasticity ○ Anxiety and panic disorders ○ Insomnia ○ Status epilepticus ○ Alcohol withdrawal ○ Anesthesia induction
Cyclobenzaprine, metaxalone, tizanidine	
These medications act in the CNS to enhance GABA and produce sedative effects and depress spasticity of muscles.	Relief of muscle spasm related to muscle injury
Baclofen	
Baclofen acts in the CNS to enhance GABA, produce sedative effects, and depress spasticity of muscles.	Relief of spasticity related to cerebral palsy, spinal cord injury, and multiple sclerosis
Dantrolene	
Dantrolene is a peripherally acting muscle relaxant that acts directly on spastic muscles and inhibits muscle contraction by preventing release of calcium in skeletal muscles.	• Relief of spasticity related to cerebral palsy, spinal cord injury and multiple sclerosis • Treatment of malignant hyperthermia

Complications

SIDE/ADVERSE EFFECTS	NURSING INTERVENTIONS/CLIENT EDUCATION
All muscle relaxants and antispasmodics	
CNS depression (sleepiness, lightheadedness, fatigue)	• Start at low doses. • Inform clients of potential side effects. • Advise clients to avoid hazardous activities, such as driving, and concurrent use of other CNS depressants, such as alcohol.
Centrally acting agents: Diazepam, cyclobenzaprine, metaxalone, tizanidine	
Hepatic toxicity with metaxalone, tizanidine, (anorexia, nausea, vomiting, abdominal pain, jaundice)	• Obtain the client's baseline liver function and perform periodic follow-up liver function tests. • Observe clients for signs of toxicity, and notify the provider if they occur. • Start at low dose.
Physical dependence from chronic long-term use	• Advise clients not to discontinue medication abruptly.
Baclofen	
Nausea, constipation, and urinary retention	• Advise clients of side effects and notify the provider if symptoms occur. • Monitor the client's I&O. • Advise clients to increase intake of high-fiber foods.
Peripherally acting agent: Dantrolene	
Hepatic toxicity (anorexia, nausea, vomiting, abdominal pain, jaundice)	• Obtain the client's baseline liver function studies and perform periodic follow-up liver function tests. • Observe clients for signs of toxicity and notify the provider if symptoms occur. • Start at low doses.
Muscle weakness	• Monitor effectiveness of medication.

Contraindications/Precautions

- Baclofen and dantrolene
  - Pregnancy Risk Category C
- Diazepam
  - Pregnancy Risk Category D
- Use both of these medications cautiously in clients with impaired liver and renal function.

Interactions

MEDICATION/FOOD INTERACTIONS	NURSING INTERVENTIONS/CLIENT EDUCATION
CNS depressants (alcohol, opioids, antihistamines) have additive CNS depressant effects.	• Advise clients to avoid concurrent use.

Nursing Administration

- Instruct clients to take medications as prescribed.
- Advise clients not to stop taking medication abruptly to avoid withdrawal reaction.
- Advise clients to avoid CNS depressants while using these medications.
- Provide assistance as needed in self-administration of medication and performance of ADLs.

Nursing Evaluation of Medication Effectiveness

- Depending on therapeutic intent, effectiveness may be evidenced by:
  - Absence of muscle rigidity and spasms, good range of motion
  - Absence of pain
  - Increased ability to perform ADLs

MEDICATION CLASSIFICATION: MUSCARINIC AGONISTS

- Select Prototype Medication: bethanechol (Urecholine)

Purpose

- Expected Pharmacological Action
  - Stimulation of muscarine receptors of the GU tract, thereby causing relaxation of the trigone and sphincter muscles and contraction of the detrusor muscle
- Therapeutic Uses
  - Nonobstructive urinary retention, usually postoperatively or postpartum

Complications

SIDE/ADVERSE EFFECTS	NURSING INTERVENTIONS/CLIENT EDUCATION
Extreme muscarinic stimulation may result in sweating, tearing, urinary urgency, bradycardia and hypotension	Instruct clients to report symptoms if they occur.

Contraindications/Precautions

- Contraindicated in clients with urinary or gastrointestinal obstruction, peptic ulcer disease, coronary insufficiency, asthma and hyperthyroidism

Nursing Administration

- Administer by oral route, 1 hr before or 2 hr after meals.
- Monitor I & O.

Nursing Evaluation of Medication Effectiveness

- Depending on therapeutic intent, effectiveness may be evidenced by:
    - Relief of urinary retention

MEDICATION CLASSIFICATION: MUSCARINIC ANTAGONISTS

- Select Prototype Medication:
    - M3 receptor selective: oxybutynin (Ditropan)
- Other Medications:
    - M3 receptor selective: Darifenacin (Enablex)
    - Nonselective: tolterodine (Detrol)

Purpose

- Expected Pharmacological Action
    - Inhibiting muscarinic receptors of the detrusor muscle of the bladder, which prevents contractions of the bladder and the urge to void
- Therapeutic Uses
    - Overactive bladder

Complications

SIDE/ADVERSE EFFECTS	NURSING INTERVENTIONS/CLIENT EDUCATION
Anticholinergic effects (constipation, dry mouth, blurred vision, photophobia, dry eyes)	Instruct clients to increase dietary fiber, consume 2 to 3 L/day of fluid from beverage and food sources, sip fluids, and avoid hazardous activities if vision is impaired.
CNS effects (hallucinations, confusion, insomnia, nervousness)	Instruct clients to report symptoms to the provider. The medication may need to be discontinued

 Contraindications/Precautions

- These medications are contraindicated in clients who have glaucoma, myasthenia gravis, paralytic ileus, GI or GU obstruction, or urinary retention.
- Use cautiously in children and older adults.
- Use cautiously in clients who have gastroesophageal reflux disease (GERD), heart failure, or kidney or liver impairment.

Interactions

MEDICATION/FOOD INTERACTIONS	NURSING INTERVENTIONS/CLIENT EDUCATION
Antihistamines, tricyclic antidepressants, or phenothiazines used concurrently can result in extreme muscarinic blockage.	Concurrent use is not recommended.

Nursing Administration

- Administer by oral route. Use extended-release formulations to minimize anticholinergic effects.
- Advise clients to swallow extended-release tablets and to avoid chewing or crushing the tablets.
- Instruct clients that the shell of extended-release tablets will be eliminated whole in the stool.
- The transdermal patch is administered two times a week. Instruct clients to apply to dry skin of hip, abdomen, or buttock and to rotate sites.

Nursing Evaluation of Medication Effectiveness

- Depending on therapeutic intent, effectiveness may be evidenced by:
    - Decrease of urinary urgency and frequency, nocturia, and urge incontinence

CHAPTER 15: MISCELLANEOUS CENTRAL NERVOUS SYSTEM MEDICATIONS

Application Exercises

1. A nurse is caring for a client who received a bolus dose of succinylcholine (Anectine) IV before an endoscopy procedure. During the procedure, the client suddenly develops rigidity, and his body temperature begins to rise. Which of the following should the nurse administer?

    A. A second dose of succinylcholine (Anectine)

    B. Naloxone (Narcan) as an antagonist at receptor sites

    C. Dantrolene (Dantrium) to slow metabolic activity of muscles

    D. Vecuronium (Norcuron) as an adjunct to muscle relaxation

2. Which of the following laboratory values should the nurse recognize as a possible adverse reaction to the administration of succinylcholine?

    A. Serum sodium 130 mEq/L

    B. Serum sodium 150 mEq/L

    C. Serum potassium 3.0 mEq/L

    D. Serum potassium 5.2 mEq/L

3. A nurse is teaching a client who has begun taking oral baclofen (Lioresal) three times daily to treat muscle spasms caused by a spinal cord injury. Which of the following statements by the client indicates to the nurse a need for further teaching?

    A. "I will stop taking this medication right away if I develop dizziness."

    B. "I know the doctor will gradually increase my dose of this medication for awhile."

    C. "I'll make sure that I empty my bladder completely while taking this medication."

    D. "I won't be able to drink alcohol while I'm taking this medication."

4. A nurse is caring for a client who has been prescribed oxybutynin (Ditropan). Which of the following outcomes should the nurse add to this client's plan of care while he is taking this medication?

    A. The client will experience less pain and muscle soreness.

    B. The client will have an increase in range of motion.

    C. The client will experience less constipation.

    D. The client will have fewer episodes of nocturia.

CHAPTER 15: MISCELLANEOUS CENTRAL NERVOUS SYSTEM MEDICATIONS

Application Exercises Answer Key

1.A nurse is caring for a client who received a bolus dose of succinylcholine (Anectine) IV before an endoscopy procedure. During the procedure, the client suddenly develops rigidity, and his body temperature begins to rise. Which of the following should the nurse administer?

A. A second dose of succinylcholine (Anectine)

B. Naloxone (Narcan) as an antagonist at receptor sites

C. Dantrolene (Dantrium) to slow metabolic activity of muscles

D. Vecuronium (Norcuron) as an adjunct to muscle relaxation

Dantrolene is administered for clients who develop malignant hyperthermia, which can be caused by succinylcholine. Dantrolene decreases fever and rigidity through direct action on skeletal muscles to slow their metabolic activity. A second dose of succinylcholine would further exacerbate the problem. Naloxone is used to reverse the effects of opioids, but is not effective for malignant hyperthermia. Vecuronium is an intermediate-acting nondepolarizing neuromuscular blocker, which can be used for muscle relaxation during surgery, but is not useful in treating malignant hyperthermia.

NCLEX® Connection: Pharmacological and Parenteral Therapies: Adverse Effects/ Contraindications/Side Effects/Interactions

2. Which of the following laboratory values should the nurse recognize as a possible adverse reaction to the administration of succinylcholine?

A. Serum sodium 130 mEq/L

B. Serum sodium 150 mEq/L

C. Serum potassium 3.0 mEq/L

D. Serum potassium 5.2 mEq/L

Serum potassium level of 5.2 mEq/L indicates hyperkalemia, which is an adverse reaction to the administration of succinylcholine. The administration of succinylcholine does not result in hyponatremia, hypernatremia, or hypokalemia.

NCLEX® Connection: Pharmacological and Parenteral Therapies: Adverse Effects/ Contraindications/Side Effects/Interactions

3. A nurse is teaching a client who has begun taking oral baclofen (Lioresal) three times daily to treat muscle spasms caused by a spinal cord injury. Which of the following statements by the client indicates to the nurse a need for further teaching?

    A. "I will stop taking this medication right away if I develop dizziness."

    B. "I know the doctor will gradually increase my dose of this medication for awhile."

    C. "I'll make sure that I empty my bladder completely while taking this medication."

    D. "I won't be able to drink alcohol while I'm taking this medication."

    Abrupt withdrawal from baclofen may cause some severe reactions, such as seizures. If the client stops taking the medication, withdrawal should be done gradually over 7 to 14 days. The initial dosage of baclofen is usually low and gradually increased to prevent CNS depression. Urinary retention is an adverse reaction that may occur with baclofen, and the client should be taught to empty the bladder when urinating. Alcohol and other CNS depressants may potentiate the effects of baclofen and cause decreased level of consciousness or respiratory depression.

NCLEX® Connection: Pharmacological and Parenteral Therapies: Medication Administration

4. A nurse is caring for a client who has been prescribed oxybutynin (Ditropan). Which of the following outcomes should the nurse add to this client's plan of care while he is taking this medication?

    A. The client will experience less pain and muscle soreness.

    B. The client will have an increase in range of motion.

    C. The client will experience less constipation.

    D. The client will have fewer episodes of nocturia.

    Oxybutynin is prescribed to decrease the urge to void by inhibiting muscarinic receptors of the detrusor muscle, which contracts the bladder. Expected outcomes might include a decrease of nocturia, voiding fewer times during the day, and/or decreasing incontinence. Oxybutynin will not decrease skeletal muscle pain or increase range of motion. Constipation is a possible adverse reaction to this medication, which the client should be taught to prevent.

NCLEX® Connection: Pharmacological and Parenteral Therapies: Expected Actions/ Outcomes

UNIT 2 MEDICATIONS AFFECTING THE NERVOUS SYSTEM

Chapter 16 Sedative-Hypnotics

Overview

- Sedatives are CNS depressants that induce a sense of calm and decrease anxiety. Hypnotics are CNS depressants that induce sleep.
- The three types of sedative-hypnotics are benzodiazepines, barbiturates, and benzodiazepine-like medications. The most commonly used are benzodiazepines and benzodiazepine-like medications.
- IV anesthetics are usually administered during induction of general anesthesia. Most have a quick onset of action and short duration. These medications may be nonopioids or opioids.

MEDICATION CLASSIFICATION: BENZODIAZEPINES

- Select Prototype Medication: diazepam (Valium)
- Other Medications:
    - Alprazolam (Xanax)
    - Lorazepam (Ativan)
    - Chlordiazepoxide (Librium)
    - Temazepam (Restoril)

Purpose

- Expected Pharmacological Action
    - These medications enhance the action of gamma-amino butyric acid (GABA) in the CNS.
- Therapeutic Uses
    - These medications are used to treat:
        - Anxiety disorders
        - Seizure disorders
        - Insomnia
        - Muscle spasm
        - Alcohol withdrawal
        - Panic disorder
        - Induction of anesthesia

Complications

SIDE/ADVERSE EFFECTS	NURSING INTERVENTIONS/CLIENT EDUCATION
CNS depression (lightheadedness, drowsiness, incoordination)	• Advise clients to observe for symptoms and notify the provider if they occur. • Advise clients to avoid hazardous activities such as driving or operating heavy equipment/machinery.
Anterograde amnesia	• Advise clients to observe for symptoms and notify the provider if they occur.
Paradoxical response such as insomnia, excitation, euphoria, anxiety, rage	• Advise clients to observe for symptoms. If symptoms occur, instruct the client to notify the provider and stop the medication.
Respiratory depression, especially with IV administration	• Monitor the client's vital signs. • Have resuscitation equipment available.
Physical dependence • Withdrawal following short-term therapy manifests as anxiety, insomnia, tremors and dizziness. • Withdrawal following long-term therapy manifests as delirium, paranoia, panic, hypertension and seizures.	• Discontinue medication slowly by tapering dose over weeks to months.
Acute toxicity; oral toxicity (drowsiness, lethargy, confusion); IV toxicity (respiratory depression)	• For oral toxicity, gastric lavage can be used, followed by the administration of activated charcoal or saline cathartics. • For IV toxicity, administer flumazenil (Romazicon) to counteract sedation and reverse side effects. • Monitor the client's vital signs, maintain patent airway, and provide fluids to maintain blood pressure. • Have resuscitation equipment available.

Contraindications/Precautions

- These medications are Pregnancy Risk Category D.
- These medications are contraindicated in clients who have sleep apnea, respiratory depression, organic brain disease, or lactation.
- Use cautiously in clients who have a history of substance abuse, liver dysfunction, and renal failure.

Interactions

MEDICATION/FOOD INTERACTIONS	NURSING INTERVENTIONS/CLIENT EDUCATION
CNS depressants such as alcohol, barbiturates, opioids cause additive CNS depressant effects with concurrent use.	• Take complete medication history to identify concurrent use of other CNS depressants. • Advise clients to avoid alcohol and other CNS depressants.

Nursing Administration

- Ensure proper route of administration.
  - All agents may be given by oral route.
  - IV administration is acceptable with diazepam, lorazepam, and chlordiazepoxide.
  - Lorazepam is the agent of choice for IM injection.
- Advise clients to take the medication as prescribed and to avoid abrupt discontinuation of treatment to prevent withdrawal symptoms.
- When discontinuing benzodiazepines, taper dose over several weeks.
- Administer medication with meals. Advise clients to swallow sustained-release tablets and to avoid chewing or crushing the tablet.
- Inform clients about possible development of dependency during and after treatment, and to notify the provider if symptoms occur.

Nursing Evaluation of Medication Effectiveness

- Depending on therapeutic intent, effectiveness may be evidenced by:
  - Improvement of symptoms as evidenced by absence of panic attacks, decrease or absence of anxiety, normal sleep pattern, absence of seizures, absence of withdrawal symptoms from alcohol, and relaxation of muscles.

MEDICATION CLASSIFICATION: NONBENZODIAZEPINES

- Select Prototype Medication: zolpidem (Ambien)
- Other Medications:
  - Zaleplon (Sonata)
  - Eszopiclone (Lunesta)
  - Trazodone (Desyrel)

Purpose

- Expected Pharmacological Action
  - These medications enhance the action of gamma-amino butyric acid (GABA) in the CNS. This results in prolonged sleep duration and decreased awakenings. These medications do not function as antianxiety, muscle relaxant, or antiepileptic agents. There is a low risk of tolerance, abuse, and dependence.
- Therapeutic Uses
  - Management of insomnia

Complications

SIDE/ADVERSE EFFECTS	NURSING INTERVENTIONS/CLIENT EDUCATION
Daytime sleepiness and lightheadedness	• Administer medication at bedtime. • Advise clients to take medication allowing for at least 8 hr of sleep.

Contraindications/Precautions

- Pregnancy Risk Category B
- Contraindicated in clients who are breastfeeding
- Use cautiously in older adult clients and in clients with impaired kidney, liver, and/or respiratory function.

Interactions

MEDICATION/FOOD INTERACTIONS	NURSING INTERVENTIONS/CLIENT EDUCATION
CNS depressants such as alcohol, barbiturates, opioids cause additive CNS depression.	• Advise clients to avoid alcohol and other CNS depressants.

Nursing Administration

- Advise clients to take the medication just before bedtime.
- Administer all agents by oral route.

Nursing Evaluation of Medication Effectiveness

- Depending on therapeutic intent, effectiveness may be evidenced by:
  - Effective sleep pattern

MEDICATION CLASSIFICATION: MELATONIN AGONIST

- Select Prototype Medication: ramelteon (Rozerem)

Purpose

- Expected Pharmacological Action
  - Activation of melatonin receptors
- Therapeutic Uses
  - Management of insomnia

Complications

SIDE/ADVERSE EFFECTS	NURSING INTERVENTIONS/CLIENT EDUCATION
Sleepiness, dizziness, fatigue	• Ramelteon is generally well tolerated. Instruct clients to notify the provider if symptoms occur. • Advise clients to avoid activities such as driving if symptoms occur.
Hormonal effects (amenorrhea, decreased libido, difficulty with fertility, galactorrhea)	• Instruct clients to notify the provider if symptoms occur. Medication may be discontinued

Contraindications/Precautions

- Contraindicated in pregnancy and lactation
- Use cautiously in clients with liver disease

Interactions

MEDICATION/FOOD INTERACTIONS	NURSING INTERVENTIONS/CLIENT EDUCATION
High-fat foods decrease absorption.	Take medication on an empty stomach.
Concurrent use of fluvoxamine (Luvox) can increase levels of ramelteon.	Avoid concurrent use.
CNS depressants such as opioids, alcohol can cause additive CNS depression.	Avoid concurrent use.

Nursing Administration

- Administer by oral route.
- Instruct clients to take medication 30 min prior to bedtime.
- Instruct clients to take medication on an empty stomach.

Nursing Evaluation of Medication Effectiveness

- Depending on therapeutic intent, effectiveness may be evidenced by:
  - Improvement in sleep patterns

MEDICATION CLASSIFICATION: INTRAVENOUS ANESTHETICS

- Intravenous nonopioid agents
  - Select Prototype Medications:
    - Barbiturates: thiopental (Pentothal)
    - Benzodiazepines: midazolam (Versed), diazepam (Valium)
  - Other Medications: propofol (Diprivan), Ketamine (Ketalar)
- Intravenous opioid agents
  - Select Prototype Medication: fentanyl (Sublimaze)
  - Other Medications: alfentanil (Alfenta), sufentanil (Sufenta)

Purpose

- Expected Pharmacological Action
  - These medications produce loss of consciousness and elimination of response to painful stimuli.
- Therapeutic Uses
  - Induction and maintenance of anesthesia
  - Conscious sedation (usually an IV nonopioid agent combined with an opioid agent)
  - Intubation and mechanical ventilation

Complications

SIDE/ADVERSE EFFECTS	NURSING INTERVENTIONS/CLIENT EDUCATION
Respiratory and cardiovascular depression with high risk for hypotension	• Provide continuous monitoring of vital signs and ECG. • Maintain mechanical ventilation during procedure. • Have equipment ready for resuscitation.
Bacterial infection (with propofol)	• Use opened vials within 6 hr. • Monitor for signs of infection such as fever, malaise after surgery.
Psychologic reactions (with ketamine) • Hallucinations, mental confusion • Children less than 15 years of age and adults older than 65 years of age are at lower risk.	• Avoid use in clients with a history of mental illness. • Maintain a quiet, low-stimulus environment during recovery. • Give diazepam prior to ketamine.

Contraindications/Precautions

- Avoid use in clients who have a history of mental illness.
- Use cautiously in clients who have respiratory and cardiovascular disease.

Interactions

MEDICATION/FOOD INTERACTIONS	NURSING INTERVENTIONS/CLIENT EDUCATION
CNS depressants (alcohol, barbiturates, opioids) create additive CNS depression.	• Clients may require lower dose • Provide continuous monitoring of vital signs and ECG. • Have equipment ready for resuscitation.
CNS stimulants, (amphetamines, cocaine) create additive CNS stimulation.	• Clients may require higher doses. • Provide continuous monitoring of vital signs and ECG. • Have equipment ready for resuscitation.
Opioid analgesics (fentanyl) provide analgesia and cough suppression.	• Monitor bladder and bowel function. • Encourage early ambulation and assist clients to void.

Nursing Administration

- Administer midazolam slowly over 2 min. Additional doses should be given at 2 min intervals.
- Inject propofol into large vein to decrease pain at injection site.
- Instruct clients to arrange for a ride home following outpatient procedure.

Nursing Evaluation of Medication Effectiveness

- Depending on therapeutic intent, effectiveness may be evidenced by:
  - Surgical procedure occurs with loss of consciousness and elimination of pain.
  - Postoperative recovery as demonstrated by the following:
    - Vital signs return to baseline.
    - Client is oriented to time, place, and person.
    - Bowel sounds return.
    - Voiding occurs within 8 hr.
    - Nausea and vomiting are controlled.

CHAPTER 16: SEDATIVE-HYPNOTICS

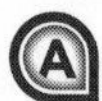

Application Exercises

1. A nurse is preparing to care for a client in the surgical unit who will be receiving diazepam (Valium) IV. For which of the following should the nurse monitor this client?

    A. Status epilepticus

    B. Respiratory depression

    C. Malignant hyperthermia

    D. Acute facial dystonia

2. A nurse is caring for a client who is receiving moderate sedation with diazepam (Valium) IV. The client's respiration decreases to 10/min. Which of the following medications should the nurse anticipate administering to this client?

    A. Ketamine (Ketalar)

    B. Naltrexone (ReVia)

    C. Flumazenil (Romazicon)

    D. Fluvoxamine (Luvox)

3. A nurse is teaching a client about possible adverse effects of her new prescription for ramelteon (Rozerem). For which of the following should the nurse teach the client to notify the provider?

    A. Decreased libido

    B. Blurred vision

    C. Productive cough

    D. Dry mouth

4. A client is admitted to undergo a surgical procedure. The nurse should be aware that which of the following pre-existing conditions may be a contraindication for the use of ketamine (Ketalar) as an intravenous anesthetic for this client?

    A. Peptic ulcer disease

    B. Breast cancer

    C. Diabetes

    D. Schizophrenia

CHAPTER 16: SEDATIVE-HYPNOTICS

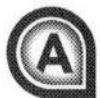

Application Exercises Answer Key

1. A nurse is preparing to care for a client in the surgical unit who will be receiving diazepam (Valium) IV. For which of the following should the nurse monitor this client?

   A. Status epilepticus

   B. Respiratory depression

   C. Malignant hyperthermia

   D. Acute facial dystonia

   The nurse should monitor this client for respiratory depression, which may occur when the medication is administered intravenously or taken orally along with other CNS depressant medications or alcohol. Diazepam is used to treat seizures, therefore, this is not an adverse reaction to the medication. Malignant hyperthermia and facial dystonia are not caused by administration of benzodiazepines, such as diazepam.

NCLEX® Connection: Pharmacological and Parenteral Therapies: Adverse Effects/ Contraindications/Side Effects/Interactions

2. A nurse is caring for a client who is receiving moderate sedation with diazepam (Valium) IV. The client's respiration decreases to 10/min. Which of the following medications should the nurse anticipate administering to this client?

   A. Ketamine (Ketalar)

   B. Naltrexone (ReVia)

   C. Flumazenil (Romazicon)

   D. Fluvoxamine (Luvox)

   Flumazenil reverses toxicity caused by benzodiazepines, such as diazepam. Ketamine is an anesthetic agent, which will potentiate the effects of diazepam. Naltrexone is used to decrease the effects of alcohol, but is not used for benzodiazepine toxicity. Fluvoxamine is an SSRI antidepressant, which will also not be useful to treat benzodiazepine toxicity.

NCLEX® Connection: Pharmacological and Parenteral Therapies: Adverse Effects/ Contraindications/Side Effects/Interactions

3. A nurse is teaching a client about possible adverse effects of her new prescription for ramelteon (Rozerem). For which of the following should the nurse teach the client to notify the provider?

    A. Decreased libido

    B. Blurred vision

    C. Productive cough

    D. Dry mouth

    Amenorrhea, decreased libido, galactorrhea, and problems with fertility are adverse effects of ramelteon for which the client should be taught to notify the provider. Blurred vision, productive cough, and dry mouth are not adverse effects of this medication.

NCLEX® Connection: Pharmacological and Parenteral Therapies: Adverse Effects/ Contraindications/Side Effects/Interactions

4. A client is admitted to undergo a surgical procedure. The nurse should be aware that which of the following pre-existing conditions may be a contraindication for the use of ketamine (Ketalar) as an intravenous anesthetic for this client?

    A. Peptic ulcer disease

    B. Breast cancer

    C. Diabetes

    D. Schizophrenia

    Ketamine is contraindicated for clients with a history of mental illness, such as schizophrenia, because this anesthetic can cause psychologic reactions such as hallucinations. There is no contraindication to the use of ketamine for clients with peptic ulcer disease, breast cancer, or diabetes.

NCLEX® Connection: Pharmacological and Parenteral Therapies: Adverse Effects/ Contraindications/Side Effects/Interactions

UNIT 3: MEDICATIONS AFFECTING THE RESPIRATORY SYSTEM

- Airflow Disorders
- Upper Respiratory Disorders

NCLEX® CONNECTIONS

When reviewing the chapters in this unit, keep in mind the relevant sections of the NCLEX® outline, in particular:

CLIENT NEEDS: PHARMACOLOGICAL AND PARENTERAL THERAPIES

Relevant topics/tasks include:

- Adverse Effects/Contraindications/Side Effects/Interactions
  - Provide information to the client on common side effects/adverse effects/potential interactions of medications and when to notify the provider.
- Expected Actions/Outcomes
  - Use clinical decision making/critical thinking when addressing expected effects/outcomes of medications.
- Medication Administration
  - Educate the client on medication self-administration procedures.

UNIT 3 MEDICATIONS AFFECTING THE RESPIRATORY SYSTEM

Chapter 17 Airflow Disorders

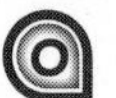

Overview

- Asthma is a chronic inflammatory disorder of the airways. It is an intermittent and reversible airflow obstruction that affects the bronchioles. The obstruction occurs either by inflammation or airway hyper-responsiveness leading to bronchoconstriction.
- Medication management usually addresses both inflammation and bronchoconstriction. These same medications may be used in symptomatic treatment of chronic obstructive pulmonary disease (COPD).
- Medications include:
  - Bronchodilator agents such as $beta_2$-adrenergic agonists, methylxanthines, inhaled anticholinergics, and anti-inflammatory agents such as glucocorticoids, mast cell stabilizers, and leukotriene modifiers.

MEDICATION CLASSIFICATION: $BETA_2$-ADRENERGIC AGONISTS

- Select Prototype Medication: albuterol (Proventil, Ventolin)
- Other Medications:
  - Formoterol (Foradil Aerolizer)
  - Salmeterol (Serevent)
  - Terbutaline (Brethine)

Purpose

- Expected Pharmacological Action
  - $Beta_2$-adrenergic agonists act by selectively activating the $beta_2$-receptors in the bronchial smooth muscle, resulting in bronchodilation. As a result of this:
    - Bronchospasm is relieved.
    - Histamine release is inhibited.
    - Ciliary motility is increased.

- Therapeutic Uses

MEDICATION	ROUTE	THERAPEUTIC USES
Albuterol (Proventil, Ventolin)	• Inhaled, short-acting • Oral, long-acting	• Prevention of asthma attack (exercise-induced) • Treatment for ongoing asthma attack • Long-term control of asthma
Formoterol (Foradil Aerolizer) Salmeterol (Serevent)	• Inhaled, long-acting	• Long-term control of asthma
Terbutaline (Brethine)	• Oral, long-acting	• Long-term control of asthma

Complications

SIDE/ADVERSE EFFECTS	NURSING INTERVENTIONS/CLIENT EDUCATION
Inhaled agents (short and long acting) have minimal adverse effects.	
Oral agents can cause tachycardia and angina because of activation of $alpha_1$ receptors in the heart	• Advise clients to observe for signs and symptoms (chest, jaw, or arm pain or palpitations) and to notify the provider if they occur. • Instruct clients on how to check pulse and to report an increase of greater than 20 to 30 beats/min. • Advise clients to avoid caffeine. • Dosage may need to be lowered.
Tremors caused by activation of $beta_2$ receptors in skeletal muscle	• Tremors usually resolve with continued medication use. • Dosage may need to be reduced.

Contraindications/Precautions

- $Beta_2$-adrenergic agonists are Pregnancy Risk Category C.
- These agents are contraindicated in clients with tachydysrhythmia.
- Use cautiously in clients who have diabetes, hyperthyroidism, heart disease, hypertension, and angina.

Interactions

MEDICATION/FOOD INTERACTIONS	NURSING INTERVENTIONS/CLIENT EDUCATION
Use of beta-adrenergic blockers (propranolol) can negate effects of both medications.	• Beta-adrenergic blockers should not be used concurrently.
MAOIs and tricyclic antidepressants can increase the risk of tachycardia and angina.	• Instruct clients to report changes in heart rate and chest pain.

Nursing Administration

- Instruct clients to follow manufacturer's instructions for use of device: metered-dose inhaler (MDI), dry-powder inhaler(DPI), and nebulizer.
- When a client is prescribed an inhaled beta$_2$-agonist and an inhaled glucocorticoid, advise the client to inhale the beta$_2$-agonist before inhaling the glucocorticoid. The beta$_2$-agonist promotes bronchodilation and enhances absorption of the glucocorticoid.
- Advise clients not to exceed prescribed dosages.
- Ensure that clients know the appropriate dosage schedule (if the medication is to be taken on a fixed or a when-necessary schedule).
- Formoterol and salmeterol are both long-acting beta$_2$-agonist inhalers. These inhalers are used every 12 hr for long-term control and are not to be used to abort an asthma attack. A short-acting beta$_2$-agonist should be used if clients need to treat an acute attack.
- Advise clients to observe for signs of an impending asthma attack and to keep a log of the frequency and intensity of attacks.
- Instruct clients to notify the provider if there is an increase in the frequency and intensity of asthma attacks.

Nursing Evaluation of Medication Effectiveness

- Depending on therapeutic intent, effectiveness may be evidenced by:
  - Long-term control of asthma attacks.
  - Prevention of exercise-induced asthma attack.
  - Resolution of asthma attack as evidenced by absence of shortness of breath, clear breath sounds, absence of wheezing, return of respiratory rate to baseline.

MEDICATION CLASSIFICATION: METHYLXANTHINES

- Select Prototype Medication: theophylline (Theolair, Theo-24)

Purpose

- Expected Pharmacological Action
  - Theophylline causes relaxation of bronchial smooth muscle, resulting in bronchodilation.

- Therapeutic Uses
  - Oral theophylline is used for long-term control of chronic asthma.
  - Route of administration: oral or IV (emergency use only)

Complications

SIDE/ADVERSE EFFECTS	NURSING INTERVENTIONS/CLIENT EDUCATION
• Mild toxicity reaction may include GI distress and restlessness. • More severe reactions can occur with higher therapeutic levels and can include dysrhythmias and seizures	• Monitor theophylline serum levels to keep within therapeutic range (5 to 15 mcg/mL). Side effects are unlikely to occur at levels less than 20 mcg/mL. • If symptoms occur, stop the medication. If necessary, activated charcoal can be used to decrease absorption, lidocaine can be used to treat dysrhythmias, and diazepam can be used to control seizures. • Instruct client that periodic blood levels will be needed. Advise client to report any symptoms of nausea, diarrhea, or restlessness that may indicate toxicity.

Contraindications/Precautions

- Pregnancy Risk Category C
- Use cautiously in clients who have heart disease, hypertension, liver and renal dysfunction, and diabetes.
- Use cautiously in children and older adults.

Interactions

MEDICATION/FOOD INTERACTIONS	NURSING INTERVENTIONS/CLIENT EDUCATION
• Caffeine increases CNS and cardiac adverse effects of theophylline. • Caffeine can also increase theophylline levels.	• Advise clients to avoid consuming caffeinated beverages (coffee, caffeinated colas).
• Phenobarbital and phenytoin decrease theophylline levels.	• When theophylline is used concurrently with these medications, increase the dosage of theophylline.
• Cimetidine (Tagamet), ciprofloxacin (Cipro), and other fluoroquinolone antibiotics increase theophylline levels.	• When theophylline is used concurrently with these medications, decrease the dosage of theophylline.

Nursing Administration

- Advise clients to take the medication as prescribed. If a dose is missed, the following dose should not be doubled.
- Instruct clients not to chew or crush sustained-release preparations. These medications should be swallowed whole.

Nursing Evaluation of Medication Effectiveness

- Depending on therapeutic intent, effectiveness may be evidenced by:
  - Long-term control of asthma attacks

MEDICATION CLASSIFICATION: INHALED ANTICHOLINERGICS

- Select Prototype Medication: ipratropium (Atrovent)
- Other Medications: tiotropium (Spiriva)

Purpose

- Expected Pharmacological Action
  - These medications block muscarinic receptors of the bronchi, resulting in bronchodilation.
- Therapeutic Uses
  - These medications are used to relieve bronchospasm associated with chronic obstructive pulmonary disease.
  - These medications are used for allergen-induced and exercise-induced asthma.
  - Route of administration: inhalation

Complications

SIDE/ADVERSE EFFECTS	NURSING INTERVENTIONS/CLIENT EDUCATION
Local anticholinergic effects (dry mouth, hoarseness)	Advise clients to sip fluids and suck on hard candies to control dry mouth.

Contraindications/Precautions

- Inhaled anticholinergics are Pregnancy Risk Category B.
- These agents are contraindicated in clients who have an allergy to peanuts because the medication preparations may contain soy lecithin.
- Use cautiously in clients who have narrow-angle glaucoma and benign prostatic hypertrophy (due to anticholinergic effects).

Nursing Administration

- Advise clients to rinse the mouth after inhalation to decrease unpleasant taste.
- Usual adult dosage is two puffs. Instruct clients to wait the length of time directed between puffs.
- If clients are prescribed two inhaled medications, instruct clients to wait at least 5 min between medications.

Nursing Evaluation of Medication Effectiveness

- Depending on therapeutic intent, effectiveness may be evidenced by:
  - Control of bronchospasm in clients with chronic obstructive pulmonary disease
  - Prevention of allergen-induced and exercise-induced asthma attack

MEDICATION CLASSIFICATION: GLUCOCORTICOIDS

- Select Prototype Medication:
  - Inhalation: beclomethasone dipropionate (QVAR)
  - Oral: prednisone (Deltasone)
- Other Medications:
  - Inhalation:
    - Budesonide (Pulmicort Flexhaler)
    - Fluticasone propionate and salmeterol (Advair)
    - Fluticasone propionate (Flovent)
    - Triamcinolone acetonide (Azmacort)
  - Oral: Prednisolone (Prelone)
  - IV:
    - Hydrocortisone sodium succinate (Solu-Cortef)
    - Methylprednisolone sodium succinate (Solu-Medrol)

Purpose

- Expected Pharmacological Action
  - These medications prevent inflammation, suppress airway mucus production, and promote responsiveness of $beta_2$ receptors in the bronchial tree.
  - The use of glucocorticoids does not provide immediate effects, but rather promotes decreased frequency and severity of exacerbations and acute attacks.
- Therapeutic Uses
  - Short-term IV agents are used for status asthmaticus.
  - Inhaled agents are used for long-term prophylaxis of asthma.
  - Short-term oral therapy is used to treat symptoms following an acute asthma attack.
  - Long-term oral therapy is used to treat chronic asthma.
  - Replacement therapy is used for primary adrenocortical insufficiency.
  - Promote lung maturity and decrease respiratory distress in fetuses at risk for preterm birth.

Complications

SIDE/ADVERSE EFFECTS	NURSING INTERVENTIONS/CLIENT EDUCATION
Beclomethasone dipropionate	
Difficulty speaking, hoarseness, and candidiasis	• Advise clients to use a spacer with MDI. • Advise clients to rinse mouth or gargle with water or salt water after use. • Advise clients to monitor for redness, sores, or white patches and to report to provider if they occur. Candidiasis may be treated with nystatin oral suspension.
Prednisone when used for 10 days or more can result in:	
Suppression of adrenal gland function, such as a decrease in the ability of the adrenal cortex to produce glucocorticoids: Can occur with inhaled agents and oral agents	• Administer oral glucocorticoid on an alternate-day dosing schedule. • Monitor the client's blood glucose levels. • Taper the client's dose.
Bone loss (can occur with inhaled agents and oral agents)	• Advise clients to perform weight-bearing exercises. • Advise clients to consume a diet with sufficient calcium and vitamin D intake. • Use the lowest dose possible to control symptoms. • Oral medications should be given on an alternate-day dosing schedule.
Hyperglycemia and glucosuria	• Clients with diabetes should have their blood glucose monitored. • Clients may need an increase in insulin dosage.
Myopathy as evidenced by muscle weakness	• Instruct clients to report signs of muscle weakness. • Medication dosage should be decreased.
Peptic ulcer disease	• Advise clients to avoid NSAIDs. • Advise clients to report black, tarry stools. Check stool for occult blood periodically. • Administer with food or meals.
Infection	• Advise clients to notify the provider if early signs of infection occur (sore throat, weakness, malaise).
Disturbances of fluid and electrolytes (fluid retention as evidenced by weight gain, and edema and hypokalemia as evidenced by muscle weakness)	• Instruct clients to observe for symptoms and report to the provider.

Contraindications/Precautions

- Pregnancy risk category C
- Contraindicated in clients who have received a live virus vaccine
- Contraindicated in clients with systemic fungal infections
- Use cautiously in children, and in clients who have diabetes, hypertension, peptic ulcer disease, and/or renal dysfunction.
- Use cautiously in clients taking NSAIDs.

Interactions

MEDICATION/FOOD INTERACTIONS	NURSING INTERVENTIONS/CLIENT EDUCATION
Prednisone	
Concurrent use of potassium-depleting diuretics increases the risk of hypokalemia.	• Monitor potassium level and administer supplements as needed.
Concurrent use of NSAIDs increases the risk of GI ulceration.	• Advise clients to avoid use of NSAIDs. If GI distress occurs, instruct clients to notify the provider.
Concurrent use of glucocorticoids and hypoglycemic agents (oral and insulin) will counteract the effects.	• Clients should notify the provider if hyperglycemia occurs. The client may need increased dosage of insulin or oral hypoglycemics.

Nursing Administration

- Instruct clients to use glucocorticoid inhalers on a regular, fixed schedule for long-term therapy of asthma. Glucocorticoids are not to be used to treat an acute attack.
- Administer using an MDI device, DPI, or nebulizer.
- Clients should use a spacer with all preparations except beclomethasone.
- When a client is prescribed an inhaled beta$_2$-agonist and an inhaled glucocorticoid, advise the client to inhale the beta$_2$-agonist before inhaling the glucocorticoid. The beta$_2$-agonist promotes bronchodilation and enhances absorption of the glucocorticoid.
- Oral glucocorticoids are used short-term, 3 to 10 days following an acute asthma attack.
- If client is on long-term oral therapy, additional dosages of oral glucocorticoids are required in times of stress (infection, trauma).
- Clients who discontinue oral glucocorticoid medications or switch from oral to inhaled agents require additional doses of glucocorticoids during periods of stress.

Nursing Evaluation of Medication Effectiveness

- Depending on therapeutic intent, effectiveness may be evidenced by:
  - Long-term control of asthma attacks
  - Resolution of acute attack as demonstrated by absence of shortness of breath, clear breath sounds, absence of wheezing, and return of respiratory rate to baseline

MEDICATION CLASSIFICATION: MAST CELL STABILIZERS (ANTI-INFLAMMATORIES)

- Select Prototype Medication: cromolyn sodium (Intal)
- Other Medication: nedocromil sodium (Tilade)

Purpose

- Expected Pharmacological Action
  - Anti-inflammatory action
    - These medications stabilize mast cells, which inhibits the release of histamine and other inflammatory mediators.
    - These medications suppress inflammatory cells (eosinophils, macrophages).
- Therapeutic Uses
  - Management of chronic asthma
  - Prophylaxis of exercise-induced asthma
  - Prevention of allergen-induced attack
  - Allergic rhinitis by intranasal route
  - Route of administration: inhalation

Complications

- Safest of all asthma medications
- Safe to use for children

Contraindications/Precautions

- These agents are Pregnancy Risk Category B.
- Fluorocarbons in aerosols make this medication contraindicated for clients who have coronary artery disease, dysrhythmias, and status asthmaticus.
- Use cautiously in clients with liver and kidney impairment.

Nursing Administration

- Advise clients to take medication 15 min before exercise or exposure to allergen.
- Advise clients that long-term prophylaxis may take several weeks for full therapeutic effects to be established.
- Advise clients that this is not a bronchodilator and is not intended for aborting an asthmatic attack.
- Instruct clients in the proper use of administration devices (nebulizer, MDI).

Nursing Evaluation of Medication Effectiveness

- Depending on therapeutic intent, effectiveness may be evidenced by:
  - Prevention of exercise- or allergen-induced bronchospasm
  - Decreased episodes of allergic rhinitis
  - Long-term control of asthma

MEDICATION CLASSIFICATION: LEUKOTRIENE MODIFIERS

- Select Prototype Medication: montelukast (Singulair)
- Other Medication: zileuton (Zyflo), zafirlukast (Accolate)

Purpose

- Expected Pharmacological Action
  - Leukotriene modifiers prevent the effects of leukotrienes, thereby suppressing inflammation, bronchoconstriction, airway edema, and mucus production.
- Therapeutic Uses
  - Leukotriene modifiers are used for long-term therapy of asthma in adults and children 15 years and older and to prevent exercise-induced bronchospasm.
  - Route of administration: oral

Complications

SIDE/ADVERSE EFFECTS	NURSING INTERVENTIONS/CLIENT EDUCATION
Liver injury with use of zileuton (Zyflo) and zafirlukast (Accolate)	• Obtain baseline liver function tests and monitor periodically. • Advise clients to monitor for signs of liver damage (nausea, anorexia, abdominal pain). • Instruct clients to notify the provider if symptoms occur.

 Contraindications/Precautions

- Use cautiously in clients with liver dysfunction.

Interactions

MEDICATION/FOOD INTERACTIONS	NURSING INTERVENTIONS/CLIENT EDUCATION
Zileuton and zafirlukast inhibit metabolism of warfarin (Coumadin), leading to increased warfarin levels.	• Advise clients to observe for signs of bleeding and to notify the provider. • Monitor prothrombin time (PT) and INR levels.
Zileuton and Zafirlukast inhibit metabolism of theophylline, leading to increased theophylline levels.	• Monitor theophylline levels. • Advise clients to observe for signs of theophylline toxicity (nausea, vomiting, seizures), and to notify the provider.

Nursing Administration

- Advise clients to take zileuton as prescribed. Zileuton can be given with or without food.
- Advise clients that zafirlukast should not be given with food, and to administer it 1 hr before or 2 hr after meals.
- Advise clients to take montelukast once daily at bedtime.

Nursing Evaluation of Medication Effectiveness

- Depending on therapeutic intent, effectiveness may be evidenced by:
  - Long-term control of asthma

CHAPTER 17: AIRFLOW DISORDERS

 Application Exercises

1. A nurse is providing teaching to a client with asthma about how to use cromolyn (Intal). Which of the following should the nurse include in her teaching? (Select all that apply.)

    _____ Take the medication 15 min before exercising.

    _____ Follow a fixed-dosage schedule for long-term control of asthma.

    _____ Expect to lose weight while taking this medication.

    _____ Observe for adverse effects such as tremors, restlessness, and palpitations.

    _____ Do not crush or chew tablets.

2. What information should the nurse provide to a client who is starting beclomethasone dipropionate (QVAR) for long-term management of asthma?

3. Which of the following instructions should be given to a client who has been prescribed albuterol (Proventil) and beclomethasone dipropionate (QVAR) inhalers for the control of asthma?

    A. Alternate which inhaler is used so that both are not taken the same time of day.

    B. Use the albuterol inhaler 5 min before using the beclomethasone inhaler.

    C. Only use beclomethasone if experiencing an acute attack.

    D. Use the beclomethasone inhaler first and immediately follow with the albuterol inhaler.

4. Albuterol (Proventil) is used in the treatment of asthma to

    A. decrease inflammation.

    B. promote bronchodilation.

    C. decrease airway mucus production.

    D. suppress the effects of leukotriene compounds.

5. A client is prescribed oral prednisone for treatment of chronic asthma. The nurse should instruct the client to watch for which of the following?

    A. Weight gain and fluid retention

    B. Nervousness and insomnia

    C. Chest pain and tachycardia

    D. Drowsiness and activity intolerance

6. Match the following pharmacologic agents with the appropriate client instructions.

______	Theophylline	A. Take this short-acting $beta_2$-agonist to abort an acute asthma attack.
______	Albuterol	B. Take this medication once daily at bedtime.
______	Salmeterol	C. Avoid caffeine when using this oral methylxanthine medication.
______	Montelukast	D. Take this inhaled $beta_2$-agonist every 12 hr.

CHAPTER 17: AIRFLOW DISORDERS

Application Exercises Answer Key

1. A nurse is providing teaching to a client with asthma about how to use cromolyn (Intal). Which of the following should the nurse include in her teaching? (Select all that apply.)

   __X__ **Take the medication 15 min before exercising.**

   __X__ **Follow a fixed-dosage schedule for long-term control of asthma.**

   _____ Expect to lose weight while taking this medication.

   _____ Observe for adverse effects such as tremors, restlessness, and palpitations.

   _____ Do not crush or chew tablets.

   Cromolyn is used for prophylactic treatment of asthma. It should not be used to abort an asthma attack but can be used to prevent exercise induced bronchospasm. For long-term control, cromolyn should be taken on a fixed-dose schedule. Cromolyn does not promote weight loss, has no significant side effects, and is only given by inhalation.

NCLEX® Connection: Pharmacological and Parenteral Therapies, Medication Administration

2. What information should the nurse provide to a client who is starting beclomethasone dipropionate (QVAR) for long-term management of asthma?

   Inhaled glucocorticoids are generally safe. Use a spacer during administration by MDI.

   Rinse mouth and gargle after inhaling the dose (prevents oropharyngeal candidiasis).

   Engage in weight-bearing exercises and ensure adequate intake of calcium and vitamin D (inhaled glucocorticoids promote bone loss).

NCLEX® Connection: Pharmacological and Parenteral Therapies, Medication Administration

3. Which of the following instructions should be given to a client who has been prescribed albuterol (Proventil) and beclomethasone dipropionate (QVAR) inhalers for the control of asthma?

   A. Alternate which inhaler is used so that both are not taken the same time of day.

   B. Use the albuterol inhaler 5 min before using the beclomethasone inhaler.

   C. Only use beclomethasone if experiencing an acute attack.

   D. Use the beclomethasone inhaler first and immediately follow with the albuterol inhaler.

   When a client is prescribed an inhaled beta$_2$-agonist, such as albuterol, and an inhaled glucocorticoid, such as beclomethasone, the beta$_2$-agonist should be administered first. The beta$_2$-agonist promotes bronchodilation and enhances absorption of the glucocorticoid.

NCLEX® Connection: Pharmacological and Parenteral Therapies, Medication Administration

4. Albuterol (Proventil) is used in the treatment of asthma to

   A. decrease inflammation.

   B. promote bronchodilation.

   C. decrease airway mucus production.

   D. suppress the effects of leukotriene compounds.

   Beta$_2$-adrenergic agonists promote bronchodilation; glucocorticoids and cromolyn decrease inflammation; montelukast (Singulair), a leukotriene modifier, decreases airway mucus production and suppresses the effects of leukotriene compounds.

NCLEX® Connection: Pharmacological and Parenteral Therapies, Expected Actions/Outcomes

5. A client is prescribed oral prednisone for treatment of chronic asthma. The nurse should instruct the client to watch for which of the following?

   A. Weight gain and fluid retention

   B. Nervousness and insomnia

   C. Chest pain and tachycardia

   D. Drowsiness and activity intolerance

   Weight gain and fluid retention can result from oral glucocorticoid use. Nervousness, insomnia, chest pain, tachycardia, drowsiness, and activity intolerance are not side effects of oral glucocorticoids.

NCLEX® Connection: Pharmacological and Parenteral Therapies, Adverse Effects/Contraindications/Side Effects/Interactions

6. Match the following pharmacologic agents with the appropriate client instructions.

C	Theophylline	A. Take this short-acting beta$_2$-agonist to abort an acute asthma attack.
A	Albuterol	B. Take this medication once daily at bedtime.
D	Salmeterol	C. Avoid caffeine when using this oral methylxanthine medication.
B	Montelukast	D. Take this inhaled beta$_2$-agonist every 12 hr.

NCLEX® Connection: Pharmacological and Parenteral Therapies, Medication Administration

UNIT 3 MEDICATIONS AFFECTING THE RESPIRATORY SYSTEM

Chapter 18 Upper Respiratory Disorders

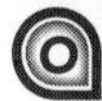

Overview

- The medications in this section work on the CNS, nasal passages, or other parts of the respiratory system to treat the effects of allergic rhinitis or coughs from the common cold, influenza, and other disorders.
  - Antihistamines, often prescribed for allergic rhinitis, may also be used to treat nausea, motion sickness, allergic reactions, and insomnia.
  - Acetylcysteine, a mucolytic, is frequently prescribed as an antidote for acetaminophen toxicity.
- This section includes opioid and nonopioid antitussives, expectorants, mucolytics, decongestants, and antihistamine medications.
- Medications in this section are frequently combined for increased effectiveness. For example, an antitussive may be combined with an expectorant to better control a cough.

MEDICATION CLASSIFICATION: ANTITUSSIVES — OPIOIDS

- Select Prototype Medication: codeine
- Other Medication: hydrocodone

Purpose

- Expected Pharmacological Action
  - Codeine suppresses cough through its action on the central nervous system.
- Therapeutic Uses
  - Codeine is used for chronic nonproductive cough.

Complications

SIDE/ADVERSE EFFECTS	NURSING INTERVENTIONS/CLIENT EDUCATION
CNS effects (dizziness, lightheadedness, drowsiness, respiratory depression)	• Obtain the client's baseline vital signs. • Monitor clients when ambulating. • Advise clients to lie down if feeling lightheaded. • Observe for signs of respiratory depression such as respiratory rate less than 12/min. Stimulate the client to breathe if respiratory depression occurs. It may be necessary to stop the medication and administer naloxone (Narcan). • Advise clients to avoid driving while taking codeine.
GI distress (nausea, vomiting, constipation)	• Instruct clients to take oral codeine with food. • Advise clients to increase fluids and dietary fiber.
Potential for abuse	• Advise clients of the potential for abuse. • Use for short duration.

Contraindications/Precautions

- Codeine is Pregnancy Category Risk C.
- This medication is contraindicated in clients who have acute asthma, head trauma, liver and renal dysfunction, and acute alcoholism.

- Use cautiously in children, older adults, and clients with a history of substance abuse.

Nursing Administration

- Advise clients to avoid hazardous activities, such as driving while taking codeine.
- Advise clients to change positions slowly and to lie down if feeling dizzy.
- Advise clients to avoid alcohol and other CNS depressants while taking codeine.

MEDICATION CLASSIFICATION: ANTITUSSIVES — NON-OPIOIDS

- Select Prototype Medication: dextromethorphan (found in many different products for cough, such as Robitussin and others)
- Other Medications: benzonatate (Tessalon), diphenhydramine (Benadryl)

Purpose

- Expected Pharmacological Action
  - Dextromethorphan suppresses cough through its action on the CNS. Although not an opioid, it is derived from opioids.

- Therapeutic Uses
  - Cough suppression

Complications

- This medication has few adverse effects.
- Some mild nausea, dizziness, and sedation may occur.
- There is some potential for abuse.

Contraindications/Precautions

- Pregnancy Category Risk C

Interactions

- May cause high fever when used within 2 weeks of MAOI antidepressants

Nursing Administration

- Some formulations may contain alcohol and/or sucrose.
- Available forms include capsules, lozenges (for clients older than 12 years), liquids, and syrups.

Nursing Evaluation of Medication Effectiveness

- Depending on therapeutic intent, effectiveness may be evidenced by:
  - Absence or decreased episodes of coughing.

MEDICATION CLASSIFICATION: EXPECTORANTS

- Select Prototype Medication: guaifenesin (Mucinex)

Purpose

- Expected Pharmacological Action
  - Guaifenesin promotes increased cough production through increasing mucous secretion. These actions allow clients to decrease chest congestion by coughing out secretions.
- Therapeutic Uses
  - Although guaifenesin is available as an expectorant alone (Mucinex), it is most often combined with antitussives (either opioid or nonopioid), or a decongestant for treating symptoms of colds, allergic rhinitis, or for cough caused by lower respiratory disorders.

Complications

SIDE/ADVERSE EFFECTS	NURSING INTERVENTIONS/CLIENT EDUCATION
GI upset	• Take with food if GI upset occurs.
Drowsiness, dizziness	• Do not take prior to driving or activities if these reactions occur.
Allergic reaction (rash)	• Stop taking guaifenesin and obtain medical care if rash or other symptoms of allergy occur.

Contraindications/Precautions

- Guaifenesin is Pregnancy Risk Category C.
- Advise clients who are breastfeeding to talk to the provider before taking medications containing guaifenesin.
- Depending on the formulation and medication combinations, preparations containing guaifenesin may not be recommended for children.

Nursing Administration

- Advise clients to increase fluid intake when taking guaifenesin, in order to promote liquefying secretions.
- This medication is available in tablets (which should not be crushed) and capsules, which may be opened to sprinkle on foods.
- Advise clients to read over-the-counter labels carefully to discover what medications have been combined in the preparation used. Guaifenesin is frequently combined with other medications (antitussives, decongestants) as a liquid or syrup (for example, Mucinex D combines guaifenesin with the sympathomimetic decongestant, pseudoephedrine).

Nursing Evaluation of Medication Effectiveness

- Depending on therapeutic intent, effectiveness may be evidenced by the following:
    - Cough is more productive and mucous is easier to expectorate
    - Chest congestion is decreased

MEDICATION CLASSIFICATION: MUCOLYTICS

- Select Prototype Medication: acetylcysteine (Mucomyst, Acetadote)
- Other Medication: hypertonic saline

Purpose

- Expected Pharmacological Action
    - Mucolytics enhance the flow of secretions in the respiratory passages.

- Therapeutic uses
  - Mucolytics are used in clients with acute and chronic pulmonary disorders exacerbated by large amounts of secretions.
  - Mucolytics are used in clients with cystic fibrosis.
  - Acetylcysteine is the antidote for acetaminophen poisoning.

Complications

SIDE/ADVERSE EFFECTS	NURSING INTERVENTIONS/CLIENT EDUCATION
Aspiration and bronchospasm when administered orally	• Monitor clients for signs of aspiration and bronchospasm. Stop medication immediately and notify the provider.

Contraindications/Precautions

- Acetylcysteine is Pregnancy Risk Category B.
- This medication should not be used in clients at risk for GI hemorrhage.
- Use cautiously in clients who have peptic ulcer disease, esophageal varices, and severe liver disease.

Nursing Administration

- Advise clients that acetylcysteine has an odor that smells like rotten eggs.
- Acetylcysteine is administered by inhalation to liquefy nasal and bronchial secretions and facilitate coughing.
- The medication is administered orally or IV for acetaminophen overdose.
  - Oral doses are mixed with fruit juice, cola drinks, or water. Doses are administered every 4 hr for 72 hr.
  - Three IV doses are administered starting with loading dose, followed by the next dose to be infused over 4 hr, followed by the last dose infused over 16 hr.
- Be prepared to suction clients if aspiration occurs with oral administration.

Nursing Evaluation of Medication Effectiveness

- Depending on therapeutic intent, effectiveness may be evidenced by:
  - Improvement of symptoms as demonstrated by regular respiratory rate, clear lung sounds, and increased ease of expectoration

MEDICATION CLASSIFICATION: DECONGESTANTS

- Select Prototype Medication: phenylephrine
- Other Medications:
  - Ephedrine
  - Naphazoline
  - Phenylpropanolamine

Purpose

- Expected Pharmacological Action
  - Sympathomimetic decongestants stimulate alpha$_1$-adrenergic receptors causing reduction in the inflammation of the nasal membranes.
- Therapeutic Uses
  - This medication can be used to treat allergic rhinitis by relieving nasal stuffiness.
  - This medication acts as a decongestant for clients with sinusitis and the common cold.

Complications

SIDE/ADVERSE EFFECTS	NURSING INTERVENTIONS/CLIENT EDUCATION
Rebound congestion secondary to prolonged use of topical agents	• Advise clients to use for short-term therapy, no more than 3 to 5 days. • Taper use and discontinue medication using one nostril at a time.
CNS stimulation (agitation, nervousness, uneasiness)	• CNS stimulation is rare with the use of topical agents • Advise clients to observe for signs of CNS stimulation, and to notify the provider if symptoms occur. • Stop medication.
Vasoconstriction	• Advise clients who have hypertension and coronary artery disease to avoid using these medications.

Contraindications/Precautions

- These medications are contraindicated in clients who have chronic rhinitis.
- Use cautiously in clients who have coronary artery disease and hypertension.

Nursing Administration

- When administering nasal drops, instruct clients to be in the lateral, head low position to increase the desired effect and to prevent swallowing the medication.
- Drops are preferred for children because they can be administered precisely and toxicity can be prevented.
- Educate clients in the differences between topical and oral agents.
    - Topical agents are usually more effective and work faster.
    - Topical agents have a shorter duration.
    - Vasoconstriction and CNS stimulation are uncommon with topical agents, but are a concern with oral agents.
    - Oral agents do not lead to rebound congestion.
- Advise clients to use topical decongestions for no longer than 3 to 5 days to avoid rebound congestion.
- Instruct clients not to exceed recommended doses.

Nursing Evaluation of Medication Effectiveness

- Depending on therapeutic intent, effectiveness may be evidenced by:
    - Improvement of symptoms (relief of congestion, increased ease of breathing, ability to sleep comfortably)

MEDICATION CLASSIFICATION: ANTIHISTAMINES

- Select Prototype Medications:
    - 1st generation H_1 antagonists:
        - Diphenhydramine (Benadryl)
        - Promethazine (Phenergan)
        - Dimenhydrinate (Dramamine)
- Other Medications:
    - 2nd generation H_1 antagonists:
        - Loratadine (Claritin)
        - Cetirizine (Zyrtec)
        - Fexofenadine (Allegra)
        - Desloratadine (Clarinex)

Purpose

- Expected Pharmacological Action
  - Antihistamine action is on the H_1 receptors, which results in the blocking of histamine release in the small blood vessels, capillaries, and nerves during allergic reactions. When used for upper respiratory infections, antihistamines relieve symptoms by suppressing mucous secretion because of their anticholinergic effect.
- Therapeutic Uses
  - 1st generation H_1 antagonists are used for:
    - Mild allergic reactions (seasonal allergic rhinitis, urticaria, mild transfusion reaction)
    - Anaphylaxis (hypotension, acute laryngeal edema, bronchospasm)
    - Motion sickness
    - Insomnia

Complications

SIDE/ADVERSE EFFECTS	NURSING INTERVENTIONS/CLIENT EDUCATION
1st generation H_1 antagonists	
Sedation	• Advise clients to take the medication at night to minimize daytime sedative effect. • Avoid driving, hazardous activities, consumption of alcohol, and other CNS depressant medications (barbiturates, benzodiazepines, opioids).
Anticholinergic effects (dry mouth, constipation)	• Advise clients to take sips of water, suck on sugarless candies, and maintain 2 to 3 L of water each day from food and beverage sources.
Gastrointestinal discomfort (nausea, vomiting, constipation)	• Advise clients to take antihistamine with meals.
Acute toxicity (flushed face, high fever, tachycardia, dry mouth, urinary retention, pupil dilation): Children have symptoms of excitation, hallucinations, incoordination and seizures.	• Advise clients to notify the provider if symptoms occur. • Induce vomiting to remove the antihistamine. • Administer activated charcoal and cathartic to decrease absorption of antihistamine. • Administer acetaminophen for fever. • Apply ice packs or sponge baths.

Contraindications/Precautions

- Antihistamines are contraindicated during the third trimester of pregnancy, for mothers who are breastfeeding, and for newborns. Newborns are sensitive to the adverse effects, such as sedation, of these medications.

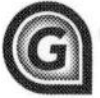

- Use cautiously in children and older adults (impact of adverse effects).
- Use cautiously in clients who have asthma, urinary retention, open angle glaucoma, hypertension, and prostate hypertrophy (impact of anticholinergic medications).

Interactions

MEDICATION/FOOD INTERACTIONS	NURSING INTERVENTIONS/CLIENT EDUCATION
CNS depressants/alcohol cause additive CNS depression.	• Advise clients to avoid alcohol and medications causing CNS depression (opioids, barbiturates, and benzodiazepines).

Nursing Administration

- Advise clients taking 1st generation medications to be aware of sedating effects.

Nursing Evaluation of Medication Effectiveness

- Depending on therapeutic intent, effectiveness may be evidenced by:
    - Improvement of allergic reaction (absence of rhinitis, urticaria)
    - Relief of symptoms of motion sickness (decreased nausea and vomiting)

CHAPTER 18: UPPER RESPIRATORY DISORDERS

Application Exercises

1. A nurse is caring for a client who states she has been taking phenylephrine (Neo-Synephrine) nasal drops for the past 10 days for her upper respiratory symptoms. For which of the following adverse effects should the nurse assess?

    A. Sedation

    B. Nasal congestion

    C. Productive cough

    D. Constipation

2. A nurse is teaching a client to self-administer nasal drops for allergic rhinitis symptoms. The nurse should teach the client to lie in which of the following positions to obtain the best effect of the medication?

    A. Supine with head flexed

    B. Sitting with head in neutral position

    C. Lateral with head in low position

    D. Prone with head extended

3. A preschool child recently diagnosed with cystic fibrosis has a new prescription for acetylcysteine (Mucomyst). The nurse teaches the client and her family that the purpose of this medication is to do which of the following?

    A. Suppress cough

    B. Decrease pain

    C. Minimize nasal congestion

    D. Loosen secretions

4. An adult client is taking diphenhydramine (Benadryl) for symptoms of allergic rhinitis. For which of the following adverse reactions should the nurse teach the client to watch? (Select all that apply)

    _____ Dry mouth

    _____ Nonproductive cough

    _____ Skin rash

    _____ Diarrhea

    _____ Urinary hesitation

CHAPTER 18: UPPER RESPIRATORY DISORDERS

Application Exercises Answer Key

1. A nurse is caring for a client who states she has been taking phenylephrine (Neo-Synephrine) nasal drops for the past 10 days for her upper respiratory symptoms. For which of the following adverse effects should the nurse assess?

   A. Sedation

   B. Nasal congestion

   C. Productive cough

   D. Constipation

   When used for over 5 days, rebound nasal congestion may occur when taking topical sympathomimetic medications, such as phenylephrine. Insomnia, rather than sedation, is a possible adverse effect of this medication. Productive cough is not an expected adverse effect. Constipation, an anticholinergic adverse effect, is not caused by sympathomimetic medications such as phenylephrine.

NCLEX® Connection: Pharmacological and Parenteral Therapies: Adverse Effects/ Contraindications /Side Effects/Interactions

2. A nurse is teaching a client to self-administer nasal drops for allergic rhinitis symptoms. The nurse should teach the client to lie in which of the following positions to obtain the best effect of the medication?

   A. Supine with head flexed.

   B. Sitting with head in neutral position

   C. Lateral with head in low position.

   D. Prone with head extended.

   Lying on the side with the head in a low position helps spread the nasal drops, allows the medication to be more effective, and prevents swallowing the medication. None of the other positions will allow the medication to spread as well to affected areas.

NCLEX® Connection: Pharmacological and Parenteral Therapies: Medication Administration

3. A preschool child recently diagnosed with cystic fibrosis has a new prescription for acetylcysteine (Mucomyst). The nurse teaches the client and her family that the purpose of this medication is to do which of the following?

   A. Suppress cough

   B. Decrease pain

   C. Minimize nasal congestion

   D. Loosen secretions

   Acetylcysteine, when administered by inhalation, is a mucolytic medication that liquefies secretions and allows them to be expectorated more easily. The medication does not suppress cough, minimize nasal congestion, or decrease pain.

NCLEX® Connection: Pharmacological and Parenteral Therapies: Expected Actions/Outcomes

4. An adult client is taking diphenhydramine (Benadryl) for symptoms of allergic rhinitis. For which of the following adverse reactions should the nurse teach the client to watch? (Select all that apply)

   __X__ **Dry mouth**

   _____ Nonproductive cough

   _____ Skin rash

   _____ Diarrhea

   __X__ **Urinary hesitation**

   Dry mouth and urinary hesitation are anticholinergic symptoms that can occur when a client takes diphenhydramine. Constipation, rather than diarrhea, is an adverse reaction of this medication. Neither cough nor a skin rash are expected adverse reactions to this medication. Diphenhydramine is sometimes prescribed to treat nonproductive cough and also is prescribed for skin rash caused by allergies.

NCLEX® Connection: Pharmacological and Parenteral Therapies: Adverse Effects/ Contraindications/Side Effects/Interactions

UNIT 4: MEDICATIONS AFFECTING THE CARDIOVASCULAR SYSTEM

- Medications Affecting Urinary Output
- Medications Affecting Blood Pressure
- Cardiac Glycosides and Heart Failure
- Angina
- Medications Affecting Cardiac Rhythm
- Antilipemic Agents

NCLEX® CONNECTIONS

When reviewing the chapters in this unit, keep in mind the relevant sections of the NCLEX® outline, in particular:

CLIENT NEEDS: PHARMACOLOGICAL AND PARENTERAL THERAPIES

Relevant topics/tasks include:

- Adverse Effects/Contraindications/Side Effects/Interactions
  - Notify the provider of side effects, adverse effects, and contraindications of medications and parenteral therapy.
- Dosage Calculation
  - Use clinical decision making/critical thinking when calculating dosages.
- Medication Administration
  - Titrate dosage of medication based on assessment and ordered parameters.

UNIT 4 MEDICATIONS AFFECTING THE CARDIOVASCULAR SYSTEM

Chapter 19 Medications Affecting Urinary Output

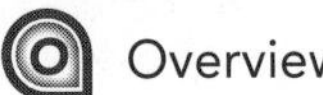

Overview

- Indications for medications that affect urinary output include management of blood pressure, excretion of edematous fluid related to heart failure, kidney and liver disease, and prevention of renal failure.
- Medications include high-ceiling loop diuretics, thiazide diuretics, potassium-sparing diuretics, and osmotic diuretics.

MEDICATION CLASSIFICATION: HIGH CEILING LOOP DIURETICS

- Select Prototype Medication: furosemide (Lasix)
- Other Medications:
  - Ethacrynic acid (Edecrin)
  - Bumetanide (Bumex)
  - Torsemide (Demadex)

Purpose

- Expected Pharmacological Action
  - High ceiling loop diuretics work in the ascending limb of loop of Henle to:
    - Block reabsorption of sodium and chloride and to prevent reabsorption of water
    - Cause extensive diuresis even with severe renal impairment
- Therapeutic Uses
  - High ceiling loop diuretics are used when there is an emergent need for rapid mobilization of fluid such as:
    - Pulmonary edema caused by heart failure
    - Conditions not responsive to other diuretics such as edema caused by liver, cardiac, or kidney disease; hypertension
  - These medications may also be used to treat hypercalcemia related to kidney stone formation.
- Route of administration: Oral, IV, IM.

Complications

SIDE/ADVERSE EFFECTS	NURSING INTERVENTIONS/CLIENT EDUCATION
Dehydration, hyponatremia, hypochloremia	• Assess/monitor clients for signs of dehydration: dry mouth, increased thirst, minimal urine output, and weight loss. • Monitor electrolytes. • Report urine output less than 30 mL/hr. Stop medication and notify the provider. • If signs of headache and/or chest, calf, or pelvic pain occur, notify the provider. This may be an indication of thrombosis or embolism. • Minimize the risk for dehydration by starting clients on low doses and monitoring daily weights.
Hypotension	• Monitor the client's blood pressure. • Instruct clients about signs of postural hypotension (lightheadedness, dizziness). If these occur, advise clients to sit or lie down. • Advise clients to avoid sudden changes of position and arise slowly from lying down or sitting.
Ototoxicity (transient with furosemide and irreversible with ethacrynic acid)	• Advise clients to notify the provider of tinnitus, which may indicate ototoxicity. • Avoid use with other ototoxic medications, such as gentamicin.
Hypokalemia (K+ less than 3.5 mEq/L)	• Monitor the client's cardiac status and potassium levels. • Report a decrease in potassium level (K+ less than 3.5 mEq/L). • Teach clients to consume high-potassium foods such as bananas, potatoes. • Teach clients signs of hypokalemia such as nausea/vomiting, general weakness.
Other adverse effects (hyperglycemia, hyperuricemia, and decrease in calcium and magnesium levels)	• Monitor the client's blood glucose, uric acid, and calcium and magnesium levels. • Report elevated levels.

Contraindications/Precautions

- Pregnancy Risk Category C
- Avoid using these medications during pregnancy unless absolutely required.
- Use cautiously in clients who have diabetes and/or gout.

Interactions

MEDICATION/FOOD INTERACTIONS	NURSING INTERVENTIONS/CLIENT EDUCATION
Digoxin (Lanoxin) toxicity can occur in the presence of hypokalemia.	• Monitor the client's cardiac status and potassium and digoxin levels. • Potassium-sparing diuretics are often used in conjunction with loop diuretics to reduce the risk of hypokalemia.
Concurrent use of antihypertensives can have additive hypotensive effect.	• Monitor the client's blood pressure.
Hyponatremia can lead to decrease in lithium carbonate (Eskalith) excretion, which may lead to toxicity.	• Monitor the client's lithium levels. Dosage may need to be adjusted.
NSAIDs reduce diuretic effect.	• Watch for a decrease in the effectiveness of the diuretic, such as a decrease in urine output.

Nursing Administration

- Obtain the client's baseline data to include orthostatic blood pressure, weight, electrolytes, and location and extent of edema.
- Weigh clients at the same time each day; usually upon awakening.
- Monitor the client's blood pressure and I&O.
- Avoid administering the medication late in the day to prevent nocturia. Usual dosing time is 0800 and 1400.
- Administer furosemide orally, IV bolus dose, or continuous IV infusion. Infuse IV doses at 20 mg/min or slower to avoid abrupt hypotension and hypovolemia.
- If potassium level drops below 3.5 mEq/L, clients should be placed on a potassium supplement.
- If the medication is used for hypertension, teach clients to self-monitor blood pressure and weight by keeping a log.
- Advise clients to get up slowly to minimize postural hypotension. If faintness or dizziness occurs, instruct clients to sit or lie down.
- Teach clients to report significant weight loss, lightheadedness, dizziness, GI distress, and/or general weakness to the provider.
- Encourage clients to consume foods high in potassium, such as avocados and strawberries.
- Instruct clients with diabetes to monitor for elevated blood glucose levels.
- Instruct clients to observe for signs of low magnesium levels such as muscle twitching and tremors.

Nursing Evaluation of Medication Effectiveness

- Depending on therapeutic intent, effectiveness may be evidenced by:
  - Decrease in pulmonary or peripheral edema
  - Weight loss
  - Decrease in blood pressure
  - Increase in urine output

MEDICATION CLASSIFICATION: THIAZIDE DIURETICS

- Select Prototype Medication: hydrochlorothiazide (Hydrodiuril)
- Other Medications:
  - Chlorothiazide (Diuril)
  - Methyclothiazide (Enduron)
  - Thiazide-type diuretics:
    - indapamide (Lozide, Lozol)
    - chlorthalidone (Hygroton)
    - metolazone (Zaroxolyn)

Purpose

- Expected Pharmacological Action
  - Thiazide diuretics work in the early distal convoluted tubule to:
    - Block the reabsorption of sodium and chloride, and prevent the reabsorption of water at this site
    - Promote diuresis when renal function is not impaired
- Therapeutic Uses
  - Thiazide diuretics are often the medication of first choice for essential hypertension.
  - These medications may be used for edema of mild-to-moderate heart failure and liver and kidney disease.

Complications

SIDE/ADVERSE EFFECTS	NURSING INTERVENTIONS/CLIENT EDUCATION
Dehydration	• Assess/monitor clients for signs of dehydration (dry mouth, increased thirst, minimal urine output, weight loss). • Monitor electrolytes and weight. • Report urine output less than 30 mL/hr. Stop medication and notify the provider.
Hypokalemia (K+ less than 3.5 mEq/L)	• Monitor the client's cardiac status and K+ levels. • Report a decrease in K+ level (less than 3.5 mEq/L). • Teach clients to consume foods high in potassium, such as spinach and tomatoes. • Teach clients to recognize signs and symptoms of hypokalemia (nausea/vomiting, general weakness).
Hyperglycemia	• Monitor clients for an increase in blood glucose levels.

Contraindications/Precautions

- Thiazide diuretics are Pregnancy Risk Category B. Avoid use during pregnancy and lactation. If a thiazide diuretic is indicated, advise clients not to breastfeed.

Interactions

MEDICATION/FOOD INTERACTIONS	NURSING INTERVENTIONS/CLIENT EDUCATION
Digoxin (Lanoxin) toxicity can occur in the presence of hypokalemia.	• Monitor the client's cardiac status and potassium and digoxin levels. • A potassium-sparing diuretic is used in conjunction with thiazide diuretics to reduce the risk of hypokalemia.
Antihypertensives have additive hypotensive effects.	• Monitor the client's blood pressure.
Hyponatremia can lead to decrease in lithium carbonate (Eskalith) excretion, which may lead to toxicity.	• Monitor the client's lithium levels. Dosage may need to be adjusted.
NSAIDs reduce diuretic effect.	• Watch for a decrease in the effectiveness of the diuretic, such as reduced urine output.

Nursing Administration

- Chlorothiazide may be administered orally and IV, all others can only be given orally.
- Obtain the client's baseline data to include orthostatic blood pressure, weight, electrolytes, and location and extent of edema.
- Monitor the client's potassium levels.

- Instruct clients to take the medication first thing in the morning; if twice-a-day dosing is prescribed, be sure the second dose is taken by 1400 to prevent nocturia.
- Encourage clients to consume foods high in potassium and maintain adequate fluid intake (1,500 mL per day, unless contraindicated).
- If GI upset occurs, clients should take the medication with or after meals.
- Alternate-day dosing can decrease electrolyte imbalances.

Nursing Evaluation of Medication Effectiveness

- Depending on therapeutic intent, effectiveness may be evidenced by:
  - Decrease in blood pressure
  - Decrease in edema
  - Increase in urine output

MEDICATION CLASSIFICATION: POTASSIUM-SPARING DIURETICS

- Select Prototype Medication: spironolactone (Aldactone)
- Other Medications: triamterene (Dyrenium), amiloride (Midamor)

Purpose

- Expected Pharmacological Action
  - Potassium-sparing diuretics block the action of aldosterone (sodium and water retention), which results in potassium retention and the secretion of sodium and water.
- Therapeutic Uses
  - Potassium-sparing diuretics are combined with other diuretics for potassium-sparing effects.
  - Potassium-sparing diuretics are used for heart failure.
  - In primary hyperaldosteronism, potassium-sparing diuretics block actions of aldosterone.
- Route of administration: Oral

Complications

SIDE/ADVERSE EFFECTS	NURSING INTERVENTIONS/CLIENT EDUCATION
Hyperkalemia (K+ greater than 5.0 mEq/L)	• Monitor potassium level. Initiate cardiac monitoring for serum potassium greater than 5 mEq/L. • Treat hyperkalemia by discontinuing medication, restricting potassium in the diet, and insulin injections to drive potassium back into the cell.
Endocrine effects (impotence in male clients; irregularities of menstrual cycle in female clients)	• Advise clients to observe for side effects. • Clients should notify the provider if these responses occur.

Contraindications/Precautions

- Do not administer to clients who have hyperkalemia.
- Potassium-sparing diuretics are contraindicated in clients who have severe renal failure and anuria.

Interactions

MEDICATION/FOOD INTERACTIONS	NURSING INTERVENTIONS/CLIENT EDUCATION
Concurrent use of ACE inhibitors increases the risk of hyperkalemia.	• Monitor the client's K+ levels. Notify the provider if K+ is greater than 5.0 mEq/L.
Concurrent use of potassium supplements increases the risk of hyperkalemia.	• Clients should not take this medication and a potassium supplement concurrently.

Nursing Administration

- Obtain the client's baseline data.
- Monitor the client's potassium levels regularly.
- Can only be given orally.
- Teach clients to avoid salt substitutes that contain potassium.
- Teach clients to self-monitor blood pressure.
- Instruct clients to keep a log of blood pressure and weight.
- Warn clients that triamterene may turn urine a bluish color.

Nursing Evaluation of Medication Effectiveness

- Depending on therapeutic intent, effectiveness may be evidenced by:
  - Maintenance of normal potassium levels: between 3.5 mEq/L and 5.0 mEq/L
  - Weight loss
  - Decrease in blood pressure and edema.

MEDICATION CLASSIFICATION: OSMOTIC DIURETICS

- Select Prototype Medication: mannitol (Osmitrol)

Purpose

- Expected Pharmacological Action
  - Osmotic diuretics reduce intracranial pressure and intraocular pressure by raising serum osmolality and drawing fluid back into the vascular and extravascular space.
- Therapeutic Uses
  - Osmotic diuretics prevent renal failure in specific situations, such as hypovolemic shock and severe hypotension.
  - These medications decrease intracranial pressure (ICP) caused by cerebral edema.
  - These medications decrease intraocular pressure (IOP).
  - Osmotic diuretics promote sodium retention and water excretion in clients with hyponatremia and fluid volume excess.

Complications

SIDE/ADVERSE EFFECTS	NURSING INTERVENTIONS/CLIENT EDUCATION
Heart failure, pulmonary edema	• If signs of heart failure develop (dyspnea, weakness, fatigue, distended neck veins, and/or weight gain), stop the medication immediately and notify the provider.
Renal failure	• If signs of renal failure develop (urine output less than 30 mL/hr, increased serum creatinine [greater than 1.2 mg/dL] and BUN [greater than 20 mg/dL]), stop the medication immediately and notify the provider.
Fluid and electrolyte imbalances	• Monitor the client's laboratory values.

Contraindications/Precautions

- Use extreme caution in clients with heart failure.

Interactions

- Furosemide contributes to therapeutic effect by promoting renal excretion of fluid drawn into vasculature by osmotic diuretics.

Nursing Administration

- Administer mannitol by continuous IV infusion.
- To prevent administering microscopic crystals, use a filter needle when drawing from the vial and a filter in the IV tubing.
- Monitor daily weight, I & 0, and serum electrolytes.
- Monitor for signs of dehydration, acute renal failure, and edema.
- Use of furosemide may help prevent rebound fluid retention; this contributes to therapeutic effect.

Nursing Evaluation of Medication Effectiveness

- Depending on therapeutic intent, effectiveness may be evidenced by:
  - Normal renal function as demonstrated by:
    - Urine output of at least 30 mL/hr
    - Serum creatinine between 0.6 to 1.2 mg/dL for men and 0.5 to 1.1 mg/dL for women
    - BUN levels between 10 to 20 mg/dL
  - Decrease in intracranial pressure
  - Decrease in intraocular pressure

CHAPTER 19: MEDICATIONS AFFECTING URINARY OUTPUT

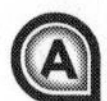

Application Exercises

1. A nurse is caring for a client prescribed hydrochlorothiazide (Hydrodiuril) for a client with hypertension. Which of the following instructions should the nurse include in the client's teaching?

    A. "Your diet should include foods high in potassium."

    B. "Take the medication right before bedtime."

    C. "You may notice some swelling in your feet."

    D. "Avoid drinking liquids early in the morning."

2. For which of the following side effects should a client taking furosemide (Lasix) for hypertension be assessed?

    A. Visual disturbances

    B. Hearing loss

    C. Tremors

    D. Restlessness

3. A client has a new prescription for spironolactone (Aldactone). Which of the following laboratory values should the nurse recognize as a reason to hold the morning dose of this medication and notify the provider?

    A. Serum sodium 148 mEq/L

    B. Serum potassium 5.2 mEq/L

    C. Serum creatinine 1.2 mg/dL

    D. Serum chloride 106 mEq/L

4. A nurse is administering mannitol (Osmitrol) to a client who has increased intracranial pressure. For which of the following findings should the nurse discontinue the medication and notify the provider?

    A. Blood glucose 150 mg/dL

    B. Dyspnea

    C. Urine output 40 mL/hr

    D. Headache

CHAPTER 19: MEDICATIONS AFFECTING URINARY OUTPUT

Application Exercises Answer Key

1. A nurse is caring for a client who is prescribed hydrochlorothiazide (Hydrodiuril) for hypertension. Which of the following instructions should the nurse include in the client's teaching?

   A. "Your diet should include foods high in potassium."

   B. "Take the medication right before bedtime."

   C. "You may notice some swelling in your feet."

   D. "Avoid drinking liquids early in the morning."

   Clients who take hydrochlorothiazide are at risk for potassium loss. Eating foods high in potassium (bananas, cantaloupe, white potatoes) can help prevent this. Diuretics should be taken early in the morning and usually no later than 1400. Clients should notice decreased swelling. Clients need adequate fluid intake to promote urine output. Fluids are best taken in the morning.

NCLEX® Connection: Pharmacological and Parenteral Therapies: Adverse Effects/ Contraindications/Side Effects/Interactions

2. For which of the following side effects should a client taking furosemide (Lasix) for hypertension be assessed?

   A. Visual disturbances

   B. Hearing loss

   C. Tremors

   D. Restlessness

   Furosemide is ototoxic and may cause hearing loss. Visual disturbances, tremors, and restlessness are not side effects of furosemide.

NCLEX® Connection: Pharmacological and Parenteral Therapies: Adverse Effects/ Contraindications/Side Effects/Interactions

3. A client has a new prescription for spironolactone (Aldactone). Which of the following laboratory values should the nurse recognize as a reason to hold the morning dose of this medication and notify the provider?

   A. Serum sodium 148 mEq/L

   B. Serum potassium 5.2 mEq/L

   C. Serum creatinine 1.2 mg/dL

   D. Serum chloride 106 mEq/L

   The nurse should not administer spironolactone, a potassium-sparing diuretic, if the serum potassium is higher than 5.0 mEq/L. A serum sodium of 148 mEq/L is elevated, but this would not be a contraindication to giving the medication. The serum creatinine and serum chloride levels are within expected reference ranges.

NCLEX® Connection: Pharmacological and Parenteral Therapies: Expected Actions/Outcomes

4. A nurse is administering mannitol (Osmitrol) to a client who has increased intracranial pressure. For which of the following findings should the nurse discontinue the medication and notify the provider?

    A. Blood glucose 150 mg/dL

    B. Dyspnea

    C. Urine output 40 mL/hr

    D. Headache

    Dyspnea may be an indication that the client is developing heart failure. The medication should be discontinued and the provider notified immediately. A blood glucose of 150 mg/dL is not an indication to discontinue the medication. Urine output of 40 mL/hr indicates adequate urine output. Headache may be a indication of increased intracranial pressure for which the medication is being administered.

NCLEX® Connection: Pharmacological and Parenteral Therapies: Adverse Effects/Contraindications/Side Effects/Interactions

UNIT 4 MEDICATIONS AFFECTING THE CARDIOVASCULAR SYSTEM

Chapter 20 Medications Affecting Blood Pressure

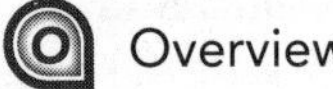

Overview

- Blood pressure may be controlled in a variety of ways with a variety of agents that may be used alone or in combination. Guidelines for pharmacological management of hypertension can be found in The Seventh Report of the Joint National Committee on Prevention, Detection, Evaluation, and Treatment of High Blood Pressure (JNC 7) prepared by the US Department of Health and Human Services.
- The classifications of medications used to control blood pressure include:
  - Thiazide diuretics
  - Angiotensin-converting enzyme (ACE) inhibitors
  - Angiotensin II receptor blockers (ARBS)
  - Calcium channel blockers (CCB)
  - Alpha adrenergic blockers
  - Centrally acting $alpha_2$ agonists
  - Beta adrenergic blockers
  - Vasodilators

MEDICATION CLASSIFICATION: ANGIOTENSIN-CONVERTING ENZYME (ACE) INHIBITORS

- Select Prototype Medication: captopril (Capoten)
- Other Medications:
  - Enalapril (Vasotec)
  - Enalaprilat (Vasotec IV)
  - Fosinopril (Monopril)
  - Lisinopril (Prinivil)
  - Ramipril (Altace)

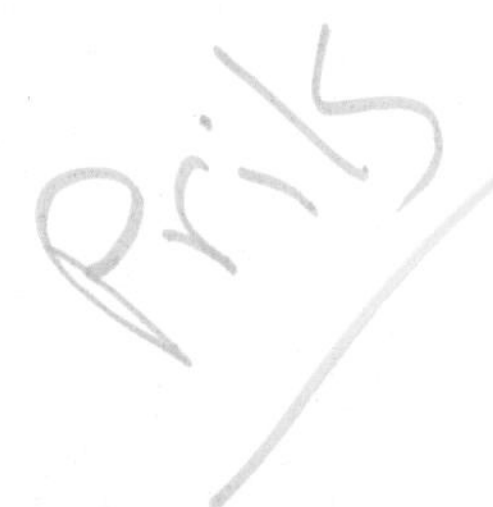

Purpose

- Expected Pharmacological Action
  - ACE inhibitors produce their effects by blocking the production of angiotensin II, leading to:
    - Vasodilation (mostly arteriole)
    - Excretion of sodium and water, and retention of potassium by actions in the kidneys
    - Reduction in pathological changes in the blood vessels and heart that result from the presence of angiotensin II and aldosterone
- Therapeutic Uses
  - Hypertension
  - Heart failure
  - Myocardial infarction (To decrease mortality and to decrease risk of heart failure and left ventricular dysfunction)
  - Diabetic and nondiabetic nephropathy
  - For clients at high risk for a cardiovascular event, ramipril can be used to prevent MI, stroke, or death.

Complications

SIDE/ADVERSE EFFECTS	NURSING INTERVENTIONS/CLIENT EDUCATION
First-dose orthostatic hypotension	• If the client is already taking a diuretic, the medication should be stopped temporarily for 2 to 3 days prior to the start of an ACE inhibitor. • Start treatment with a low dosage of the medication. • Monitor the client's blood pressure for 2 hr after initiation of treatment. • Instruct clients to change positions slowly and to lie down if feeling dizzy, lightheaded, or faint.
Cough related to inhibition of kinase II (alternative name for ACE) which results in increase in bradykinin	• Inform clients of the possibility of experiencing a dry cough and to notify the provider. The medication should be discontinued.
Hyperkalemia	• Monitor potassium levels to maintain a level within the expected reference range of 3.5 to 5 mEq/L. • Advise clients to avoid the use of salt substitutes containing potassium.
Rash and dysgeusia (altered taste), primarily with captopril	• Clients should inform the provider if these effects occur. • Symptoms will stop with discontinuation of the medication.

SIDE/ADVERSE EFFECTS	NURSING INTERVENTIONS/CLIENT EDUCATION
Angioedema	• Manifested as swelling of the tongue and oral pharynx. • Treat severe effects with subcutaneous injection of epinephrine. • Medication should be discontinued.
Neutropenia (rare but serious complication of captopril)	• Monitor the client's WBC counts every 2 weeks for 3 months, then periodically. • This condition is reversible when detected early. • Inform clients to notify the provider at the first signs of infection, (fever, sore throat) because medication should be discontinued.

 Contraindications/Precautions

- These medications are Pregnancy Risk Category D during the second and third trimester, related to fetal injury.
- ACE inhibitors are contraindicated in clients with renal stenosis when present bilaterally or in a single remaining kidney.
- These medications are contraindicated in clients with a history of angioedema following use of ACE inhibitor.
- Use cautiously in clients with renal impairment and collagen vascular disease because they are at greater risk for developing neutropenia. Closely monitor these clients for signs of infection.

Interactions

MEDICATION/FOOD INTERACTIONS	NURSING INTERVENTIONS/CLIENT EDUCATION
Diuretics can contribute to first-dose hypotension.	Clients should be advised to temporarily stop taking diuretics 2 to 3 days before the start of therapy with an ACE inhibitor.
Antihypertensive medications may have an additive hypotensive effect.	Advise clients that dosage of medication may need to be adjusted if ACE inhibitors are added to the treatment regimen.
Potassium supplements and potassium-sparing diuretics increase the risk of hyperkalemia.	Clients should only take potassium supplements if prescribed by the provider. Clients should avoid salt substitutes that contain potassium.
ACE inhibitors can increase levels of lithium carbonate (Eskalith).	Monitor the client's lithium levels to avoid toxicity.
Use of NSAIDs may decrease the antihypertensive effect of ACE inhibitors.	Avoid concurrent use.

Nursing Administration

- Administer ACE inhibitors orally except enalaprilat, which is the only ACE inhibitor for IV use.
- Advise clients that the medication may be prescribed as a single formulation or in combination with hydrochlorothiazide.
- Advise clients that blood pressure has to be monitored after the first dose for at least 2 hr to detect hypotension.
- Instruct clients that captopril should be taken at least 1 hr before meals. All other ACE inhibitors can be taken with or without food.
- Advise clients to notify the provider if cough, rash, dysgeusia (lack of taste), and/or signs of infection occur.

MEDICATION CLASSIFICATION: ANGIOTENSIN II RECEPTOR BLOCKERS (ARBs)

- Select Prototype Medication: losartan (Cozaar)
- Other Medications:
  - Valsartan (Diovan)
  - Irbesartan (Avapro)
  - Candesartan (Atacand)
  - Olmesartan (Benicar)

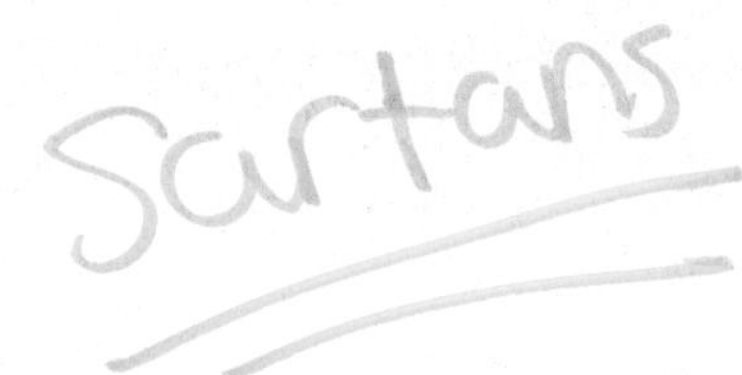

Purpose

- Expected Pharmacological Action
  - These medications block the action of angiotensin II in the body. This results in:
    - Vasodilation (mostly arteriole)
    - Excretion of sodium and water, and retention of potassium (through effects on the kidney)
- Therapeutic Uses
  - Hypertension
  - Heart failure and prevention of mortality following MI
  - Stroke prevention
  - Delay progression of diabetic nephropathy

Complications

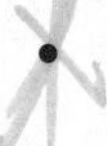

- The major difference between ARBs and ACE inhibitors is that cough and hyperkalemia are not side effects of ARBs.

SIDE/ADVERSE EFFECTS	NURSING INTERVENTIONS/CLIENT EDUCATION
Angioedema	• Advise clients to observe for signs and symptoms (skin wheals, swelling of tongue) and to notify provider. • Treat severe effects with subcutaneous injection of epinephrine. • Medication should be discontinued.
Fetal injury	• Advise women of risk during the second and third trimester of pregnancy.

Contraindications/Precautions

- ARBs are contraindicated in second and third trimester related to fetal injury (Pregnancy Risk Category D).
- These medications are contraindicated in clients with renal stenosis when present bilaterally or in a single remaining kidney
- Use cautiously in clients who experienced angioedema with ACE inhibitor (not an absolute contraindication).

Interactions

MEDICATION/FOOD INTERACTIONS	NURSING INTERVENTIONS/CLIENT EDUCATION
Antihypertensive medications may have an additive effect when used with ARBs.	• Advise clients that dosage of medication may need to be adjusted if ACE inhibitors are added to the treatment regimen.

Nursing Administration

- Administer medications by oral route.
- Advise clients that medication may be prescribed as a single formulation or in combination with hydrochlorothiazide.
- Advise clients that ARBs can be taken with or without food.

MEDICATION CLASSIFICATION: CALCIUM CHANNEL BLOCKERS

- Select Prototype Medications:
  - Nifedipine (Adalat, Procardia)
  - Verapamil (Calan)
  - Diltiazem (Cardizem)
- Other Medications:
  - Amlodipine (Norvasc)
  - Felodipine (Plendil)
  - Nicardipine (Cardene, Cleviprex)

Purpose

- Expected Pharmacological Action

MEDICATION	EXPECTED PHARMACOLOGICAL ACTION	SITE OF ACTION AT THERAPEUTIC DOSES
Nifedipine	• Blocking of calcium channels in blood vessels leads to vasodilation of peripheral arterioles and arteries/arterioles of the heart.	• Nifedipine acts primarily on arterioles. • Veins are not significantly affected.
Verapamil, diltiazem	• Blocking of calcium channels in blood vessels leads to vasodilation of peripheral arterioles and arteries/arterioles of the heart. • Blocking of calcium channels in the myocardium, the SA node, and the AV node leads to a decreased force of contraction, a decreased heart rate, and slowing of the rate of conduction through the AV node.	• These medications act on arterioles and the heart at therapeutic doses. • Veins are not significantly affected.

- Therapeutic Uses

MEDICATION	ANGINA PECTORIS	HYPERTENSION	CARDIAC DYSRHYTHMIAS (ATRIAL FIBRILLATION, ATRIAL FLUTTER, SVT)
Nifedipine	X	X	
Amlodipine	X	X	
Nicardipine	X	X	
Felodipine		X	
Verapamil, diltiazem	X	X	X

Complications

SIDE/ADVERSE EFFECTS	NURSING INTERVENTIONS/CLIENT EDUCATION
Nifedipine	
Reflex tachycardia	• Monitor clients for an increased heart rate. • A beta-blocker (metoprolol [Lopressor]) can be administered to counteract tachycardia.
Peripheral edema	• Inform clients to observe for swelling in lower extremities and notify the provider if this occurs. • A diuretic may be prescribed to control edema.
Acute toxicity	• With excessive doses, the heart, in addition to blood vessels, is affected. • Monitor the client's vital signs and ECG. Gastric lavage and cathartic may be indicated. • Administer medications (norepinephrine, calcium, isoproterenol, lidocaine, and IV fluids). • Have equipment for cardioversion and cardiac pacer available.
Verapamil, diltiazem	
Orthostatic hypotension and peripheral edema	• Monitor the client's blood pressure, edema, and weight daily. • Instruct clients to observe for swelling in the lower extremities, and notify the provider if it occurs. • A diuretic may be prescribed to control edema. • Instruct clients about the signs of postural hypotension (lightheadedness, dizziness). If these occur, advise clients to sit or lie down. Can be minimized by getting up slowly.
Constipation (primarily verapamil)	• Advise clients to increase intake of high fiber food and oral fluids, if not restricted.
Suppression of cardiac function (bradycardia, heart failure)	• Monitor the client's ECG, pulse rate, and rhythm. • Advise clients to observe for suppression of cardiac function (slow pulse, activity intolerance), and to notify provider if these occur. Medication may be discontinued.
Dysrhythmias (QRS complex is widened and QT interval is prolonged)	• Monitor the client's vital signs and ECG.
Acute toxicity resulting in hypotension, bradycardia, AV block and ventricular tachydysrhythmias.	• Monitor the client's vital signs and ECG. Gastric lavage and cathartic may be indicated. • Administer medications (norepinephrine, calcium, isoproterenol, lidocaine, and IV fluids). • Have equipment for cardioversion and cardiac pacer available.

Contraindications/Precautions

- Pregnancy Risk Category C
- Use cautiously with women who are lactating.
- These medications are contraindicated in clients who have heart block, hypotension, bradycardia, aortic stenosis, or severe heart failure.
- Use verapamil and diltiazem cautiously in clients receiving digoxin and beta-blockers.

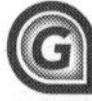

- Use cautiously in older adults and clients who have kidney disorders, liver disorders, or mild to moderate heart failure.

Interactions

MEDICATION/FOOD INTERACTIONS	NURSING INTERVENTIONS/CLIENT EDUCATION
Nifedipine	
Beta-blockers, such as metoprolol (Lopressor), are used to decrease reflex tachycardia.	• Monitor clients for excessive slowing of heart rate.
Consuming grapefruit juice and nifedipine can lead to toxicity.	• Monitor clients for signs of decrease in blood pressure, increase in heart rate, and flushing. • Advise clients to avoid drinking grapefruit juice.
Verapamil, diltiazem	
Verapamil can increase digoxin (Lanoxin) levels, increasing the risk of digoxin toxicity. Digoxin can cause an additive effect and intensify AV conduction suppression.	• Digoxin levels should be monitored to maintain therapeutic range between 0.5 to 2.0 ng/mL. • Monitor vital signs for bradycardia and for signs of AV block, such as a reduced ventricular rate.
Concurrent use of beta-blockers can lead to heart failure, AV block, and bradycardia.	• Allow several hours between administration of IV verapamil (Calan) and beta-blockers.
Consuming grapefruit juice and verapamil or diltiazem can lead to toxicity.	• Monitor clients for signs of constipation, a decrease in blood pressure, a decrease in heart rate, and AV block. • Advise clients to avoid drinking grapefruit juice.

Nursing Administration

- Advise clients not to chew or crush sustained-release tablets.
- For intravenous administration, administer injections slowly over a period of 2 to 3 min.
- Advise clients who have angina to record pain frequency, intensity, duration, and location. The provider should be notified if attacks increase in frequency, intensity, and/or duration.
- Teach clients to monitor blood pressure and heart rate, as well as keep a blood pressure record.

MEDICATION CLASSIFICATION: ALPHA ADRENERGIC BLOCKERS (SYMPATHOLYTICS)

- Select Prototype Medication: prazosin (Minipress)
- Other Medication: doxazosin mesylate (Cardura)

Purpose

- Expected Pharmacological Action
  - Selective $alpha_1$ blockade results in:
    - Venous and arterial dilation
    - Smooth muscle relaxation of the prostatic capsule and bladder neck
- Therapeutic uses
  - Primary hypertension.
  - Doxazosin mesylate (Cardura) may be used to decrease symptoms of benign prostatic hypertrophy (BPH), which include urgency, frequency, and dysuria.

Complications

SIDE/ADVERSE EFFECTS	NURSING INTERVENTIONS/CLIENT EDUCATION
First-dose orthostatic hypotension	• Start treatment with low dosage of medication. • First dose may be given at night. • Monitor blood pressure for 2 hr after the initiation of treatment. • Instruct clients to avoid activities requiring mental alertness for the first 12 to 24 hr. • Instruct clients to change positions slowly and to lie down if feeling dizzy, lightheaded, or faint.

Contraindications/Precautions

- Pregnancy Risk Category C
- Contraindicated in clients with hypersensitivity to medication

Interactions

MEDICATION/FOOD INTERACTIONS	NURSING INTERVENTIONS/CLIENT EDUCATION
Antihypertensive medications may have an additive hypotensive effect	• Instruct clients to observe for signs of hypotension (dizziness, lightheadedness, faintness). • Instruct clients to lie down if these symptoms occur, and to change positions slowly.
NSAIDs and clonidine may decrease the antihypertensive effects of prazosin.	• Advise clients to avoid OTC NSAIDs.

Nursing Administration

- Obtain baseline blood pressure and heart rate.
- Instruct clients that the medication can be taken with food.
- Recommend that clients take the initial dose at bedtime to decrease "first-dose" hypotensive effect.

MEDICATION CLASSIFICATION: CENTRALLY ACTING ALPHA$_2$ AGONISTS

- Select Prototype Medication: clonidine (Catapres)
- Other Medications: guanfacine HCl (Tenex), methyldopa (Aldomet)

Purpose

- Expected Pharmacological Action
  - These medications act within the CNS to decrease sympathetic outflow resulting in decreased stimulation of the adrenergic receptors (both alpha and beta receptors) of the heart and peripheral vascular system.
    - Decrease in sympathetic outflow to the myocardium results in bradycardia and decreased cardiac output (CO).
    - Decrease in sympathetic outflow to the peripheral vasculature results in vasodilation, which leads to decreased blood pressure.
- Therapeutic Uses
  - Primary hypertension (administered alone, with a diuretic, or with another antihypertensive agent)
  - Severe cancer pain (administered parenterally by epidural infusion)
  - Investigational use
    - Migraine headache
    - Flushing from menopause
    - Management of ADHD and Tourette's syndrome
    - Management of withdrawal symptoms from alcohol, tobacco, and opioids

Complications

SIDE/ADVERSE EFFECTS	NURSING INTERVENTIONS/CLIENT EDUCATION
Drowsiness and sedation	• Drowsiness will diminish as use of medication continues. • Advise clients to avoid activities that require mental alertness until symptoms subside.
Dry mouth	• Advise clients to be compliant with medication regimen. • Reassure clients that symptoms usually resolve in 2 to 4 weeks. • Encourage clients to chew gum or suck on hard candy, and to take small amounts of water or ice chips.
Rebound hypertension	• Advise clients not to discontinue treatment without consulting the provider. • Clonidine should be discontinued gradually over the course of 2 to 4 days.

Contraindications/Precautions

- Clonidine is Pregnancy Risk Category C.
- Avoid use during lactation.
- This medication is contraindicated for clients taking anticoagulant medications
- Avoid use of transdermal patch on affected skin in scleroderma and systemic lupus erythematosus (SLE).
- Use cautiously in clients with cerebrovascular disease, recent MI, diabetes mellitus, major depressive disorder, or chronic renal failure.

Interactions

MEDICATION/FOOD INTERACTIONS	NURSING INTERVENTIONS/CLIENT EDUCATION
Antihypertensive medications may have an additive hypotensive effect.	• Instruct clients to observe for signs of hypotension (dizziness, lightheadedness, faintness). • Instruct clients to lie down if feeling dizzy, lightheaded, or faint, and change positions slowly.
Concurrent use of prazosin (Minipress), MAOIs, and tricyclic antidepressants can counteract the antihypertensive effect of clonidine.	• Monitor clients for therapeutic effect. Monitor blood pressure. Do not use concurrently.
Additive CNS depression can occur with concurrent use of other CNS depressants, such as alcohol.	• Advise clients of additive CNS depression with alcohol, and encourage clients to avoid use.

Nursing Administration

- Administer medication by oral, epidural, and transdermal routes.
- Medication is usually administered twice a day in divided doses. Take larger dose at bedtime to decrease the occurrence of daytime sleepiness.
- Transdermal patches are applied every seven days. Advise clients to apply patch on hairless, intact skin on torso or upper arm.

MEDICATION CLASSIFICATION: BETA ADRENERGIC BLOCKERS (SYMPATHOLYTICS)

- Select Prototype Medications:
  - Cardioselective: $Beta_1$
    - Metoprolol (Lopressor)
    - Atenolol (Tenormin)
    - Metoprolol succinate (Toprol XL)
    - Esmolol HCL (Brevibloc)
  - Nonselective: ($Beta_1$ and $Beta_2$)
    - Propranolol (Inderal)
    - Nadolol (Corgard)
    - Labetalol (Normodyne)

Purpose

- Expected Pharmacological Action
  - In cardiac conditions, the primary effects of beta-adrenergic blockers are a result of $beta_1$-adrenergic blockade in the myocardium and in the electrical conduction system of the heart.
    - Decreased heart rate (chronotropic [rate] action)
    - Decreased myocardial contractility (inotropic [force] action)
    - Decreased rate of conduction through the AV node
- Therapeutic Uses
  - Primary hypertension (Exact mechanism unknown: may be related to long-term use causing reduction in peripheral vascular resistance)
  - Angina, tachydysrhythmias, heart failure and myocardial infarction.
  - Other uses may include:
    - Treatment of hyperthyroidism, migraine headache, stage fright, pheochromocytoma, and glaucoma

Complications

SIDE/ADVERSE EFFECTS	NURSING INTERVENTIONS/CLIENT EDUCATION
Beta$_1$ Blockade – metoprolol, propranolol	
Bradycardia	• Monitor the client's pulse. If below 60/min, hold medication, and notify the provider. • Use cautiously in clients with diabetes. This medication can mask tachycardia, an early sign of low blood glucose in clients with diabetes. Advise clients to monitor blood glucose to detect hypoglycemia.
Decreased cardiac output	• Use cautiously with clients in heart failure. Doses are started very low and titrated to the desired level. • Advise clients to observe for signs of worsening heart failure (shortness of breath, edema, fatigue). • The provider should be notified if symptoms occur.
AV block	• Obtain a baseline ECG and monitor.
Orthostatic hypotension	• Advise clients to sit or lie down if experiencing dizziness or faintness. • Clients should avoid sudden changes of position and rise slowly.
Rebound myocardium excitation	• The myocardium becomes sensitized to catecholamines with long-term use of beta-blockers. • Advise clients not to stop taking beta-blockers abruptly, but to follow the provider's instructions. • Use of beta-blockers should be discontinued over 1 to 2 weeks.
Beta$_2$ Blockade – propranolol	
Bronchoconstriction	• Avoid in clients with asthma. • Clients with asthma should be administered a beta$_1$ selective agent.
Glycogenolysis is inhibited	• Clients with diabetes rely on the breakdown of glycogen into glucose to manage low blood glucose (can happen with insulin overdose). • In addition, a decreased heart rate can further mask symptoms of impending low blood glucose level. Clients with diabetes should be administered a beta$_1$ selective agent.

Contraindications/Precautions

- Beta-adrenergic blockers are contraindicated in clients with AV block and sinus bradycardia.
- Nonselective beta-adrenergic blockers are contraindicated in clients with asthma, bronchospasm, and heart failure.
- Use cardioselective beta-adrenergic blockers cautiously in clients with heart failure, asthma, bronchospasm, diabetes, with history of severe allergies, and depression.

Interactions

MEDICATION/FOOD INTERACTIONS	NURSING INTERVENTIONS/CLIENT EDUCATION
Beta$_1$ Blockade – metoprolol, propranolol	
Calcium channel blockers (CCB): verapamil (Calan) and diltiazem (Cardizem) intensify the effects of beta-blockers • Decreased heart rate • Decreased myocardial contractility • Decreased rate of conduction through the AV node	• Monitor ECG and blood pressure. • Monitor clients closely if taking a CCB and beta-blocker concurrently. Reduce dose if needed.
Concurrent use of antihypertensive medications with beta-blockers can intensify the hypotensive effect of both medications.	• Monitor clients for a drop in blood pressure.
Beta$_2$ Blockade – propranolol	
Propranolol use can mask the hypoglycemic effect of insulin and prevent the breakdown of fat in response to hypoglycemia.	• Monitor blood glucose levels.

Nursing Administration

- Administer medications orally, usually once or twice a day.
- Administer the following medications by IV route: atenolol, metoprolol, labetalol, propranolol.
- Advise clients not to discontinue medication without consulting the provider.
- Advise clients to avoid sudden changes in position to prevent occurrence of orthostatic hypotension.
- Instruct clients not to crush or chew extended release tablets.
- Teach clients to self monitor heart rate and blood pressure at home on a daily basis.

Nursing Evaluation of Medication Effectiveness

- Depending on therapeutic intent, effectiveness may be evidenced by:
  - Absence of chest pain.
  - Absence of cardiac dysrhythmias.
  - Normotensive blood pressure readings.
  - Control of heart failure signs and symptoms.

MEDICATIONS FOR HYPERTENSIVE CRISIS

- Select Prototype Medication: nitroprusside sodium (Nitropress)
- Other Medications:
    - Nitroglycerin (Nitrostat IV)
    - Nicardipine (Cardene)
    - Clevidipine (Cleviprex)
    - Enalaprilat (Vasotec IV)
    - Esmolol HCL (Brevibloc)

Purpose

- Expected Pharmacological Action
    - Direct vasodilation of arteries and veins resulting in rapid reduction of blood pressure (decreased preload and afterload)
- Therapeutic Uses
    - Hypertensive emergencies

Complications

SIDE/ADVERSE EFFECTS	NURSING INTERVENTIONS/CLIENT EDUCATION
Excessive hypotension	• Administer medication slowly because rapid administration will cause blood pressure to go down rapidly. • Monitor the client's blood pressure and ECG.
Cyanide poisoning (headache and drowsiness, and may lead to cardiac arrest)	• Clients who have liver dysfunction are at increased risk. • Risk of cyanide poisoning may be reduced by administering medication at a rate of 5 mcg/kg/min or less, and giving thiosulfate concurrently. Medication should be discontinued if cyanide toxicity occurs.
Thiocyanate poisoning	• This effect can be manifested as altered mental status. • Avoid prolonged use of nitroprusside. Monitor plasma levels if used for more than 3 days. Level should be maintained at less than 0.1 mg/mL.

Contraindications/Precautions

- Pregnancy Risk Category C

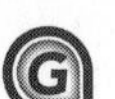

- Use cautiously in clients who have liver and kidney disease or fluid and electrolyte imbalances, and in older adults.

Interactions

- Nitroprusside should not be administered in the same infusion as any other medication.

Nursing Administration

- Prepare medication by adding to diluent for IV infusion.
- Note color of solution. Solution may be light brown in color. Discard solution of any other color.
- Protect IV container and tubing from light.
- Discard medication after 24 hr.
- Monitor vital signs and ECG continuously.

Nursing Evaluation of Medication Effectiveness

- Depending on therapeutic intent, effectiveness may be evidenced by:
    - Decrease in blood pressure and maintenance of normotensive blood pressure
    - Improvement of heart failure such as ability to perform activities of daily living, improved breath sounds, absence of edema
    - Improvement in renal function and delay of further progression of renal disease

CHAPTER 20: MEDICATIONS AFFECTING BLOOD PRESSURE

Application Exercises

1. Propranolol (Inderal) is contraindicated for a client who has which of the following conditions?

   A. Asthma
   B. Diabetes
   C. Angina
   D. Dementia

2. When providing teaching to a client taking verapamil (Calan) for control of hypertension, which of the following should the nurse include?

   A. Increase the amount of dietary fiber in the diet.
   B. Drink at least one glass of grapefruit juice each day.
   C. Decrease the amount of calcium in the diet.
   D. Withhold food for 1 hr after the medication is taken.

3. A client receiving captopril (Capoten) and spironolactone (Aldactone), a potassium-sparing diuretic, should be monitored for which of the following adverse effects? (Select all that apply.)

   _____ Hyperkalemia
   _____ Hypotension
   _____ Reflex tachycardia
   _____ Headache
   _____ Drowsiness

4. Match the medications with their corresponding side effects.

_____	enalapril (Vasotec)	A. Drowsiness
_____	nifedipine (Adalat)	B. Dry cough
_____	clonidine (Catapres)	C. Inhibition of glycogenolysis
_____	labetalol (Normodyne)	D. Reflex tachycardia

CHAPTER 20: MEDICATIONS AFFECTING BLOOD PRESSURE

Application Exercises Answer Key

1. Propranolol (Inderal) is contraindicated for a client who has which of the following conditions?

    A. Asthma

    B. Diabetes

    C. Angina

    D. Dementia

    Propranolol is a nonselective beta-adrenergic blocker and blocks both $beta_1$ and $beta_2$ receptors. Blockade of $beta_2$ receptors in the lungs causes bronchoconstriction, so it is contraindicated in clients with asthma. Use propranolol cautiously with clients who have diabetes, but it is not contraindicated. Propranolol can be used to treat angina. It is not contraindicated in dementia.

NCLEX® Connection: Pharmacological and Parenteral Therapies: Expected Actions/Outcomes

2. When providing teaching to a client taking verapamil (Calan) for control of hypertension, which of the following should the nurse include?

    A. Increase the amount of dietary fiber in the diet.

    B. Drink at least one glass of grapefruit juice each day.

    C. Decrease the amount of calcium in the diet.

    D. Withhold food for 1 hr after the medication is taken.

    Constipation is a side effect of verapamil. Increasing dietary fiber can help prevent constipation. Clients should avoid drinking grapefruit juice when taking verapamil because concurrent use can lead to toxicity. There is no restriction on calcium intake when taking verapamil. There is no restriction regarding food intake after taking verapamil.

NCLEX® Connection: Pharmacological and Parenteral Therapies: Medication Administration

3. A client receiving captopril (Capoten) and spironolactone (Aldactone), a potassium-sparing diuretic, should be monitored for which of the following adverse effects? (Select all that apply.)

    __X__ **Hyperkalemia**

    __X__ **Hypotension**

    _____ Reflex tachycardia

    _____ Headache

    _____ Drowsiness

    ACE inhibitors can lead to hyperkalemia. Using a potassium-sparing diuretic with an ACE inhibitor will further increase the potassium. Both captopril and spironolactone can lower blood pressure, therefore taking them together can have an additive effect, leading to hypotension. Reflex tachycardia, headache, and drowsiness are not side effects of either medication.

NCLEX® Connection: Pharmacological and Parenteral Therapies: Adverse Effects/Contraindications/Side Effects/Interactions

4. Match the medications with their corresponding side effects.

B	enalapril (Vasotec)	A. Drowsiness
D	nifedipine (Adalat)	B. Dry cough
A	clonidine (Catapres)	C. Inhibition of glycogenolysis
C	labetalol (Normodyne)	D. Reflex tachycardia

Enalapril (Vasotec) and other ACE inhibitors may cause a dry cough related to inhibition of kinase II, which results in increase in bradykinin. Nifedipine (Adalat) may cause reflex tachycardia and increased angina. Clonidine (Catapres), a central acting Alpha$_2$ agonist, may cause drowsiness and sedation. Nonselective beta-adrenergic blockers may inhibit glycogenolysis, causing hypoglycemia.

NCLEX® Connection: NCLEX connection: Pharmacological and Parenteral Therapies: Adverse Effects/Contraindications/Side Effects/Interactions

UNIT 4 MEDICATIONS AFFECTING THE CARDIOVASCULAR SYSTEM

Chapter 21 Cardiac Glycosides and Heart Failure

Overview

- Heart failure, cardiac failure, or pump failure results from the inability of the heart muscle to pump enough blood to supply the whole body.
- The different determinants of cardiac output such as heart rate, stroke volume, preload, and afterload are affected in heart failure.
- Inability to pump sufficient blood results in:
    - Decreased tissue perfusion as evidenced by fatigue, weakness, and activity intolerance
    - Pulmonary and systemic congestion or volume overload as evidenced by jugular venous distention, peripheral edema, and dyspnea.
- Diuretics, ACE inhibitors, angiotensin II receptor blockers (ARBs), and beta adrenergic blockers are the medications of choice for treatment of heart failure. Cardiac glycosides are indicated if these medications are unable to control symptoms.

MEDICATION CLASSIFICATION: CARDIAC GLYCOSIDES

- Select Prototype Medication: digoxin (Lanoxin, Lanoxicaps, and Digitek)

Purpose

- Expected Pharmacological Action
    - Positive inotropic effect = increased force of myocardial contraction
        - Increased force and efficiency of myocardial contraction improves the heart's effectiveness as a pump, improving stroke volume and cardiac output.
    - Negative chronotropic effect = decreased heart rate
        - At therapeutic levels, digoxin slows the rate of SA node depolarization and the rate of impulses through the conduction system of the heart.
        - A decreased heart rate gives the ventricles more time to fill with blood coming from the atria, which leads to increased SV and increased CO.
- Therapeutic Uses
    - Treatment of heart failure
    - Dysrhythmias (atrial fibrillation)

Complications

SIDE/ADVERSE EFFECTS	NURSING INTERVENTIONS/CLIENT EDUCATION
• Dysrhythmias (caused by interfering with the electrical conduction in the myocardium) • Cardiotoxicity leading to bradycardia	• Conditions that increase the risk of developing digoxin-induced dysrhythmias include hypokalemia, increased serum digoxin levels, and heart disease. • Monitor serum levels of K+ to maintain a level between 3.5 to 5.0 mEq/L. • Instruct clients to report signs of hypokalemia (nausea/vomiting, general weakness). Potassium supplements may be prescribed if clients are concurrently taking a diuretic. • Teach clients to consume high-potassium foods (spinach, bananas, potatoes). • Monitor the client's digoxin level. ○ Therapeutic serum levels may vary, but usually range from 0.5 to 2.0 ng/mL. ○ Signs of toxicity may appear at levels less than 1.75 ng/mL. ○ Clients with heart failure respond best with serum medication levels between 0.5 to 0.8 ng/mL. ○ Dosages should be based on serum levels and client response to medication. • Teach clients to monitor pulse rate, and recognize and report changes. The rate may be irregular with early or extra beats noted.
• GI effects include anorexia (usually the first sign), nausea, vomiting, and abdominal pain.	• Teach clients to monitor for these effects and report to the provider if they occur.
• CNS effects include fatigue, weakness, vision changes (diplopia, blurred vision, yellow-green or white halos around objects).	• Teach clients to monitor for these effects and report to the provider if they occur.

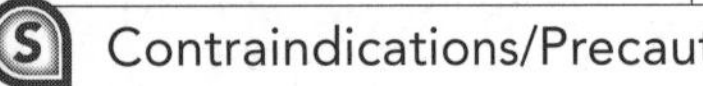

Contraindications/Precautions

- Cardiac glycosides are Pregnancy Risk Category C.
- These agents are contraindicated in clients with disturbances in ventricular rhythm, including ventricular fibrillation, ventricular tachycardia, and second- and third-degree heart block.
- Use cautiously in clients who have hypokalemia, partial AV block, advanced heart failure, and renal insufficiency.

Interactions

MEDICATION/FOOD INTERACTIONS	NURSING INTERVENTIONS/CLIENT EDUCATION
• Thiazide diuretics, such as hydrochlorothiazide (HCTZ), and loop diuretics, such as furosemide (Lasix), may lead to hypokalemia, which increases the risk of developing dysrhythmias	• Monitor K+ level and maintain between 3.5 to 5.0 mEq/L. • Hypokalemia can be treated with potassium supplements or a potassium-sparing diuretic.
• ACE inhibitors and ARBs increase the risk of hyperkalemia, which can lead to decreased therapeutic effects of digoxin.	• Use cautiously if these medications are used with potassium supplements or a potassium-sparing diuretic. • Maintain K+ between 3.5 to 5.0 mEq/L.
• Sympathomimetic medications such as dopamine (Intropin) complement the inotropic action of digoxin and increase the rate and force of heart muscle contraction. • These medications may be beneficial, but also may increase the risk of tachydysrhythmias.	• Monitor ECG. Instruct clients to measure heart rate and report palpitations.
• Quinidine increases the risk of digoxin toxicity when used concurrently.	• Avoid concurrent use.
• Verapamil (Calan) increases plasma levels of digoxin.	• If used concurrently, digoxin dose should be decreased. Concurrent use is usually avoided because of verapamil cardiosuppression action counteracting the action of digoxin.

Nursing Administration

- Advise clients to take the medication as prescribed. If a dose is missed, the next dose should not be doubled.
- Check pulse rate and rhythm before administration of digoxin and record. Notify the provider if heart rate is less than 60/min in an adult, less than 70/min in children, and less than 90/min in infants.
- Administer digoxin at the same time daily.
- Monitor digoxin levels periodically during treatment and maintain therapeutic levels between 0.5 to 2.0 ng/mL to prevent digoxin toxicity.
- Avoid taking OTC medications to prevent adverse and side effects and medication interactions.
- Instruct clients to observe symptoms of hypokalemia, such as muscle weakness, and to notify the provider if symptoms occur.
- Instruct clients to observe symptoms of digoxin toxicity (anorexia, fatigue, weakness), and to notify the provider if symptoms occur.

- Management of digoxin toxicity
  - Digoxin and potassium-sparing medication should be stopped immediately.
  - Monitor K+ levels. For levels less than 3.5 mEq/L, administer potassium intravenously or by mouth. Do not give any further K+ if the level is greater than 5.0 mEq/L.
  - Treat dysrhythmias with phenytoin (Dilantin) or lidocaine.
  - Treat bradycardia with atropine.
  - For excessive overdose, activated charcoal, cholestyramine, or Digibind can be used to bind digoxin and prevent absorption.

Nursing Evaluation of Medication Effectiveness

- Depending on therapeutic intent, effectiveness may be evidenced by:
  - Control of heart failure signs and symptoms.
  - Absence of cardiac dysrhythmias.

MEDICATION CLASSIFICATION: ADRENERGIC AGONISTS

- Select Prototype Medication:
  - Catecholamines:
    - Epinephrine (Adrenaline)
    - Dopamine (Intropin)
    - Dobutamine (Dobutrex)
- Other Medications:
  - Isoproterenol: catecholamine
  - Terbutaline: noncatecholamine

Purpose

RECEPTORS	SITE/RESPONSE
$Alpha_1$	• Activation of receptors in arterioles of skin, viscera and mucous membranes, and veins leads to vasoconstriction.
$Beta_1$	• Heart stimulation leads to increased heart rate, increased myocardial contractility, and increased rate of conduction through the AV node. • Activation of receptors in the kidney lead to the release of renin.
$Beta_2$	• Activation of receptors in the arterioles of the heart, lungs, and skeletal muscles leads to vasodilation. • Bronchial stimulation leads to bronchodilation. • Activation of receptors in uterine smooth muscle causes relaxation. • Activation of receptors in the liver cause glycogenolysis. • Skeletal muscle receptor activation leads to muscle contraction.
Dopamine	• Activation of receptors in the kidney cause the renal blood vessels to dilate.

RECEPTORS	PHARMACOLOGICAL ACTION	THERAPEUTIC USE
	Epinephrine	
$Alpha_1$	• Vasoconstriction	• Slows absorption of local anesthetics • Manages superficial bleeding • Decreased congestion of nasal mucosa • Increased blood pressure
$Beta_1$	• Increased heart rate • Increased myocardial contractility • Increased rate of conduction through the AV node	• Treatment of AV block and cardiac arrest
$Beta_2$	• Bronchodilation	• Asthma
	Dopamine	
Low dose: • Dopamine	• Renal blood vessel dilation	• Shock • Heart failure
Moderate dose: • Dopamine • $Beta_1$	• Renal blood vessel dilation • Increased heart rate • Increased myocardial contractility • Increased rate of conduction through the AV node	
High dose: • Dopamine • $Beta_1$ • $Alpha_1$	• Renal blood vessel dilation • Increased heart rate • Increased myocardial contractility • Increased rate of conduction through the AV node • Vasoconstriction	
	Dobutamine	
$Beta_1$	• Increased heart rate • Increased myocardial contractility • Increased rate of conduction through the AV node	• Heart failure

Complications

SIDE/ADVERSE EFFECTS	NURSING INTERVENTIONS/CLIENT EDUCATION
Epinephrine	
Vasoconstriction from activation of $alpha_1$ receptors in the heart can lead to hypertensive crisis.	• Provide for continuous cardiac monitoring. • Report changes in vital signs to the provider.
$Beta_1$ receptor activation in the heart can cause dysrhythmias. $Beta_1$ receptor activation also increases the workload of the heart and increases oxygen demand leading to the development of angina.	• Provide for continuous cardiac monitoring. • Monitor clients closely for dysrhythmias, change in HR and chest pain. • Notify the provider of signs of dysrhythmias, increased heart rate and chest pain, and treat per protocol.
Dopamine	
$Beta_1$ receptor activation in the heart can cause dysrhythmias. $Beta_1$ receptor activation also increases the workload of the heart and increases oxygen demand leading to development of angina.	• Provide for continuous cardiac monitoring. • Monitor clients closely for dysrhythmias, change in HR, and chest pain. • Notify the provider of signs of dysthymias, increased HR, and chest pain, and treat per protocol.
Necrosis can occur from extravasation of high doses of dopamine.	• Monitor IV site carefully. • Discontinue infusion at first sign of irritation.
Dobutamine	
Increased HR	• Provide for continuous cardiac monitoring. • Report changes in vital signs to the provider.

Contraindications/Precautions

- Epinephrine and dopamine are Pregnancy Risk Category C.
- Dobutamine is Pregnancy Risk Category B.
- These medications are contraindicated in clients who have tachydysrhythmias and ventricular fibrillation.
- Use cautiously in clients who have hyperthyroidism, angina, history of myocardial infarction, hypertension, and diabetes.

Interactions

MEDICATION/FOOD INTERACTIONS	NURSING INTERVENTIONS/CLIENT EDUCATION
MAOIs prevent inactivation of epinephrine and therefore prolong the effects of epinephrine.	• Avoid use of MAOIs in clients receiving epinephrine.
Tricyclic antidepressants block uptake of epinephrine, which will prolong and intensify effects of epinephrine.	• Clients taking these medications concurrently may need a lowered dosage of epinephrine.
General anesthetics can cause the heart to become hypersensitive to the effects of epinephrine, leading to dysrhythmias.	• Perform continuous ECG monitoring. • Notify the provider of signs of chest pain, dysrhythmias, and increased heart rate.
Alpha-adrenergic blocking agents, such as phentolamine, block action at alpha receptors.	• Phentolamine may be used to treat epinephrine toxicity.
Beta-adrenergic blocking agents, such as propranolol block action at beta receptors.	• Propranolol may be used to treat chest pain and dysrhythmias.
Diuretics promote beneficial effects of dopamine.	• Monitor for therapeutic effects.

Nursing Administration

- This medication must be administered IV by continuous infusion.
- Use an IV pump to control infusion.
- Dosage is titrated based on blood pressure response.
- Stop the infusion at first evidence of infiltration. Extravasation can be treated with local injection of an alpha-adrenergic blocking agent, such as phentolamine.
- Assess/monitor clients for chest pain. Notify the provider if chest pain occurs.
- Provide continuous ECG monitoring. Notify the provider of signs of tachycardia or dysrhythmias.

Nursing Evaluation of Medication Effectiveness

- Depending on therapeutic intent, effectiveness may be evidenced by:
    - Improved perfusion as evidenced by urine output of ≥ 30 mL/hr (with normal renal function), improved mental status, and systolic blood pressure maintained at ≥ 90 mm Hg

CHAPTER 21: CARDIAC GLYCOSIDES AND HEART FAILURE

 Application Exercises

1. A nurse is monitoring serum electrolytes for a client prescribed digoxin (Lanoxin). Which of the following laboratory values should the nurse report to the provider?

   A. Sodium 135 mg/dL
   B. Potassium 2.8 mEq/L
   C. Chloride 101 mEq/L
   D. Calcium 9.6 mEq/L

2. A nurse is providing teaching to a client who is prescribed digoxin (Lanoxin). Which of the following may indicate digoxin toxicity and should be reported to the provider? (Select all that apply)

   _____ Fatigue
   _____ Constipation
   _____ Anorexia
   _____ Rash
   _____ Diplopia

3. A nurse is providing teaching to a client about foods high in potassium. Which of the following foods has the highest potassium content?

   A. 1 cup of spinach
   B. 0.5 cup raisins
   C. 1 cup of orange juice
   D. 0.5 cup of nonfat milk

CHAPTER 21: CARDIAC GLYCOSIDES AND HEART FAILURE

Application Exercises Answer Key

1. A nurse is monitoring serum electrolytes for a client prescribed digoxin (Lanoxin). Which of the following laboratory values should the nurse report to the provider?

   A. Sodium 135 mg/dL

   B. Potassium 2.8 mEq/L

   C. Chloride 101 mEq/L

   D. Calcium 9.6 mEq/L

   Hypokalemia can result in fatal dysrhythmias. Digoxin works by binding to and inhibiting the enzyme Na+K+-ATPase. Potassium and digoxin compete for the same binding sites on this enzyme. With hypokalemia, digoxin has more opportunity to bind to Na+K+-ATPase and can lead to cardiotoxicity.

NCLEX® Connection: Pharmacological and Parenteral Therapies: Medication Administration

2. A nurse is providing teaching to a client who is prescribed digoxin (Lanoxin). Which of the following may indicate digoxin toxicity and should be reported to the provider? (Select all that apply)

   __X__ **Fatigue**

   _____ Constipation

   __X__ **Anorexia**

   _____ Rash

   __X__ **Diplopia**

   Fatigue, anorexia, and diplopia are side effects indicating possible digoxin toxicity. Constipation and rash are not side effects of digoxin toxicity.

NCLEX® Connection: Pharmacological and Parenteral Therapies: Adverse Effects/ Contraindications/Side Effects/Interactions

3. A nurse is providing teaching to a client about foods high in potassium. Which of the following foods has the highest potassium content?

   A. 1 cup of spinach

   B. 0.5 cup raisins

   C. 1 cup of orange juice

   D. 0.5 cup of nonfat milk

   A cup of spinach contains 839 mg of potassium, which is the highest content of these foods; 0.5 cup of raisins has 544 mg of potassium, 1 cup of orange juice contains 496 mg of potassium, and 0.5 cup of nonfat milk has 376 mg of potassium.

NCLEX® Connection: Pharmacological and Parenteral Therapies: Medication Administration

UNIT 4 MEDICATIONS AFFECTING THE CARDIOVASCULAR SYSTEM

Chapter 22 Angina

Overview

- Anginal pain is a result of an imbalance between myocardial oxygen supply and demand. Pharmacological management is aimed at prevention of myocardial ischemia and pain as well as prevention of myocardial infarction and death.
- Anginal pain is managed with organic nitrates, beta adrenergic blocking agents, calcium channel blockers, and ranolazine. In addition, clients with chronic stable angina should concurrently take an antiplatelet agent, such as aspirin or clopidogrel (Plavix), a cholesterol-lowering agent, and an ACE inhibitor to prevent myocardial infarction and death.

MEDICATION CLASSIFICATION: ORGANIC NITRATES

- Select Prototype Medication:
  - Nitroglycerin
    - Sublingual tablet: Nitrostat
    - Translingual spray: Nitrolingual
    - Topical ointment: Nitro-Bid
    - Transderm patch: Nitro-Dur
    - Intravenous: Nitro-Bid IV
- Other Medications:
  - Sublingual: isosorbide dinitrate (Isordil)
  - Oral: isosorbide mononitrate (Imdur)

Purpose

- Expected Pharmacological Action
  - In chronic stable exertional angina, nitroglycerin (NTG) dilates veins and decreases venous return (preload), which decreases cardiac oxygen demand.
  - In variant (Prinzmetal's or vasospastic) angina, nitroglycerin prevents or reduces coronary artery spasm, thus increasing oxygen supply.
- Therapeutic Uses
  - Treatment of acute angina attack
  - Prophylaxis of chronic stable angina or variant angina

Complications

SIDE/ADVERSE EFFECTS	NURSING INTERVENTIONS/CLIENT EDUCATION
Headache	• Instruct clients to use aspirin or acetaminophen to relieve pain. • Clients should notify the provider if symptoms do not resolve in a few weeks. Dosage may need to be reduced.
Orthostatic hypotension	• Advise clients to sit or lie down if experiencing dizziness or faintness. • Clients should avoid sudden changes of position and rise slowly.
Reflex tachycardia	• Monitor the client's vital signs. • Administer a beta-blocker such as metoprolol (Lopressor) if symptoms occur.
Tolerance	• Use lowest dose needed to achieve effect. • All long-acting forms of nitroglycerin should be taken with a medication-free period each day (usually 8 hr).

Contraindications/Precautions

- Nitroglycerin is Pregnancy Risk Category C.
- This medication is contraindicated in clients with hypersensitivity to nitrates.
- Nitroglycerin is contraindicated in clients with traumatic head injury because the medication can increase intracranial pressure.
- Use cautiously in clients taking antihypertensive medications and clients who have renal or liver dysfunction.

Interactions

MEDICATION/FOOD INTERACTIONS	NURSING INTERVENTIONS/CLIENT EDUCATION
Use of alcohol can contribute to the hypotensive effect of nitroglycerin.	• Advise clients to avoid use of alcohol.
Antihypertensive medications, such as beta-blockers, calcium channel blockers, and diuretics can contribute to hypotensive effect.	• Use nitroglycerin cautiously in clients receiving these medications.
Use of sildenafil (Viagra) and nitroglycerin can result in life-threatening hypotension.	• Instruct clients not to take sildenafil if prescribed nitroglycerin.

Nursing Administration

ROUTE	USE	NURSING INTERVENTIONS/CLIENT EDUCATION
Sublingual tablet and translingual spray • Rapid onset • Short duration	• Treat acute attack • Prophylaxis of acute attack	• Use this rapid-acting nitrate at the first sign of chest pain. Do not wait until pain is severe. • Use prior to activity that is known to cause chest pain, such as climbing a flight of stairs. • For sublingual tablet: ○ Place the tablet under the tongue and allow it to dissolve. ○ Tablets should be stored in original bottles, and in a cool, dark place. ○ Discard tablets after 24 months unless indicated on the package. • Translingual spray should be sprayed against oral mucosa and not inhaled.
Transmucosal • Rapid onset • Long duration	• Treat acute attack • Prophylaxis of acute attack • Long-term prophylaxis against anginal attacks	• Use this rapid-acting nitrate at the first sign of chest pain. Do not wait until pain is severe. • Use prior to activity that is known to cause chest pain, such as climbing a flight of stairs. • Do not chew the tablet, but place the tablet between the upper lip and gum, or between the cheek and gum to be dissolved.
Sustained-release oral capsules • Slow onset • Long duration	• Long-term prophylaxis against anginal attacks	• Swallow capsules without crushing or chewing.
Transdermal • Slow onset • Long duration	• Long-term prophylaxis against anginal attacks	• To ensure appropriate dose, patches should not be cut. • Place the patch on a hairless area of skin (chest, back, or abdomen) and rotate sites to prevent skin irritation. • Wash skin with soap and water and dry thoroughly before applying new patch. • Remove the patch at night to reduce the risk of developing tolerance to nitroglycerin. Be medication-free a minimum of 8 hr each day.

ROUTE	USE	NURSING INTERVENTIONS/CLIENT EDUCATION
Topical ointment • Slow onset • Long duration	• Long-term prophylaxis against anginal attacks	• Remove the prior dose before a new dose is applied. Measure specific dose with applicator paper and spread over 2.5 to 3.5 inches of the paper. • Apply to a clean, hairless area of the body, and cover with clear plastic wrap. • Follow same guidelines for site selection as for transdermal patch. • Avoid touching ointment with the hands.
Intravenous	• Control of angina not responding to other medications • Control of BP or induced hypotension during surgery • Heart failure resulting from acute MI	• Administer with IV tubing supplied by manufacturer using a glass IV bottle. • Administer continuously due to short duration of action. • Start at a slow rate, usually 5 mcg/min, and titrate gradually until desired response is achieved. • Provide continuous cardiac monitoring during administration.

- Treatment of Anginal Attack
  - Instruct the client to stop activity.
  - The client should take a dose of rapid-acting nitroglycerin immediately.
  - If pain is unrelieved in 5 min, the client should call 9-1-1 or be driven to an emergency department.
  - The client can take up to two more doses at 5 min intervals.
- Advise clients not to stop taking long-acting nitroglycerin abruptly and follow the provider's instructions.
- Advise clients who have angina to record pain frequency, intensity, duration, and location. The provider should be notified if attacks increase in frequency, intensity, and/or duration.

Nursing Evaluation of Medication Effectiveness

- Depending on therapeutic intent, effectiveness may be evidenced by:
  - Prevention of acute anginal attacks
  - Long-term management of stable angina
  - Control of perioperative blood pressure
  - Control of heart failure following acute MI

MEDICATION CLASSIFICATION: ANTIANGINAL AGENT

- Select Prototype Medication: ranolazine (Ranexa)

Purpose

- Expected Pharmacological Action
  - Lowers cardiac oxygen demand and thereby improves exercise tolerance and decreases pain
- Therapeutic Uses
  - Chronic stable angina in combination with amlodipine (Norvasc), a beta adrenergic blocker or an organic nitrate

Complications

SIDE/ADVERSE EFFECTS	NURSING INTERVENTIONS/CLIENT EDUCATION
QT prolongation	Monitor ECG
Elevated blood pressure	Monitor blood pressure

Contraindications/Precautions

- Ranolazine is contraindicated in clients who have QT prolongation or in clients taking other medications that can result in QT prolongation.
- This medication is contraindicated in clients who have liver dysfunction.

- Use cautiously in older adult clients.

Interactions

MEDICATION/FOOD INTERACTIONS	NURSING INTERVENTIONS/CLIENT EDUCATION
Inhibitors of CYP3A4 can increase levels of ranolazine and lead to torsades de pointes. Agents include grapefruit juice, HIV protease inhibitors, macrolide antibiotics, azole antifungals and verapamil.	• Avoid concurrent use.
Quinidine and sotalol (Betapace) can further increase QT interval	• Avoid concurrent use.
Concurrent use of digoxin (Lanoxin) and simvastatin (Zocor) increases serum levels of digoxin and simvastatin.	• Monitor digoxin level. • Instruct client to report muscle weakness.

Nursing Administration

- Administer as an extended release oral tablet, twice daily.
- Obtain baseline and monitor ECG for QT prolongation.
- Obtain baseline and monitor digoxin level with concurrent use.

Nursing Evaluation of Medication Effectiveness

- Depending on therapeutic intent, effectiveness may be evidenced by:
    - Prevention of acute anginal attacks
    - Long-term management of stable angina

CHAPTER 22: ANGINA

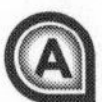

Application Exercises

1. A nurse is caring for a client who is prescribed isosorbide mononitrate (Imdur) for chronic stable angina and develops reflex tachycardia. Which of the following medications should the nurse expect to administer?

    A. Furosemide (Lasix)

    B. Captopril (Capoten)

    C. Ranolazine (Ranexa)

    D. Metoprolol (Lopressor)

2. A nurse is providing teaching to a client who is prescribed nitroglycerin (Nitrostat) for acute angina attacks. Place the following steps in the order in which the client should perform them.

    _____ Call 911 if pain is unrelieved.
    _____ Take a dose of nitroglycerin.
    _____ Wait 5 min.
    _____ Stop activity.

3. A client is prescribed a Nitro-Dur transdermal patch and is instructed to remove the patch each evening and apply a new one the following morning. Having a nitrate-free period each day will prevent which of the following side effects?

    A. Headache

    B. Tolerance

    C. Dizziness

    D. Reflex tachycardia

4. A nurse is taking a medication history from a client who has angina. The provider plans to prescribe ranolazine (Ranexa). Which of the following medications in the client's history may interact with ranolazine and should be reported to the provider? (Select all that apply)

    _____ Digoxin (Lanoxin)
    _____ Simvastatin (Zocor)
    _____ Verapamil (Calan)
    _____ Amlodipine (Norvasc)
    _____ Nitroglycerin transderm patch (Nitro-Dur)

CHAPTER 22: ANGINA

Application Exercises Answer Key

1. A nurse is caring for a client who is prescribed isosorbide mononitrate (Imdur) for chronic stable angina and develops reflex tachycardia. Which of the following medications should the nurse expect to administer?

   A. Furosemide (Lasix)

   B. Captopril (Capoten)

   C. Ranolazine (Ranexa)

   D. Metoprolol (Lopressor)

   Metoprolol, a beta blocker, may be used to manage reflex tachycardia resulting from isosorbide mononitrate. Furosemide, captopril, and ranolazine are not used for this purpose.

NCLEX® Connection: Pharmacological and Parenteral Therapies: Expected Actions/Outcomes

2. A nurse is providing teaching to a client who is prescribed nitroglycerin (Nitrostat) for acute angina attacks. Place the following steps in the order in which the client should perform them

   __**4**__ Call 911 if pain is unrelieved.

   __**2**__ Take a dose of nitroglycerin.

   __**3**__ Wait 5 min.

   __**1**__ Stop activity.

   When the client experiences an acute angina attack, he should stop all activity, take a dose of nitroglycerin, and wait 5 min, and if pain is unrelieved call 911. He can take up to 2 more doses of nitroglycerin at 5 min intervals.

NCLEX® Connection: Pharmacological and Parenteral Therapies: Expected Actions/Outcomes

3. A client is prescribed a Nitro-Dur transdermal patch and is instructed to remove the patch each evening and apply a new one the following morning. Having a nitrate-free period each day will prevent which of the following side effects?

   A. Headache

   B. Tolerance

   C. Dizziness

   D. Reflex tachycardia

   Tolerance to the vasodilation effect of nitroglycerin may develop quickly. The best way to prevent this is to have a nitrate-free period each day. This will not prevent headache, dizziness, or reflex tachycardia.

NCLEX® Connection: Pharmacological and Parenteral Therapies: Medication Administration

4. A nurse is taking a medication history from a client who has angina. The provider plans to prescribe ranolazine (Ranexa). Which of the following medications in the client's history may interact with ranolazine and should be reported to the provider? (Select all that apply)

    __X__ **Digoxin (Lanoxin)**
    __X__ **Simvastatin (Zocor)**
    __X__ **Verapamil (Calan)**
    _____ Amlodipine (Norvasc)
    _____ Nitroglycerin transderm patch (Nitro-Dur)

    Concurrent use with ranolazine increases serum levels of digoxin and simvastatin. Verapamil is an inhibitor of CYP3A4 which can increase levels of ranolazine and lead to torsades de pointes. Use of ranolazine for treatment of angina requires concurrent use with amlodipine, an organic nitrate, or a beta adrenergic blocker.

NCLEX® Connection: Pharmacological and Parenteral Therapies: Adverse Effects/ Contraindications/Side Effects/Interactions

UNIT 4 MEDICATIONS AFFECTING THE CARDIOVASCULAR SYSTEM

Chapter 23 Medications Affecting Cardiac Rhythm

Overview

- Medications affecting cardiac rhythm act by altering cardiac electrophysiologic function in order to treat or prevent dysrhythmias.
- Electrophysiological changes may include:
  - Prolonging the AV node
  - Increasing or reducing conduction speed
  - Altering ectopic pacemakers and SA node
  - Reducing myocardial excitability
  - Lengthening effective refractory period
  - Stimulating the autonomic nervous system.
- There are four main classification groups of antidysrhythmics:
  - Sodium channel blockers
  - Beta-adrenergic blockers
  - Potassium channel blockers
  - Calcium channel blockers.
- Toxicity is major concern for antidysrhythmic medications. Medication toxicity may lead to increased cardiac dysrhythmias.

MEDICATION CLASSIFICATION: ANTIDYSRHYTHMIC MEDICATIONS

<table>
<tr><th colspan="2">CLASS</th><th>SELECT PROTOTYPE MEDICATION</th><th>OTHER MEDICATIONS</th></tr>
<tr><td rowspan="3">Class I medications:
• Sodium channel blockers stabilize cardiac membranes.
• They are divided into 3 groups: 1A, 1B and 1C.</td><td>Class IA</td><td>Procainamide (Pronestyl, Procanbid) – oral and IV</td><td>• Quinidine gluconate, (Quinaglute Duratabs)
• Quinidine sulfate (Quinidex Extentabs)
• Disopyramide (Norpace)</td></tr>
<tr><td>Class IB</td><td>Lidocaine (Xylocaine) – IV</td><td>• Mexiletine (Mexitil)
• Tocainide (Tonocard)</td></tr>
<tr><td>Class IC</td><td>Propafenone (Rythmol) – Oral</td><td>• Flecainide (Tambocor)</td></tr>
<tr><td colspan="2">Class II medications
• Beta-adrenergic blockers prevent sympathetic nervous system stimulation of the heart.</td><td>• Propranolol hydrochloride (Inderal) – Oral, IV</td><td>• Esmolol hydrochloride (Brevibloc)
• Acebutolol hydrochloride (Sectral)</td></tr>
<tr><td colspan="2">Class III medications:
• Potassium channel blockers prolong the action potential and refractory period of the cardiac cycle.</td><td>• Amiodarone (Cordarone, Pacerone) – Oral, IV</td><td>• Sotalol (Betapace)
• Ibutilide (Corvert)
• Dofetilide (Tikosyn)</td></tr>
<tr><td colspan="2">Class IV medications:
• Calcium channel blockers depress depolarization and decrease oxygen demand of the heart.</td><td>• Verapamil (Calan) – Oral, IV</td><td>• Diltiazem (Cardizem)</td></tr>
</table>

- Other Medications:
  - Adenosine (Adenocard) – IV
  - Digoxin (Lanoxin) – Oral, IV

Purpose

CLASSIFICATIONS	EXPECTED PHARMACOLOGICAL ACTION	THERAPEUTIC USES
Class IA	• Decrease electrical conduction • Increase automaticity • Decrease rate of repolarization	• Supraventricular tachycardia • Ventricular tachycardia • Atrial flutter • Atrial fibrillation
Class IB	• Decrease electrical conduction • Decrease automaticity • Increase rate of repolarization	• Short-term use only for ventricular dysrhythmias
Class IC	• Decrease electrical conduction • Decrease excitability • Increase rate of repolarization	• Severe ventricular tachycardia
Class II	• Decrease heart rate • Slow rate of conduction through the SA node • Decrease atrial ectopic stimulation	• Atrial fibrillation, atrial flutter, paroxysmal SVT, hypertension, angina
Class III	• Decrease rate of repolarization • Decrease electrical conduction • Decrease contractility • Decrease automaticity	• Conversion of atrial fibrillation – oral route • Recurrent ventricular fibrillation • Recurrent ventricular tachycardia
Class IV calcium channel blockers, verapamil, diltiazem	• Decrease force of contraction • Decrease heart rate • Slow rate of conduction through the AV node	• Atrial fibrillation and flutter • SVT
Adenosine	• Decrease electrical conduction through AV node	• Paroxysmal SVT • Wolff-Parkinson-White syndrome
Digoxin	• Decrease electrical conduction through AV node • Increase myocardial contraction	• HF, atrial fibrillation and flutter, paroxysmal SVT

Complications

SIDE/ADVERSE EFFECTS	NURSING INTERVENTIONS/CLIENT EDUCATION
Procainamide	
Systemic lupus syndrome (painful, inflamed joints)	• Symptoms will resolve with discontinuation of medication. • If no alternative can be used, symptoms can be controlled with NSAIDs. • Clients should be monitored for nuclear antibody titers (ANA). If ANA titer is present and increases, medication should be discontinued.
Blood dyscrasias, such as neutropenia	• Monitor the client's weekly complete blood counts for the first 12 weeks; then periodically. • Monitor clients for signs of infection and bleeding. Medication should be stopped if there is evidence of bone marrow suppression.
Cardiotoxicity (of particular note is that the QRS complex is widened and the QT interval is prolonged)	• Monitor medication levels (therapeutic procainamide level is 4 to 8 mcg/mL). • Monitor the client's vital signs and ECG. • If dysrhythmias occur, hold medication and contact the provider.
Hypotension	• Monitor blood pressure. May need to withhold medication for hypotension.
Lidocaine	
CNS effects (drowsiness, altered mental status, paresthesias, seizures)	• Carefully monitor clients and notify the provider if symptoms occur. • Administer phenytoin (Dilantin) to control seizure activity.
Respiratory arrest	• Monitor the client's vital signs and ECG. • Ensure resuscitation equipment ready at bedside.
Propafenone	
Bradycardia, heart failure, dizziness weakness.	• Monitor heart rate. Monitor for chest pain or edema.
Propranolol hydrochloride	
Hypotension, bradycardia, heart failure, fatigue	• Monitor blood pressure and heart rate. Check apical pulse prior to dosage.

SIDE/ADVERSE EFFECTS	NURSING INTERVENTIONS/CLIENT EDUCATION
Amiodarone	
Pulmonary toxicity	• Obtain the client's baseline chest x-ray and pulmonary function tests. • Continue to monitor pulmonary function through course of therapy. • Advise clients to observe for symptoms of dyspnea, cough, and chest pain. • Notify the provider if symptoms occur.
Sinus bradycardia and AV block, which may lead to heart failure	• Monitor blood pressure and ECG. • Monitor clients for signs of heart failure (dyspnea, cough, chest pain, neck vein distention, crackles) and notify the provider if they occur. • If AV block occurs, medication should be discontinued. A pacemaker may be inserted. • Medication may be discontinued.
Visual disturbances (photophobia, blurred vision, may lead to blindness)	• Advise clients to report visual disturbances.
Other effects may include liver and thyroid dysfunction; GI disturbances, CNS effects.	• Obtain baseline liver and thyroid function and monitor periodically. • Advise clients to observe for symptoms, and report to the provider if they occur.
Phlebitis with IV administration	• Use of central venous catheter is indicated.
Hypotension, bradycardia, AV block	• Monitor cardiac status
Verapamil hydrochloride	
Bradycardia and hypotension heart failure	• Monitor ECG and blood pressure. Severe hypotension may be reversed with calcium chloride. • Clients with a history of heart failure may need a reduced dose.
Adenosine	
Sinus bradycardia (decreased conduction through AV node), hypotension, dyspnea (bronchoconstriction), flushing of face (vasodilation)	• Monitor ECG. Effects usually last 1 min or less. • Monitor clients for signs and symptoms, and notify the provider if symptoms occur.
Digoxin	
Bradycardia, hypotension, toxicity: nausea, vomiting, dysrhythmias	• Monitor apical heart rate. Hold dose for heart rate less than 60/min. • Monitor digoxin level. Therapeutic level is 0.5 to 2 ng/mL • Monitor serum potassium level.

Contraindications/Precautions

MEDICATION	CONTRAINDICATIONS/PRECAUTIONS
Procainamide	• Pregnancy Risk Category C • Procainamide is contraindicated in clients who have hypersensitivity to procaine or quinidine, complete heart block, atypical ventricular tachycardia, myasthenia gravis, and systemic lupus erythematosus. • Use cautiously in clients with partial AV block, liver or renal disorders, heart failure, and digoxin toxicity.
Lidocaine	• Pregnancy Risk Category B • Lidocaine is contraindicated in clients who have Stokes-Adams syndrome, Wolff-Parkinson-White syndrome, and severe heart block. • Use cautiously in clients who have liver and renal dysfunction, second degree heart block, sinus bradycardia, and heart failure.
Propafenone	• Pregnancy Risk Category C • Propafenone is contraindicated in clients who have AV block, severe heart failure, severe hypotension, and cardiogenic shock. • Use cautiously in clients who have liver or kidney dysfunction or those taking cardiac depressants.
Propranolol hydrochloride	• Pregnancy Risk Category C • Propranolol hydrochloride is contraindicated in clients who have greater than first degree AV block, heart failure, and bradycardia. • Use cautiously in clients who have Wolff-Parkinson-White syndrome, diabetes mellitus, or liver, thyroid and respiratory dysfunction.
Amiodarone	• Pregnancy Risk Category D • Amiodarone is contraindicated in clients who have AV block and bradycardia, newborns, and infants. • Use cautiously in clients with liver, thyroid, respiratory dysfunction, heart failure, and fluid and electrolyte imbalances.
Verapamil	• Pregnancy Risk Category C • Verapamil is contraindicated in clients with greater than first degree AV block (unless they have a working pacemaker), atrial fib/flutter, and severe hypotension. • IV form is contraindicated in ventricular tachycardia and for clients taking beta blockers. • Use cautiously in clients who have liver or kidney dysfunction or increased intracranial pressure.

MEDICATION	CONTRAINDICATIONS/PRECAUTIONS
Adenosine	• Pregnancy Risk Category C • Adenosine is contraindicated in clients who have second- and third-degree heart block, AV block, atrial flutter, and atrial fibrillation • Use cautiously in older adults and clients who have asthma.
Digoxin	• Pregnancy Risk Category C • Digoxin is contraindicated in clients who have ventricular tachycardia or ventricular fibrillation not caused by heart failure. • Use cautiously in clients who have AV block, bradycardia, renal disease, hypothyroidism, and cardiomyopathy.

Interactions

MEDICATION/FOOD INTERACTIONS	NURSING INTERVENTIONS/CLIENT EDUCATION
Procainamide	
Antidysrhythmics have additive effects and may increase the risk for toxicity.	• Monitor heart rate and rhythm. • Notify the provider of change or start of new dysrhythmia.
Anticholinergic medications may increase anticholinergic effects (dry mouth, urinary retention, constipation, and tachycardia).	• Monitor heart rate. • Sucking on hard candy or chewing gum can help relieve dry mouth. • Administer stool softeners, such as docusate sodium (Colace), to prevent constipation.
Antihypertensives have an additive hypotensive effect.	• Monitor the client's blood pressure and notify the provider if there is a significant drop.
Lidocaine	
Cimetidine, beta blockers, and phenytoin may decrease metabolism of lidocaine, increasing chance of toxicity.	• Monitor the client for side effects, such as drowsiness. • Monitor lidocaine level. Reduce dosage.
Propafenone	
Antidysrhythmics may induce heart failure.	• Use with caution. Monitor for heart failure.
Propafenone may slow medication metabolism and cause an increase in the levels of digoxin, oral anticoagulants, and propranolol.	• Monitor for medication toxicity. • Monitor coagulation.
Quinidine may slow metabolism of propafenone.	• Do not use together.

MEDICATION/FOOD INTERACTIONS	NURSING INTERVENTIONS/CLIENT EDUCATION
Propranolol	
Verapamil (Calan) and diltiazem (Cardizem) have additive cardiosuppression effects.	• Monitor ECG, heart rate, and blood pressure.
Propranolol use can mask the hypoglycemic effect of insulin and prevent the breakdown of fat in response to hypoglycemia.	• Use with caution. Monitor blood glucose levels.
Amiodarone	
Amiodarone may increase plasma levels of quinidine, procainamide, digoxin, diltiazem, and warfarin.	• Dosages of these medications should be lowered. Monitor ECG.
Cholestyramine decreases levels of amiodarone.	• Monitor for therapeutic effects.
Diuretics, other antidysrhythmics, and antibiotics (erythromycin, azithromycin [Zithromax]) may increase the risk of dysrhythmias	• Use cautiously with clients taking these medications.
Concurrent use of beta blockers, verapamil, and diltiazem can lead to bradycardia.	• Monitor clients closely.
Propranolol may increase digoxin level.	• Monitor digoxin level. Monitor heart rate.
Consuming grapefruit juice can lead to toxicity.	• Advise clients to avoid drinking grapefruit juice.
Verapamil	
Concurrent use of atenolol, esmolol, or propanol may cause additive effects of both medications.	• Monitor ECG. Reduce dosages if needed.
Verapamil may potentiate carbamazepine and digoxin.	• Monitor medication levels.
Beta blockers may cause heart failure.	• Monitor for heart failure. Use caution.
Adenosine	
Methylxanthines, such as theophylline and caffeine, block receptors for adenosine and therefore prevent therapeutic effect.	• Concurrent use should be avoided.
Cellular uptake of dipyridamole (Persantine) is blocked, leading to intensification of effects.	• Monitor clients for signs of excessive dosage, and notify the provider if these occur.
Digoxin	
Amiodarone, diltiazem, nifedipine, quinidine, and verapamil may increase digoxin levels.	• Monitor for medication level and for toxicity. Reduce medication dosage if needed.
Corticosteroids, diuretics, thiazides, and amphotericin B may cause decreased potassium level.	• Monitor potassium and monitor medication levels for toxicity.
Antacids and metoclopramide may decrease digoxin absorption.	• Monitor blood levels and effective response. Give dosages at wide intervals.

Nursing Administration

MEDICATION	NURSING INTERVENTION/CLIENT EDUCATION
Procainamide	• Advise clients to take medications as prescribed. • Advise clients not crush or chew sustained-released preparations.
Lidocaine	• Intravenous administration is usually started with a loading dose, followed by a maintenance dose of 1 to 4 mg/min. • Adjust the rate according to cardiac response. • Usually used for no more than 24 hr. • Never administer lidocaine preparation that contains epinephrine (usually in lidocaine used for local anesthesia). Severe hypertension or dysrhythmias may occur.
Propafenone	• Monitor ECG during treatment. • Monitor for bradycardia and hypotension. Monitor for dizziness or weakness. • Instruct clients to take the medication with food.
Propranolol hydrochloride	• Instruct clients to take apical pulse daily and notify the provider of significant change. • Take medication with food to increase absorption.
Amiodarone	• Amiodarone is highly toxic. Monitor clients closely for adverse effects. • Inform clients that adverse effects may continue for an extended period of time after the medication is discontinued. • Provide clients with written information regarding potential toxicities.
Verapamil	• Verapamil may cause orthostatic hypotension. Advise clients to change positions slowly. Client may need to lie flat until dizziness subsides. • Advise clients to notify the provider for peripheral edema or shortness of breath.
Adenosine	• Adenosine has a very short half-life, so adverse reactions are mild and last for less than 1 min. • Administration should be by intravenous bolus, flushed with saline following administration.
Digoxin	• Instruct clients to take apical pulse for one minute before taking a dose. If the heart rate is less than 60/min, the client should hold the dose and notify the provider. • Advise clients to eat a high-potassium diet.

Nursing Evaluation of Medication Effectiveness

- Depending on therapeutic intent, effectiveness may be evidenced by:
  - Improvement of symptoms (chest pain, shortness of breath, bradycardia, or tachycardia)
  - Absence of dysrhythmias
  - Return to baseline ECG, pulse rate, and regular rhythm.

CHAPTER 23: MEDICATIONS AFFECTING CARDIAC RHYTHM

 Application Exercises

1. Which of the following is correct regarding toxicity associated with amiodarone (Cordarone)?

   A. Visual impairment resolves when the medication is withdrawn.

   B. Ototoxicity is irreversible.

   C. Lung damage can persist for months after the medication is discontinued.

   D. Myopathy is a common manifestation of toxicity.

2. A client presents to the emergency department with severe hypotension. The family states the client is taking verapamil (Calan) for atrial fibrillation. The nurse should prepare to give which of the following?

   A. Calcium chloride

   B. Epinephrine sodium chloride

   C. Potassium chloride

   D. Magnesium sulfate

3. A nurse is caring for four clients, each taking digoxin (Lanoxin). Which of the following clients is at risk for digoxin toxicity? A client who is taking

   A. procainamide (Pronestyl) for premature ventricular contractions.

   B. ranitidine (Zantac) for peptic ulcer disease.

   C. phenytoin (Dilantin) for a seizure disorder.

   D. furosemide (Lasix) for heart failure.

4. A nurse is providing discharge instructions for a client with a prescription for propranolol (Inderal). The nurse should which of the following instructions? (Select all that apply.)

   _____ Check apical pulse before each dose.

   _____ Hold medication for apical pulse greater than 100/min.

   _____ Take medication with food to increase absorption.

   _____ Take only as needed for chest pain.

   _____ Notify the provider for significant change in heart rate.

CHAPTER 23: MEDICATIONS AFFECTING CARDIAC RHYTHM

Application Exercises Answer Key

1. Which of the following is correct regarding toxicity associated with amiodarone (Cordarone)?

    A. Visual impairment resolves when the medication is withdrawn.

    B. Ototoxicity is irreversible.

    C. Lung damage can persist for months after the medication is discontinued.

    D. Myopathy is a common manifestation of toxicity.

    Because of a long half-life, symptoms persist for months after discontinuation. Visual impairment can be permanent. Ototoxicity is not a sign of amiodarone toxicity, and myopathy is seen in clients who are receiving statins and fibrates.

NCLEX® Connection: Pharmacological and Parenteral Therapies: Adverse Effects/ Contraindications/Side Effects/Interactions

2. A client presents to the emergency department with severe hypotension. The family states the client is taking verapamil (Calan) for atrial fibrillation. The nurse should prepare to give which of the following?

    A. Calcium chloride

    B. Epinephrine sodium chloride

    C. Potassium chloride

    D. Magnesium sulfate

    Verapamil is a calcium channel blocker used to treat atrial fibrillation, atrial flutter and paroxysmal ventricular tachycardia. Severe hypotension may be reversed with calcium chloride given slowly, IV. The other medications will not reverse the hypotension.

NCLEX® Connection: Pharmacological and Parenteral Therapies: Adverse Effects/ Contraindications/Side Effects/Interactions

3. A nurse is caring for four clients, each taking digoxin (Lanoxin). Which of the following clients is at risk for digoxin toxicity? A client who is taking

    A. procainamide (Pronestyl) for premature ventricular contractions.

    B. ranitidine (Zantac) for peptic ulcer disease.

    C. phenytoin (Dilantin) for a seizure disorder.

    D. furosemide (Lasix) for heart failure.

    Loop diuretics cause potassium to be excreted from the kidneys. Hypokalemia increases the risk for digoxin toxicity. Concurrent use with procainamide, ranitidine or phenytoin does not increase the risk of digoxin toxicity.

NCLEX® Connection: Pharmacological and Parenteral Therapies: Adverse Effects/ Contraindications/Side Effects/Interactions

4. A nurse is providing discharge instructions for a client with a prescription for propranolol (Inderal). The nurse should which of the following instructions? (Select all that apply.)

 X **Check apical pulse before each dose.**

 ___ Hold medication for apical pulse of greater than 100/min.

 X **Take medication with food to increase absorption.**

 ___ Take only as needed for chest pain.

 X **Notify the provider for significant change in heart rate.**

Propranolol is a beta blocker that is used to slow tachyarrhythmias and reduce blood pressure. Clients should be instructed to check their apical pulse before each dose and notify the provider of any significant rate change. Food may increase the absorption of propranolol (Inderal). Propranolol should be taken once or twice per day, as prescribed, not as needed.

NCLEX® Connection: Pharmacological and Parenteral Therapies: Medication Administration

UNIT 4 MEDICATIONS AFFECTING THE CARDIOVASCULAR SYSTEM

Chapter 24 Antilipemic Agents

 Overview

- Antilipemic agents work in different ways to help lower low-density lipoprotein (LDL cholesterol) levels, raise high-density lipoprotein (HDL cholesterol) levels, and possibly decrease very low-density lipoprotein (VLDL) levels. These medications should be used along with lifestyle modifications such as regular activity, diet, and weight control.
- Prior to starting these medications, obtain baseline levels of total cholesterol, LDL cholesterol level, HDL cholesterol, and triglycerides (TGs). These blood values should be monitored periodically throughout the course of therapy.
- In addition, baseline liver and renal function tests should be obtained and monitored periodically throughout the course of therapy.
- Classifications include:
    - Fibrates
    - HMG CoA reductase inhibitors (Statins)
    - Cholesterol absorption inhibitors
    - Bile-acid sequestrants
    - Nicotinic acid

MEDICATION CLASSIFICATION: FIBRATES

- Select Prototype Medication: gemfibrozil (Lopid)
- Other Medications: fenofibrate (TriCor, Lofibra), clofibrate (Atromid-S)

Purpose

- Expected Pharmacological Action
    - Decrease in triglyceride levels (increase in VLDL excretion for clients unable to lower triglyceride levels with lifestyle modification)
    - Increase in HDL levels by promoting production of precursors to HDLs
- Therapeutic Uses
    - Reduction of plasma triglycerides (VLDL)
    - Increased levels of HDL

Complications

SIDE/ADVERSE EFFECTS	NURSING INTERVENTIONS/CLIENT EDUCATION
GI distress	• Usually mild and self-limiting
Gallbladder stones	• Advise clients to observe for symptoms of gallbladder disease (right upper quadrant pain, fat intolerance, bloating). • Advise clients to notify the provider if symptoms occur.
Myopathy (muscle tenderness, pain)	• Obtain baseline creatine kinase (CK) level. • Monitor CK levels periodically during treatment. • Monitor symptoms of muscle aches, pain, and tenderness, and notify the provider if symptoms occur. • Stop medication if CK levels are elevated.
Hepatotoxicity	• Obtain baseline liver function tests and monitor periodically. • Advise clients to observe for symptoms of liver dysfunction (anorexia, vomiting, nausea, jaundice), and notify the provider if symptoms occur. • Stop medication if liver function tests are abnormal.

Contraindications/Precautions

- Pregnancy Risk Category C
- Contraindicated in clients with liver disorders, severe renal dysfunction, and gallbladder disease

Interactions

MEDICATION/FOOD INTERACTIONS	NURSING INTERVENTIONS/CLIENT EDUCATION
With concurrent use, warfarin (Coumadin) increases the risk of bleeding	• Obtain the client's baseline prothrombin time (PT) and INR, and perform periodic monitoring. • Advise clients to report signs of bleeding (bruising, bleeding gums), and notify the provider if symptoms occur.
Statins increase the risk of myopathy.	• Obtain baseline creatine kinase (CK) level. • Monitor CK levels periodically during treatment. • Advise clients to report symptoms of muscle aches and pain, • Medication may be discontinued if CK levels are elevated.
Bile acid sequestrants such as cholestyramine interfere with absorption.	• Advise clients to take gemfibrozil 1 hr before or 4 hr after taking bile sequestrants.

Nursing Administration

- Administer by oral route.
- Advise clients to take medication 30 min prior to breakfast and dinner.

MEDICATION CLASSIFICATION: HMG COA REDUCTASE INHIBITORS (STATINS)

- Select Prototype Medication: atorvastatin (Lipitor)
- Other Medications:
  - Simvastatin (Zocor)
  - Lovastatin (Mevacor)
  - Pravastatin sodium (Pravachol)
  - Rosuvastatin (Crestor)
  - Fluvastatin (Lescol, Lescol XL)

Purpose

- Expected Pharmacological Action
  - Decrease manufacture of LDL cholesterol
  - Decrease manufacture of very low-density lipoproteins (VLDL)
  - Increase manufacture of high-density lipoproteins (HDL)
  - Besides affecting lipid levels, other beneficial effects include: promotion of vasodilation, decrease in plaque site inflammation, and decreased risk of thromboembolism.
- Therapeutic uses
  - Primary hypercholesterolemia
  - Prevention of coronary events (primary and secondary)
  - Protection against MI and stroke for clients with diabetes
  - Increasing levels of HDL in clients with primary hypercholesterolemia

Complications

SIDE/ADVERSE EFFECTS	NURSING INTERVENTIONS/CLIENT EDUCATION
• Hepatotoxicity, as evidenced by increase in serum transaminase	• Obtain the client's baseline liver function. • Monitor liver function tests after 12 weeks and then every 6 months. • Advise clients to observe for symptoms of liver dysfunction (anorexia, vomiting, nausea, jaundice), and notify the provider if symptoms occur. • Advise clients to avoid alcohol. • Medication may be discontinued if liver function tests are abnormal.
• Myopathy, as evidenced by muscle aches, pain, and tenderness • May progress to myositis, or rhabdomyolysis.	• Obtain baseline CK level. • Monitor CK levels while on treatment periodically. • Advise clients to report symptoms of muscle aches, pain, and tenderness. • Medication may be discontinued if CK levels are elevated.
• Peripheral neuropathy, as evidenced by weakness, numbness, tingling, and pain in the hands and feet	• Advise clients to observe for signs and symptoms, and to notify the provider if symptoms occur.

Contraindications/Precautions

- Statins are Pregnancy Risk Category X.
- These medications are contraindicated in clients who have hepatitis induced by viral infection or alcohol.
- Rosuvastatin should be avoided for clients of Asian descent.

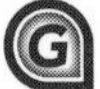

- Use cautiously in older adult clients, clients in debilitated condition, and those with chronic renal disease.

Interactions

MEDICATION/FOOD INTERACTIONS	NURSING INTERVENTIONS/CLIENT EDUCATION
Fibrates (gemfibrozil, fenofibrate) and ezetimibe (Zetia) increase the risk of myopathy	• Obtain baseline CK level. • Monitor the client's CK levels periodically during treatment. • Advise client to report symptoms of muscle aches and pain, • Medication may be discontinued if CK levels are elevated.
Medications that suppress CYP3A4, such as erythromycin and ketoconazole, can increase levels of statins when taken concurrently.	• Atorvastatin, lovastatin, and simvastatin should be avoided. • Level of statin may need to be decreased. • Advise clients to inform the provider of all medications currently taken.
Grapefruit juice suppresses CYP3A4 and can increase levels of statins.	• Advise clients to limit the amount of grapefruit juice consumed each day. Clients should not drink more than 1 qt a day.

Nursing Administration

- Administer statins by oral route.
- Administer lovastatin with evening meal; other statins can be taken without food intake but evening dosing is best.
- Atorvastatin or fluvastatin should be used in clients with renal insufficiency. For other statins, dosages will be reduced.
- Advise clients to obtain baseline cholesterol levels, HDL, LDL, and triglycerides, and monitor periodically while taking the medication.
- Advise clients to obtain baseline liver, renal function tests, and monitor periodically during treatment.

MEDICATION CLASSIFICATION: CHOLESTEROL ABSORPTION INHIBITOR

- Select Prototype Medication: Ezetimibe (Zetia)

Purpose

- Expected Pharmacological Action
    - Ezetimibe inhibits absorption of cholesterol secreted in the bile and from food.
- Therapeutic Uses
    - Clients with modified diets can use this medication as an adjunct to help lower LDL cholesterol.
    - Medication can be used alone or in combination with a statin medication.

Complications

SIDE/ADVERSE EFFECTS	NURSING INTERVENTIONS/CLIENT EDUCATION
Hepatitis	• Obtain the client's baseline liver function. • Advise clients to observe for symptoms of liver dysfunction (anorexia, vomiting, nausea, jaundice), and notify the provider if symptoms occur. • Advise clients to avoid alcohol. • Medication may be discontinued if liver function tests are abnormal.
Myopathy	• Obtain baseline CK level. • Monitor CK levels while on treatment periodically. • Advise clients to notify the provider if symptoms such as muscle aches and pains occur. • Medication may be discontinued if CK levels are elevated.

Contraindications/Precautions

- Ezetimibe is Pregnancy Risk Category X.
- Use cautiously in women who are breastfeeding.
- This medication is contraindicated in clients who have renal dysfunction.
- Use caution in clients with liver disease.

Interactions

MEDICATION/FOOD INTERACTIONS	NURSING INTERVENTIONS/CLIENT EDUCATION
Bile acid sequestrants, such as cholestyramine, interfere with absorption.	• Advise clients to take ezetimibe 1 hr before or 4 hr after taking bile sequestrants.
Statins, such as atorvastatin, can increase the risk of liver dysfunction and/or myopathy.	• Obtain baseline liver function tests and monitor periodically. Advise clients to observe for signs of liver damage (anorexia, vomiting, nausea). The provider should be notified and the medication will most likely be discontinued. • Advise clients to notify the provider of symptoms such as muscle aches and pains. • Medication may be discontinued if results of CK levels are elevated.
Concurrent use with fibrates, such as gemfibrozil, increases the risk of gallstone development and myopathy	• Ezetimibe is not recommended for use with fibrates.
Levels of ezetimibe can be increased with concurrent use of cyclosporine	• Monitor clients for side effects (liver damage, myopathy).

Nursing Administration

- Advise client to report symptoms of muscle aches and pain,
- Medication may be discontinued if CK levels are elevated.
- Advise clients to obtain baseline cholesterol levels, HDL, LDL, and triglyceride, and monitor periodically while taking the medication.
- Advise clients to obtain baseline liver, renal function tests, and monitor periodically during treatment.
- Advise clients to follow a low fat/low cholesterol diet and to get involved in a regular exercise regimen.
- Clients can take this medication in a fixed-dose combination with simvastatin as Vytorin.

MEDICATION CLASSIFICATION: BILE-ACID SEQUESTRANTS

- Select Prototype Medication: colesevelam HCL (WelChol)
- Other Medications: cholestyramine (Questran), colestipol (Colestid)

Purpose

- Expected Pharmacological Action
  - Decrease in LDL cholesterol
- Therapeutic Use
  - These medications are used as adjunct with a HMG CoA reductase inhibitor, such as atorvastatin, and with dietary measures to lower cholesterol levels.

Complications

SIDE/ADVERSE EFFECTS	NURSING INTERVENTIONS/CLIENT EDUCATION
Cholestyramine and colestipol may cause GI distress and decrease absorption of fat-soluble vitamins.	• Administer vitamin supplements.
Constipation (less with colesevelam HCL)	• Advise clients to increase the intake of high fiber food and oral fluids, if not restricted.

Contraindications/Precautions

- These medications are contraindicated in clients with biliary disease.
- Avoid use in clients with elevated VLDL.

Interactions

MEDICATION/FOOD INTERACTIONS	NURSING INTERVENTIONS/CLIENT EDUCATION
Cholestyramine and colestipol form complexes with digoxin (Lanoxin), warfarin (Coumadin), thiazides, and tetracyclines that interfere with absorption.	• Advise clients to take other medications 1 hr before or 4 hr after taking bile sequestrants. • Advise clients to inform the provider of all medications currently taken.

Nursing Administration

- Colesevelam HCL is taken orally in tablet form. Take with food and water.
- Colestipol is supplied as oral tablet, which should not be crushed or chewed. Give 30 min before a meal.
- Cholestyramine and colestipol are supplied in a powder formulation. Advise clients to use an adequate amount of fluid (4 to 8 oz) to dissolve the medication. This will prevent irritation or impaction of the esophagus.

OTHER MEDICATIONS: NICOTINIC ACID, NIACIN (NIACOR, NIASPAN)

Purpose

- Expected Pharmacological Action
  - Decrease in LDL cholesterol and triglyceride levels
- Therapeutic Uses
  - For clients at risk for pancreatitis and elevated triglyceride levels
  - To lower elevated LDL cholesterol and triglycerides, and to raise HDL levels (Niaspan)

Complications

SIDE/ADVERSE EFFECTS	NURSING INTERVENTIONS/CLIENT EDUCATION
GI distress	• Usually self-limiting. Advise client to take with food.
Facial flushing	• Advise client to take aspirin 30 min before each dose.
Hyperglycemia	• Monitor blood glucose levels
Hepatotoxicity	• Obtain baseline liver function tests and monitor periodically. • Advise clients to observe for symptoms of liver dysfunction (anorexia, vomiting, nausea, jaundice), and notify the provider if symptoms occur. • Medication may be discontinued if liver function tests are abnormal.
Hyperuricemia	• Monitor kidney function, BUN, and creatinine, I&O. • Encourage adequate fluid intake of 2 to 3 L of water each day from food and beverage sources. • Administer allopurinol if uric acid level is elevated.

 Contraindications/Precautions

- Contraindicated in clients with liver disease and gout

Nursing Administration

- Administer by oral route, either in pill or liquid form. Pill may be standard form or time-released.
- Administer standard form 3 times a day with or after meals.
- Administer time-released formulations once in the evening.
- Advise clients that dosage is much larger than dosage when taken as vitamin supplement.

Nursing Evaluation of Medication Effectiveness

- Depending on therapeutic intent, effectiveness may be evidenced by:
  - Decreased LDL cholesterol level
  - Decreased triglyceride (VLDL) levels
  - Absence of cardiovascular events such as stroke, MI, thrombosis

CHAPTER 24: ANTILIPEMIC AGENTS

Application Exercises

1. A nurse is providing teaching to a client who is prescribed lovastatin (Mevacor). Which of the following should the nurse include in the teaching?

   A. Take this medication with the evening meal.

   B. Change position slowly when rising from a chair.

   C. Maintain a steady intake of green leafy vegetables.

   D. Consume no more than 1 L of fluid/day.

2. A nurse is collecting data from a client who is taking gemfibrozil (Lopid). Which of the following assessment findings should the nurse recognize as an adverse reaction to the medication?

   A. Blurred vision

   B. Tremor

   C. Jaundice

   D. Hyperglycemia

3. A nurse is teaching a client who has a new prescription for cholestyramine (Questran). Which of the following should the nurse include in the teaching to prevent an adverse effect of this medication?

   A. Take an aspirin 30 min before taking the medication.

   B. Increase the amount of fiber and liquids in the diet while taking this medication.

   C. Creatine kinase (CK) levels should be monitored periodically while taking this medication.

   D. Do not mix this medication with water, other fluids, or foods.

CHAPTER 24: ANTILIPEMIC AGENTS

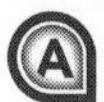

Application Exercises Answer Key

1. A nurse is providing teaching to a client who is prescribed lovastatin (Mevacor). Which of the following should the nurse include in the teaching?

    A. Take this medication with the evening meal.

    B. Change position slowly when rising from a chair.

    C. Maintain a steady intake of green leafy vegetables.

    D. Consume no more than 1 L of fluid/day.

    Lovastatin should be taken with the evening meal to increase absorption. Changing positions slowly may be necessary when taking an antihypertensive, and maintaining a steady intake of green leafy vegetables is important for clients taking warfarin. There is no indication for fluid restriction with statins.

NCLEX connection: Pharmacological and Parenteral Therapies: Adverse Effects/ Contraindications/Side Effects/Interactions

2. A nurse is collecting data from a client who is taking gemfibrozil (Lopid). Which of the following assessment findings should the nurse recognize as an adverse reaction to the medication?

    A. Blurred vision

    B. Tremor

    C. Jaundice

    D. Hyperglycemia

    Jaundice may indicate liver impairment as a result of hepatotoxicity which is a possible adverse reaction to gemfibrozil. Blurred vision, tremor, and hyperglycemia are not adverse reactions to gemfibrozil.

NCLEX® Connection: Pharmacological and Parenteral Therapies: Adverse Effects/ Contraindications/Side Effects/Interactions

3. A nurse is teaching a client who has a new prescription for cholestyramine (Questran). Which of the following should the nurse include in the teaching to prevent an adverse effect of this medication?

   A. Take an aspirin 30 min before taking the medication.

   B. Increase the amount of fiber and liquids in the diet while taking this medication.

   C. Creatine kinase (CK) levels should be monitored periodically while taking this medication.

   D. Do not mix this medication with water, other fluids, or foods.

   Cholestyramine can cause constipation. Increasing fiber and fluid intake can prevent this adverse reaction. Clients taking nicotinic acid (Niacin) should take an aspirin 30 min before taking the medication to prevent facial flushing. CK levels should be monitored for clients taking gemfibrozil (Lopid), which can cause myopathy. Cholestyramine is supplied as a powder and must be mixed with a liquid (water, fruit juice) or fruit with a high fluid content (applesauce) before administration to prevent irritation of the esophagus.

NCLEX® Connection: Pharmacological and Parenteral Therapies: Adverse Effects/ Contraindications/Side Effects/Interactions

UNIT 5: MEDICATIONS AFFECTING THE HEMATOLOGIC SYSTEM

- Medications Affecting Coagulation
- Growth Factors
- Blood and Blood Products

NCLEX® CONNECTIONS

When reviewing the chapters in this unit, keep in mind the relevant sections of the NCLEX® outline, in particular:

CLIENT NEEDS: PHARMACOLOGICAL AND PARENTERAL THERAPIES

Relevant topics/tasks include:

- Adverse Effects/Contraindications/Side Effects/Interactions
    - Evaluate and document the client's response to actions taken to counteract side effects and adverse effects of medications and parenteral therapy.
- Dosage Calculation
    - Perform calculations needed for medication administration.

UNIT 5 MEDICATIONS AFFECTING THE HEMATOLOGIC SYSTEM

Chapter 25 Medications Affecting Coagulation

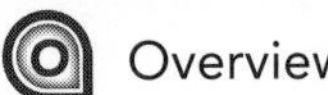

Overview

- Pharmaceutical agents that modify coagulation are used to prevent clot formation or break apart an already formed clot. These medications work in the blood to alter the clotting cascade, prevent platelet aggregation, or dissolve a clot.
- The goal of medications that alter coagulation is to increase circulation and perfusion, decrease pain and prevent further tissue damage.
- The groups of medications used include oral and parenteral anticoagulants, antiplatelet medications, and thrombolytic agents.

MEDICATION CLASSIFICATION: ANTICOAGULANTS/PARENTERAL

- Select Prototype Medication: heparin sodium
- Low molecular weight heparins (LMWH):
  - Select Prototype Medication: enoxaparin (Lovenox)
  - Other Medications: dalteparin sodium (Fragmin), tinzaparin (Innohep)
- Activated factor X (Xa) inhibitor:
  - Select Prototype Medication: fondaparinux sodium (Arixtra)

Purpose

- Expected Pharmacological Action
  - Parenteral anticoagulants prevent bleeding by inactivation of thrombin formation and factor Xa, resulting in inhibition of the formation of fibrin.
- Therapeutic Uses
  - Heparin sodium, LMWH, fondaparinux sodium
    - In conditions necessitating prompt anticoagulant activity (evolving stroke, pulmonary embolism, massive deep venous thrombosis)
    - As an adjunct for clients having open heart surgery or renal dialysis
    - As low-dose therapy for prophylaxis against postoperative venous thrombosis (for example, hip/knee replacement surgery, abdominal surgery)

- Heparin sodium, LMWH
    - In conjunction with thrombolytic therapy when treating an acute myocardial infarction
- Heparin sodium
    - Treatment of disseminated intravascular coagulation

Administration

- These medications cannot be absorbed by the intestinal tract and must be given by subcutaneous injection or IV infusion.
    - Heparin sodium: Subcutaneously every 12 hr, continuous or intermittent IV infusion
    - Enoxaparin, dalteparin sodium, tinzaparin: Subcutaneously every 12 hr for 2 to 8 days
    - Fondaparinux sodium: Subcutaneously every 12 hr for 5 to 9 days

Complications

SIDE/ADVERSE EFFECTS	NURSING INTERVENTIONS/CLIENT EDUCATION
Heparin sodium	
Hemorrhage secondary to heparin overdose	• Monitor vital signs. • Advise clients to observe for signs and symptoms of bleeding (increased heart rate, decreased blood pressure, bruising, petechiae, hematomas, black tarry stools). • In the case of heparin overdose, stop heparin, administer protamine sulfate, and avoid aspirin. • Monitor activated partial thromboplastin time (aPTT). Keep value at 1.5 to 2 times the baseline.
Heparin-induced thrombocytopenia, as evidenced by low platelet count and increased development of thrombi – mediated by antibody development (white clot syndrome)	• Monitor the client's platelet count periodically throughout treatment, especially in the first month. • Stop heparin if platelet count is less than 100,000/mm^3. Nonheparin anticoagulants, such as lepirudin (Refludan) or argatroban (Acova), can be used as a substitute if anticoagulation is still needed.
Hypersensitivity reactions (chills, fever, urticaria)	• Administer a small test dose prior to the administration of heparin.
Toxicity/overdose	• Administer protamine sulfate, which binds with heparin and forms a heparin-protamine complex that has no anticoagulant properties. • Protamine sulfate should be administered slowly intravenously, no faster than 20 mg/min or 50 mg in 10 min.

SIDE/ADVERSE EFFECTS	NURSING INTERVENTIONS/CLIENT EDUCATION
Enoxaparin	
Hemorrhage	• Monitor vital signs • Advise clients to observe for signs and symptoms of bleeding, such as increased heart rate, decreased blood pressure, bruising, petechiae, hematomas, black tarry stools. • Monitor platelet count. Instruct client to avoid aspirin.
Neurologic damage from hematoma formed during spinal or epidural anesthesia	• In clients with spinal or epidural anesthesia: Assess insertion site for signs of hematoma formation, such as redness or swelling. Monitor sensation and movement of lower extremities. Notify provider of abnormal findings.
Thrombocytopenia, as evidenced by low platelet count	• Monitor platelets. Discontinue medication for platelet count less than 100,000/mm^3.
Toxicity/overdose	• Administer protamine sulfate (heparin antagonist) • Protamine sulfate should be administered slowly intravenously, no faster than 20 mg/min, or 50 mg in 10 min.
Fondaparinux sodium	
Hemorrhage	• Monitor vital signs. • Advise clients to observe for signs and symptoms of bleeding increase (heart rate, decreased blood pressure, bruising, petechiae, hematomas, black tarry stools). • Monitor platelet count. Instruct client to avoid aspirin.
Neurologic damage from hematoma formed during spinal or epidural anesthesia.	• In clients with spinal or epidural anesthesia: Assess insertion site for signs of hematoma formation such as redness or swelling. Monitor sensation and movement of lower extremities. Notify provider of abnormal findings.
Thrombocytopenia, as evidenced by low platelet count.	• Monitor platelets. Discontinue medication for platelet count less than 100,000/mm^3.

Contraindications/Precautions

- Parenteral anticoagulants are contraindicated in clients with low platelet counts (thrombocytopenia) or uncontrollable bleeding.
- These medications should not be used during or following surgeries of the eye(s), brain, or spinal cord; lumbar puncture; or regional anesthesia.
- Use cautiously in clients who have hemophilia, increased capillary permeability, dissecting aneurysm, peptic ulcer disease, severe hypertension, hepatic or renal disease, or threatened abortion.

Interactions

MEDICATION/FOOD INTERACTIONS	NURSING INTERVENTIONS/CLIENT EDUCATION
Anti-platelet agents such as aspirin, NSAIDs, and other anticoagulants may increase risk for bleeding.	• Avoid concurrent use when possible. • Monitor carefully for evidence of bleeding. • Take precautionary measures to avoid injury (limit venipunctures and injections).

Nursing Administration

- Heparin sodium:
  - Obtain the client's baseline vital signs.
  - Obtain baseline and monitor complete blood count (CBC), platelet count, and hematocrit levels.
  - Read label carefully. Heparin is dispensed in units and in different concentrations.
  - Check dosages with another nurse before administration.
  - Use an infusion pump for continuous IV administration. Monitor rate of infusion every 30 to 60 min.
  - Monitor aPTT every 4 to 6 hr until appropriate dose is determined, then monitor daily.
  - For subcutaneous injections, use a 20 to 22 gauge needle to withdraw medication from the vial. Then, change the needle to a smaller needle (gauge 25 or 26, ½ to ⅝ in length).
  - Administer deep subcutaneous injections in the abdomen ensuring a distance of 2 inches from the umbilicus. Do not aspirate.
  - Apply pressure for 1 to 2 min after the injection. Rotate and record injection sites.
  - Instruct clients to monitor for signs of bleeding (bruising, gums bleeding, abdominal pain, nose bleeds, coffee-ground emesis and tarry stools).
  - Instruct clients not to take over-the-counter NSAIDs, aspirin, or medications containing salicylates.
  - Advise clients to use an electric razor for shaving and a soft toothbrush.
- Enoxaparin/fondaparinux sodium
  - No monitoring is required. Therefore, these medications are acceptable for home use
  - Provide instruction regarding correct self-administration. Medications may be available in pre-filled syringes.
  - For subcutaneous injections, use a 20 to 22 gauge needle to withdraw medication from the vial. Then, change to a small needle (gauge 25 or 26, ½ to ⅝ in length).
  - Deep subcutaneous injections should be administered in the abdomen, ensuring a distance of 2 inches from the umbilicus. Do not aspirate.
  - Apply pressure for 1 to 2 min after the injection. Rotate and record injection sites.

- Instruct clients to monitor for signs of bleeding such as bruising, gums bleeding, abdominal pain, nose bleeds, coffee-ground emesis, and tarry stools.
- Instruct clients not to take over-the-counter NSAIDs, aspirin, or medications containing salicylates.
- Advise client to use an electric razor for shaving and a soft toothbrush.

Nursing Evaluation of Medication Effectiveness

- Depending on therapeutic intent, effectiveness may be evidenced by the following:
  - Heparin sodium
    - Client aPTT levels of 60 to 80 seconds
  - Heparin sodium, enoxaparin, and fondaparinux sodium
    - No development or no further development of venous thrombi or emboli

MEDICATION CLASSIFICATION: ANTICOAGULANT/ORAL

- Select Prototype Medication: warfarin (Coumadin)

Purpose

- Expected Pharmacological Action
  - Oral anticoagulants antagonize vitamin K, thereby preventing the synthesis of four coagulation factors: factor VII, IX, X, and prothrombin.
- Therapeutic Uses
  - Treatment of venous thrombosis
  - Treatment of thrombus formation in clients who have atrial fibrillation or prosthetic heart valves
  - Prevention of recurrent myocardial infarction, transient ischemic attacks

Complications

SIDE /ADVERSE EFFECTS	NURSING INTERVENTIONS/CLIENT EDUCATION
Hemorrhage	• Monitor the client's vital signs. • Advise clients to observe for signs and symptoms of bleeding, such as increased heart rate, decreased blood pressure, bruising, petechiae, hematomas, black or tarry stools. • Obtain baseline prothrombin time (PT) and monitor levels of PT and International Normalized Ratio (INR) periodically. • In the case of a warfarin overdose, discontinue administration of warfarin, and administer vitamin K (Mephyton).
Hepatitis	• Monitor liver enzymes. Assess for jaundice.
Toxicity/overdose	• Administer vitamin K (Mephyton) to promote synthesis of coagulation factors VII, IX, X, and prothrombin. • Administer IV vitamin K slowly and in a diluted solution to prevent anaphylactoid-type reaction. • Use other routes of administration whenever possible. • Administer small doses of vitamin K (2.5 mg by mouth, 0.5 to 1 mg IV) to prevent development of resistance to warfarin. • If vitamin K cannot control bleeding, administer fresh frozen plasma or whole blood.

Contraindications/Precautions

- Oral anticoagulants fall into Pregnancy Risk Category X due to high risk of fetal hemorrhage, fetal death, and CNS defects. Advise clients to notify the provider if they become pregnant during warfarin therapy. If anticoagulation is needed during pregnancy, heparin can be safely used.
- Use is contraindicated in clients with low platelet counts (thrombocytopenia) or uncontrollable bleeding.
- Use is contraindicated during or following surgeries of the eye(s), brain, or spinal cord; lumbar puncture; or regional anesthesia.
- Use is contraindicated in clients with vitamin K deficiencies, liver disorders, and alcoholism due to the additive risk of bleeding.
- Use cautiously in clients who have hemophilia, dissecting aneurysm, peptic ulcer disease, severe hypertension, or threatened abortion.

Interactions

MEDICATION/FOOD INTERACTIONS	NURSING INTERVENTIONS/CLIENT EDUCATION
Concurrent use of heparin, aspirin, acetaminophen, glucocorticoids, sulfonamides, and parenteral cephalosporins increases effects of warfarin, which increases the risk for bleeding.	• Avoid concurrent use if possible. • Instruct clients to observe for inclusion of aspirin in over-the-counter medications. • If used concurrently, monitor clients carefully for signs of bleeding and increased prothrombin time (PT), INR, and aPTT levels. • Medication dosage should be adjusted accordingly.
Concurrent use of phenobarbital, carbamazepine (Tegretol), phenytoin (Dilantin), oral contraceptives, and vitamin K decreases anticoagulant effects	• Avoid concurrent use if possible. • If used concurrently, monitor clients carefully for reduced PT and INR levels. • Medication dosage should be adjusted accordingly.
Foods high in vitamin K, such as dark green leafy vegetables (lettuce, cooked spinach), cabbage, broccoli, brussel sprouts, mayonnaise, canola, and soybean oil may decrease anticoagulant effects with excessive intake	• Provide clients with a list of foods high in vitamin K. • Instruct clients to maintain a consistent intake of vitamin K to avoid sudden fluctuations that could affect the action of warfarin.

Nursing Administration

- Administration is usually oral, once daily.
- Obtain the client's baseline vital signs.
- Monitor PT levels (therapeutic level 18 to 24 sec) and INR levels (therapeutic levels 2 to 3). INR levels are the most accurate. Hold dose and notify the provider if these levels exceed therapeutic ranges.
- Obtain baseline and monitor CBC, platelet count, and Hct levels.
- Instruct clients that anticoagulant effects may take 8 to 12 hr and full therapeutic effect is not achieved for 3 to 5 days. For clients in the hospital setting, explain the need for continued heparin infusion when starting oral warfarin.
- Advise clients that anticoagulation effects can persist for up to 5 days following discontinuation of medication because of long half-life.
- Advise clients to avoid alcohol and over-the-counter and non-prescription medications to prevent adverse effects and medication interactions, such as risk of bleeding.
- Advise clients to employ nonmedication measures to avoid development of thrombi, including avoiding sitting for prolonged periods of time, not wearing constricting clothing, and elevating and moving legs when sitting.
- Advise clients to wear a medical alert bracelet indicating warfarin use.

- Be prepared to administer vitamin K for warfarin overdose.
- Teach clients to self-monitor PT and INR at home as appropriate.
- Advise clients to record dosage, route, and time of warfarin administration on a daily basis.
- Plan for frequent PT monitoring for clients who are prescribed medications that interact with warfarin. The client is at greatest risk for harm when the interacting medication is being deleted or added. Frequent PT monitoring will allow for dosage adjustments as necessary.
- Advise clients to notify the provider regarding warfarin use.
- Advise clients to use a soft-bristle toothbrush to prevent gum bleeding.

Nursing Evaluation of Medication Effectiveness

- Depending on therapeutic intent, effectiveness may be evidenced by:
  - PT 1.5 to 2 times control
  - INR of 2 to 3 for treatment of acute myocardial infarction, atrial fibrillation, pulmonary embolism, venous thrombosis, and/or tissue heart valves
  - INR of 3 to 4.5 for mechanical heart valve or recurrent systemic embolism
  - No development or no further development of venous thrombi

MEDICATION CLASSIFICATION: ANTIPLATELETS

- Antiplatelet/salicylic
  - Select Prototype Medication: aspirin (Ecotrin)
- Antiplatelet/glycoprotein inhibitors
  - Select Prototype Medication: abciximab (ReoPro)
  - Other Medications: eptifibatide (Integrilin), tirofiban (Aggrastat)
- Antiplatelet/ADP inhibitors:
  - Select Prototype Medications: clopidogrel (Plavix)
  - Other Medications: ticlopidine (Ticlid)
- Antiplatelet/arterial vasodilator:
  - Select Prototype Medication: pentoxifylline (Trental)
  - Other Medications: dipyridamole (Persantine), cilostazol (Pletal)

Purpose

- Expected Pharmacological Action
  - Antiplatelets prevent platelets from clumping together by inhibiting enzymes and factors that normally lead to arterial clotting.
  - Antiplatelet medications inhibit platelet aggregation at the onset of the clotting process. These medications alter bleeding time.
- Therapeutic Uses
  - Primary prevention of acute myocardial infarction
  - Prevention of reinfarction in clients following an acute myocardial infarction
  - Prevention of stroke
  - Acute coronary syndromes (abciximab, tirofiban, eptifibatide)
  - Intermittent claudication (cilostazol, pentoxifylline, dipyridamole)

Route of administration

- Aspirin: Oral
- Abciximab: IV
- Clopidogrel: Oral
- Pentoxifylline: Oral

Complications

SIDE/ADVERSE EFFECTS	NURSING INTERVENTIONS/CLIENT EDUCATION
Aspirin	
GI effects (nausea, vomiting, dyspepsia)	• Advise clients to use enteric-coated tablets and to take aspirin with food. • Concurrent use of a proton pump inhibitor, such as omeprazole (Prilosec), may be appropriate.
Hemorrhagic stroke	• Advise clients to observe for signs of weakness, dizziness, and headache, and to notify the provider if symptoms occur.
Prolonged bleeding time, gastric bleed, thrombocytopenia	• Monitor bleeding time. Monitor for gastric bleed, such as coffee ground emesis or bloody, tarry stools. Monitor for bruising, petechiae and bleeding gums.
Tinnitus, hearing loss	• Monitor for hearing loss. • If symptoms occur, withhold dose and notify the provider.

SIDE/ADVERSE EFFECTS	NURSING INTERVENTIONS/CLIENT EDUCATION
Abciximab	
Hypotension and bradycardia	• Monitor heart rate and blood pressure.
Prolonged bleeding time, gastric bleed, thrombocytopenia, bleed from cardiac catheterization site.	• Monitor bleeding time. • Monitor for gastric bleed (coffee-ground emesis or bloody, tarry stools). • Monitor for bruising, petechiae, and bleeding gums. • Apply pressure to cardiac catheter access site.
Clopidogrel	
Prolonged bleeding time, gastric bleed, thrombocytopenia	• Monitor bleeding time. • Monitor for gastric bleed (coffee-ground emesis or bloody, tarry stools). • Monitor for bruising, petechiae, and bleeding gums. • Apply pressure to cardiac catheter access
Pentoxifylline	
Dyspepsia, nausea, vomiting	• Take with food. • Do not crush or chew medication. • Monitor hydration if GI upset occurs.

Contraindications/Precautions

- Aspirin
  - Aspirin is Pregnancy Risk Category D in the third trimester.
  - Use is contraindicated in clients with bleeding disorders and thrombocytopenia
  - Use cautiously in clients with peptic ulcer disease and severe renal and/or hepatic disorders. Do not give to children or adolescents with fever or recent chickenpox.

  - Use with caution in older adults.
- Abciximab
  - Abciximab is Pregnancy Risk Category C.
  - Contraindications include clients with bleeding disorders, thrombocytopenia, recent stroke, AV malformation, aneurysm, uncontrolled hypertension, and recent major surgery.
  - Use cautiously in clients with peptic ulcer disease and severe renal and/or hepatic disorders.
- Clopidogrel
  - Clopidogrel is Pregnancy Risk Category B.
  - Contraindications include clients with bleeding disorders, thrombocytopenia, peptic ulcer disease, and intracranial bleed.
  - Use cautiously in clients with peptic ulcer disease and severe renal and/or hepatic disorders. Clients who are breastfeeding should not take this medication.

- Pentoxifylline
  - Pentoxifylline is Pregnancy Risk Category C.
  - Use is contraindicated in clients who have bleeding disorders or retinal or cerebral bleeds.

Interactions

MEDICATION/FOOD INTERACTIONS	NURSING INTERVENTIONS/CLIENT EDUCATION
Aspirin	
Concurrent use of other medications that enhance bleeding (NSAIDs, heparin, warfarin, thrombolytics, antiplatelets) increases risk for bleeding.	• Advise clients to avoid concurrent use. • If used concurrently, monitor the client carefully for signs of bleeding.
Urine acidifiers (ammonium chloride) may increase aspirin levels.	• Monitor for aspirin toxicity (hearing loss, tinnitus).
Concurrent use of aspirin may reduce hypertensive action of beta blockers.	• Monitor blood pressure.
Corticosteroids may increase aspirin excretion and decrease aspirin effects. These medications may increase risk for GI bleed.	• Monitor for decreased aspirin effectiveness. • Monitor for gastric bleed (coffee-ground emesis and tarry or bloody stools).
Caffeine may increase aspirin absorption.	• Monitor for toxicity.
Abciximab	
Concurrent use of other medications that enhance bleeding (NSAIDs, heparin, warfarin, thrombolytics, antiplatelets) increases risk for bleeding.	• Advise clients to avoid concurrent use. • If used concurrently, monitor the client carefully for signs of bleeding.
Clopidogrel	
Concurrent use of other medications that enhance bleeding (NSAIDs, heparin, warfarin, thrombolytics, antiplatelets) increases risk for bleeding.	• Advise clients to avoid concurrent use. • If used concurrently, monitor the client carefully for signs of bleeding.
Pentoxifylline	
Concurrent use of anticoagulants increases risk for bleeding.	• Monitor PT and INR. Clients may require reduced dosage.
Pentoxifylline may increase levels of theophylline.	• Monitor theophylline level. Clients may require reduced dosage.

Nursing Administration

- Advise clients that prevention of strokes, myocardial infarctions, and reinfarction can be accomplished with low-dose aspirin (81 mg).
- Aspirin 325 mg should be taken during initial acute episode of myocardial infarction
- Advise clients to notify the provider regarding aspirin use.

Nursing Evaluation of Medication Effectiveness

- Depending on therapeutic intent, effectiveness may be evidenced by:
  - Absence of arterial thrombosis, adequate tissue perfusion, and blood flow without occurrence of abnormal bleeding

MEDICATION CLASSIFICATION: THROMBOLYTIC MEDICATIONS

- Select Prototype Medication: streptokinase (Streptase)
- Other Medications:
  - Alteplase (Activase, tPA),
  - Tenecteplase (TNKase)
  - Reteplase (Retavase)

Purpose

- Expected Pharmacological Action
  - Thrombolytic medications dissolve clots that have already formed. Clots are dissolved by conversion of plasminogen to plasmin, which destroys fibrinogen and other clotting factors.
- Therapeutic Uses
  - Thrombolytic medications are used to treat:
    - Acute myocardial infarction
    - Deep vein thrombosis (DVT)
    - Massive pulmonary emboli
    - Ischemic stroke (alteplase)

Routes of Administration

- Streptokinase (Streptase): IV, intracoronary
- Alteplase, tenecteplase, reteplase: IV

Complications

SIDE/ADVERSE EFFECTS	NURSING INTERVENTIONS/CLIENT EDUCATION
Streptokinase	
Serious risk of bleeding from different sites (within brain, needle puncture sites, wounds)	• Limit venipunctures and injections. • Apply pressure dressings to recent wounds. • Monitor clients for changes in vital signs, alterations in level of consciousness, weakness, and signs of intracranial bleeding. • Notify the provider if symptoms occur. • Monitor aPTT and PT, Hgb and Hct.
Hypotension	• Monitor the client's blood pressure. • Give streptokinase infusion slowly to prevent hypotension.
Allergic reaction (urticaria, itching, flushing); possible severe anaphylactic reaction	• Monitor clients for symptoms of allergy, and notify the provider if symptoms occur. • Be prepared with life support equipment at bedside.

Contraindications/Precautions

- Because of the additive risk for serious bleeding, use is contraindicated in clients who have:
  - Any prior intracranial hemorrhage (hemorrhagic stroke)
  - Known structural cerebral vascular lesion (arteriovenous malformation)
  - Suspected aortic dissection
  - Active internal bleeding
  - History of significant closed head or facial trauma in the past 3 months
  - Acute pericarditis
  - Brain tumors
- Use cautiously in clients who have severe hypertension, a recent episode of ischemic stroke (6 months prior to start of treatment), or a recent major surgery (2 to 4 weeks prior to start of treatment).

Interactions

MEDICATION/FOOD INTERACTIONS	NURSING INTERVENTIONS/CLIENT EDUCATION
Concurrent use of other medications that enhance bleeding (NSAIDs, heparin, warfarin, thrombolytics, antiplatelets) increases risk for bleeding.	• If used concurrently, monitor the client carefully for signs of bleeding.

Nursing Administration

- Use of thrombolytic agents must take place within 4 to 6 hr of onset of symptoms.
- Clients receiving a thrombolytic agent should be monitored in a setting that provides for close supervision and continuous monitoring during and after administration of the medication.
- Obtain baseline platelet counts, hemoglobin (Hgb), hematocrit (Hct), aPTT, PT, INR, and fibrinogen levels, and monitor periodically.
- Obtain baseline vital signs (heart rate, blood pressure) and monitor frequently per protocol.
- Nursing care includes continuous monitoring of hemodynamic status to assess for therapeutic and adverse effects of thrombolytic (relief of chest pain, signs of bleeding). Follow facility protocol.
- Provide for client safety per facility protocol.
- Ensure adequate IV access for administration of emergency medications and availability of emergency equipment.
- Do not mix any medications in IV with thrombolytic agents.
- Minimize bruising or bleeding by limiting venipunctures and subcutaneous/intramuscular injections.
- Discontinue thrombolytic therapy if life-threatening bleeding occurs. Treat blood loss with whole blood, packed red blood cells, and/or fresh frozen plasma. IV aminocaproic acid (Amicar) should be available for administration in the event of excessive fibrinolysis.
- Following thrombolytic therapy, administer heparin or aspirin as prescribed to decrease the risk of rethrombosis.
- Following thrombolytic therapy, administer beta blockers as prescribed to decrease myocardial oxygen consumption and to reduce the incidence and severity of reperfusion arrhythmias.
- Administer H_2 antagonists, such as ranitidine (Zantac), or proton pump inhibitors, such as omeprazole (Prilosec), as prescribed to prevent GI bleeding.

Nursing Evaluation of Medication Effectiveness

- Depending on therapeutic intent, effectiveness may be evidenced by:
  - Evidence of thrombus lysis and restoration of circulation (relief of chest pain, reduction of initial ST segment injury pattern as shown on ECG 60 to 90 min after start of therapy)

CHAPTER 25: MEDICATIONS AFFECTING COAGULATION

Application Exercises

Scenario: A client is receiving heparin sodium by continuous IV infusion.

1. Which of the following laboratory values should the nurse monitor in order to evaluate the effectiveness of the heparin sodium drip?

    A. Bleeding time

    B. aPTT

    C. Hgb

    D. Platelets

2. The client begins vomiting blood. Which of the following medications should the nurse prepare to give to reverse the effects of the heparin sodium?

    A. Vitamin K

    B. Atropine sulfate

    C. Protamine sulfate

    D. Calcium gluconate

---

3. A nurse is caring for a client following thrombolytic therapy. Which of the following interventions should the nurse implement to help reduce bleeding? (Select all that apply)

    _____ Avoid IM or subcutaneous injections.

    _____ Apply pressure to bleeding puncture sites.

    _____ Reduce the maintenance IV fluid rate.

    _____ Administer furosemide (Lasix).

    _____ Administer aminocaproic acid (Amicar).

4. When caring for a client taking aspirin to reduce the risk for a myocardial infarction, the nurse should monitor for which of the following adverse effects? (Select all that apply)

    _____ Coffee-ground emesis

    _____ Hypertension

    _____ Tinnitus

    _____ Bruising

    _____ Bradycardia

    _____ Black tarry stools

CHAPTER 25: MEDICATIONS AFFECTING COAGULATION

Application Exercises Answer Key

Scenario: A client is receiving heparin sodium by continuous IV infusion.

1. Which of the following laboratory values should the nurse monitor to evaluate the effectiveness of the heparin sodium drip?

   A. Bleeding time

   B. aPTT

   C. Hgb

   D. Platelets

   The effects of heparin are evaluated by the serum activated partial thromboplastin time (aPTT). Usually an aPTT of 1.5 to 2 times the control is desired for anticoagulation. Bleeding time, Hgb, and platelets are not used to monitor the effectiveness of a heparin drip.

NCLEX® Connection: Pharmacological and Parenteral Therapies: Expected Actions/Outcomes

2. The client begins vomiting blood. Which of the following medications should the nurse prepare to give to reverse the effects of the heparin sodium?

   A. Vitamin K

   B. Atropine sulfate

   C. Protamine sulfate

   D. Calcium gluconate

   Protamine sulfate reverses the effects of heparin sodium. Vitamin K is given to reverse warfarin (Coumadin). Atropine sulfate may be used to reverse bradycardia caused by beta-adrenergic blockers. Calcium gluconate is used to treat magnesium sulfate toxicity.

NCLEX® Connection: Pharmacological and Parenteral Therapies: Adverse Effects/ Contraindications/Side Effects/Interactions

3. A nurse is caring for a client following thrombolytic therapy. Which of the following interventions should the nurse implement to help reduce bleeding. (Select all that apply)

   __X__ **Avoid IM or subcutaneous injections.**
   __X__ **Apply pressure to bleeding puncture sites.**
   _____ Reduce the maintenance IV fluid rate.
   _____ Administer furosemide (Lasix).
   __X__ **Administer aminocaproic acid (Amicar).**

   A major complication of thrombolytic therapy is bleeding. Avoid injections and additional punctures. Apply pressure to bleeding puncture sites to promote hemostasis. Aminocaproic acid may be given to reverse the thrombolytic effects. The IV fluid rate should be maintained to provide adequate fluid volume. Furosemide could further decrease vascular volume.

   NCLEX® Connection: Pharmacological and Parenteral Therapies: Adverse Effects/Contraindications/Side Effects/Interactions

4. When caring for a client taking aspirin to reduce the risk for a myocardial infarction, the nurse should monitor for which of the following adverse effects? (Select all that apply)

   __X__ **Coffee-ground emesis**
   _____ Hypertension
   __X__ **Tinnitus**
   __X__ **Bruising**
   _____ Bradycardia
   __X__ **Black tarry stools**

   Aspirin may cause prolonged bleeding time and thrombocytopenia. The client should be monitored for signs of bleeding, such as coffee ground emesis, bruising, or bloody, tarry stools. Tinnitus is a symptom of aspirin toxicity. Hypertension and bradycardia are not adverse effects of aspirin.

   NCLEX® Connection: Pharmacological and Parenteral Therapies: Adverse Effects/Contraindications/Side Effects/Interactions

UNIT 5 MEDICATIONS AFFECTING THE HEMATOLOGIC SYSTEM

Chapter 26 Growth Factors

Overview

- Blood cells and platelets are produced in the body by the biological process known as hematopoiesis. In the body this process is naturally controlled by hormones, also known as hematopoietic growth factors.
- Genetically engineered products are available for therapeutic purposes, which include:
  - Replacement of neutrophils and platelets after chemotherapy
  - Hastening of bone marrow function after a bone marrow transplant
  - Increase in RBC production for clients with chronic renal failure
- There are 3 groups of hematopoietic growth factors:
  - Erythropoietic growth factors
    - Biological name – erythropoietin
  - Leukopoietic growth factors
    - Biological name –
      - Granulocyte colony stimulating factor (G-CSF)
      - Granulocyte-macrophage colony-stimulating factor (GM-CSF)
  - Thrombopoietic growth factor
    - Interleukin-11

MEDICATION CLASSIFICATION: ERYTHROPOIETIC GROWTH FACTORS

- Select Prototype Medication: epoetin alfa (Epogen, Procrit)
- Other Medications:
  - Darbepoetin alfa (Aranesp) – long-acting erythropoietin
  - Methoxy polyethylene glycol (MGEG)-epoetin beta (Mircera) – very long-acting erythropoietin

Purpose

- Expected Pharmacological Action
  - Hematopoietic growth factors act on the bone marrow to increase production of red blood cells.
- Therapeutic Uses
  - Anemia related to chronic renal failure, use of zidovudine (Retrovir) in clients with HIV-infection, chemotherapy, and elective surgery

Complications

SIDE/ADVERSE EFFECTS	NURSING INTERVENTIONS/CLIENT EDUCATION
Hypertension secondary to elevations in hematocrit level	• This side effect occurs due to the elevation of hematocrit levels. • Monitor the client's Hgb levels and blood pressure, and if elevated, administer antihypertensive medications.
Increased risk for a cardiovascular event (MI, stroke, cardiac arrest) with an increase in Hgb above 12 g/dL or more than 1 g in 2 weeks	• Decrease dosage when these limits are reached. Therapy may be resumed when Hgb drops to acceptable level, but dosage should be reduced.

Contraindications/Precautions

- Use is contraindicated in clients with uncontrolled hypertension.
- Use is contraindicated in clients with certain cancers because of possible increase in tumor growth.
- Risk for deep vein thrombosis is higher in preoperative clients taking erythropoietic growth factors. Prophylactic use of anticoagulants decreases this risk.

Nursing Administration

- Obtain the client's baseline blood pressure. In clients with chronic renal failure, control hypertension before the start of treatment.
- Administer by subcutaneous or IV bolus injection.
- Do not agitate the vial of medication. Use each vial for one dose and do not put the needle back into the vial when withdrawing the medication.
- Do not mix medication with any other medication in syringe.
- Dosing is usually 3 times/week, but may be once a week with some types of chemotherapy.

- Monitor the client's iron levels and take measures to ensure a normal iron level. RBC growth is dependent upon adequate quantities of iron, folic acid, and vitamin B_{12}. Without adequate levels of these, erythropoietin is significantly less effective.
- Monitor the client's Hgb and Hct twice a week until target range is reached.
- Epoetin alfa should not be agitated and should not be combined with other medications.
- The longer acting forms are administered less frequently (weekly or monthly), but may be prescribed for clients with chronic renal failure only.

Nursing Evaluation of Medication Effectiveness

- Depending on therapeutic intent, effectiveness may be evidenced by:
    - Hgb level of 10 to 12 g/dL and Hct of 40%

MEDICATION CLASSIFICATION: LEUKOPOIETIC GROWTH FACTORS

- Select Prototype Medication: filgrastim (Neupogen)
- Other Medication: pegfilgrastim (Neulasta)

Purpose

- Expected Pharmacological Action
    - Stimulates the bone marrow to increase production of neutrophils
- Therapeutic Use
    - Decreases the risk of infection in clients with neutropenia, such as from cancer

Complications

SIDE/ADVERSE EFFECTS	NURSING INTERVENTIONS/CLIENT EDUCATION
Bone pain	• Monitor the client for symptoms and notify the provider. • Administer acetaminophen or opioid analgesic.
Leukocytosis	• Monitor CBC two times per week during treatment. • Decrease dose or interrupt treatment if WBC is greater than 100,000/mm³.

Contraindications/Precautions

- This medication is contraindicated in clients who are sensitive to *Escherichia coli* protein.
- Use cautiously in clients with cancer of the bone marrow.

Nursing Administration

- Administer filgrastim by short IV infusion, continuous IV, subcutaneous infusion, or subcutaneous injection.
- Do not agitate the vial of medication. Use each vial for one dose and do not combine with other medications. Do not put the needle back into the vial when withdrawing the medication.
- Pegfilgrastim is only administered IV and must be reconstituted from a powdered formulation. Infuse over 2 or 4 hr interval.
- Monitor CBC two times per week.

Nursing Evaluation of Medication Effectiveness

- Depending on therapeutic intent, effectiveness may be evidenced by:
    - Absence of infection
    - In chemotherapy for cancer treatment, an absolute neutrophil count increase to greater than 10,000/mm^3 after the chemotherapeutic-induced nadir (the peak of chemotherapeutic cell destruction usually occurring 10 to 14 days after administration)

MEDICATION CLASSIFICATION: GRANULOCYTE MACROPHAGE COLONY STIMULATING FACTOR

- Select Prototype Medication: sargramostim (Leukine)

Purpose

- Expected Pharmacological Action
    - This medication acts on the bone marrow to increase production of white blood cells (neutrophils, monocytes, macrophages, eosinophils).
- Therapeutic uses
    - Hastens bone marrow function after bone marrow transplant
    - Is used in the treatment of failed bone marrow transplant

Complications

SIDE/ADVERSE EFFECTS	NURSING INTERVENTIONS/CLIENT EDUCATION
Diarrhea, weakness, rash, malaise, and bone pain	• Monitor the client for symptoms and notify the provider if they occur. • Administer acetaminophen.
Leukocytosis, thrombocytosis	• Monitor CBC two times per week during treatment. • Reduce dose or interrupt treatment for absolute neutrophil count >20,000/mm^3, WBC >50,000/mm^3, or platelets >500,000/mm^3.

 Contraindications/Precautions

- Use is contraindicated in clients allergic to yeast products.
- Use cautiously in clients with heart disease, hypoxia, peripheral edema, or pleural or pericardial effusion.
- Use cautiously in clients with cancer of the bone marrow.

Nursing Administration

- Obtain baseline CBC, differential, and platelet count. Monitor periodically during treatment.
- Sargramostim should not be agitated and should not be combined with other medications.
- Administer by IV infusion.

Nursing Evaluation of Medication Effectiveness

- Depending on therapeutic intent, effectiveness may be evidenced by:
    - Absence of infection
    - WBC and differential within expected reference ranges

MEDICATION CLASSIFICATION: THROMBOPOIETIC GROWTH FACTORS

- Select Prototype Medication: oprelvekin (Interleukin-11, Neumega)

Purpose

- Expected Pharmacological Action
    - Increases the production of platelets
- Therapeutic Uses
    - Decreases thrombocytopenia and the need for platelet transfusions in clients receiving chemotherapy.

Complications

SIDE/ADVERSE EFFECTS	NURSING INTERVENTIONS/CLIENT EDUCATION
Fluid retention (peripheral edema, dyspnea on exertion)	• Monitor the client's I&O. • If symptoms occur, stop the medication and notify the provider.
Cardiac dysrhythmias (tachycardia, atrial fibrillation, atrial flutter)	• Use cautiously in clients with a history of cardiac dysrhythmias. • Monitor the client's vital signs, heart rate, and rhythm. • If symptoms occur, stop the medication and notify the provider.
Conjunctival injection, transient blurring of vision, papilledema	• Advise the client to observe for symptoms, and if symptoms occur, stop the medication and notify the provider.
Allergic reactions, possible anaphylaxis	• Observe the client carefully for allergic reactions; stop the medication and notify the provider if symptoms occur.

Contraindications/Precautions

- These medications are generally contraindicated in clients who have cancer of the bone marrow, because they may stimulate tumor growth.
- Use cautiously in clients with heart failure and pleural effusion.

Nursing Administration

- Obtain the client's baseline CBC, platelet count, and electrolytes.
- Oprelvekin should not be agitated and should not be combined with other medications.
- Administer oprelvekin once daily by subcutaneous injection until platelet count reaches prescribed level.

Nursing Evaluation of Medication Effectiveness

- Depending on therapeutic intent, effectiveness may be evidenced by:
  - Platelet count greater than $50,000/mm^3$

CHAPTER 26: GROWTH FACTORS

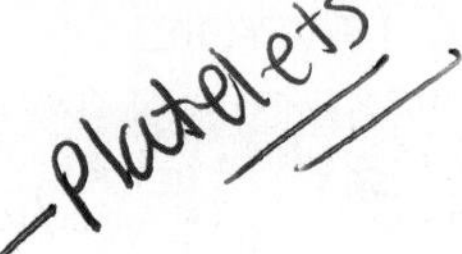

 Application Exercises

1. A client has been receiving daily doses of oprelvekin (Interleukin-11). Which of the following laboratory values should the nurse monitor to determine effectiveness of this medication?

   A. Hemoglobin

   B. Absolute neutrophil count

   C. Thrombocyte count

   D. Total white blood count

2. Which of the following interventions should the nurse implement when preparing to administer filgrastim (Neupogen) for the first time to a client who has just undergone a bone marrow transplant?

   A. Administer intramuscularly in a large muscle mass to prevent injury.

   B. Give orally with a meal or snack to prevent severe GI upset.

   C. Shake vial gently to mix well before withdrawing dose.

   D. Discard vial after removing one dose of the medication.

3. The nurse should assess for which of the following adverse reactions in a client receiving epoetin alfa (Epogen)?

   A. Leukocytosis

   B. Hypertension

   C. Fluid retention

   D. Blurred vision

CHAPTER 26: GROWTH FACTORS

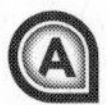

Application Exercises Answer Key

1. A client has been receiving daily doses of oprelvekin (Interleukin-11). Which of the following laboratory values should the nurse monitor to determine effectiveness of this medication?

    A. Hemoglobin

    B. Absolute neutrophil count

    C. Thrombocyte count

    D. Total white blood count

    The expected outcome for oprelvekin is an increased thrombocyte count to be greater than 50,000/mm^3. Hemoglobin levels should be monitored for a client receiving epoetin alfa (Epogen). Absolute neutrophil count should be monitored for a client receiving filgrastim (Neupogen). Total WBC should be monitored for a client receiving sargramostim (Leukine).

NCLEX® Connection: Pharmacological and Parenteral Therapies: Expected Actions/ Outcomes

2. Which of the following interventions should the nurse implement when preparing to administer filgrastim (Neupogen) for the first time to a client who has just undergone a bone marrow transplant?

    A. Administer intramuscularly in a large muscle mass to prevent injury.

    B. Give orally with a meal or snack to prevent severe GI upset.

    C. Shake vial gently to mix well before withdrawing dose.

    D. Discard vial after removing one dose of the medication.

    Filgrastim is dispensed in a vial meant for single-dose use and any unused portion should be discarded. The medication is administered by subcutaneous and IV routes only, so neither oral nor IM administration is appropriate. The vial should not be shaken before withdrawal because this may damage the medication.

NCLEX® Connection: Pharmacological and Parenteral Therapies: Medication Administration

3. The nurse should assess for which of the following adverse reactions in a client receiving epoetin alfa (Epogen)?

    A. Leukocytosis

    B. Hypertension

    C. Fluid retention

    D. Blurred vision

    Hypertension is a common adverse reaction of epoetin alfa. Leukocytosis is an adverse reaction of granulocyte colony-stimulating factor administration. Fluid retention and blurred vision are adverse reactions seen in oprelvekin administration.

NCLEX® Connection: Pharmacological and Parenteral Therapies: Adverse Effects/ Contraindications/Side Effects/Interactions

UNIT 5 MEDICATIONS AFFECTING THE HEMATOLOGIC SYSTEM

Chapter 27 Blood and Blood Products

Overview

- Blood and blood products are used to increase intravascular volume, replace clotting factors and components of blood, replace blood loss, and improve oxygen carrying capacity.
- Blood products include whole blood and components of blood, such as packed red blood cells, platelets, plasma, white blood cells, and albumin.

EXPECTED PHARMACOLOGICAL ACTION	THERAPEUTIC USES	TYPE OF REACTION
Whole blood		
Increases circulating blood volume	• Replacement therapy for acute blood loss secondary to traumatic injuries or surgical procedures • Volume expansion in clients with extensive burn injury, dehydration, shock	• Acute hemolytic reaction • Febrile nonhemolytic reaction • Anaphylactic reactions • Mild allergic reactions • Circulatory overload • Sepsis
Packed red blood cells		
Increases the number of RBCs	• Severe symptomatic anemia (Hgb < 6 g/dL) • Hemoglobinopathies • Medication-induced hemolytic anemia • Erythroblastosis fetalis	• Acute hemolytic reaction • Febrile nonhemolytic reaction • Anaphylactic reactions • Mild allergic reactions • Sepsis
Platelet concentrate		
Increases platelet counts	• Thrombocytopenia (platelet count $< 20{,}000/mm^3$) – aplastic anemia, chemotherapy-induced bone marrow suppression • Active bleeding (platelet count $< 80{,}000$ mm^3)	• Febrile nonhemolytic reaction • Mild allergic reactions • Sepsis

EXPECTED PHARMACOLOGICAL ACTION	THERAPEUTIC USES	TYPE OF REACTION
	Fresh frozen plasma	
Replaces coagulation factors	• Active bleeding or massive hemorrhage • Extensive burns • Shock • Disseminated intravascular coagulation • Antithrombin III deficiency • Thrombotic thrombocytopenic purpura • Reversal of anticoagulation effects of warfarin • Replacement therapy for coagulation factors II, V, VII, IX, X, and XI	• Acute hemolytic reaction • Febrile nonhemolytic reaction • Anaphylactic reactions • Mild allergic reactions • Circulatory overload • Sepsis
	Pheresed granulocytes	
Replaces neutrophils/granulocytes	• Severe neutropenia (ANC less than 500) • Life-threatening bacterial/fungal infection not responding to antibiotic therapy • Neonatal sepsis • Neutrophil dysfunction	• Acute hemolytic reaction • Febrile nonhemolytic reaction • Anaphylactic reactions • Mild allergic reactions • Circulatory overload • Sepsis
	Albumin	
Expands circulating blood volume by exerting oncotic pressure	• Hypovolemia • Hypoalbuminemia • Burns • Adult respiratory distress • Severe nephrosis • Cardiopulmonary bypass surgery • Hemolytic disease of the newborn	• Risk for fluid volume excess such as pulmonary edema

Complications

SIDE/ADVERSE EFFECTS	NURSING INTERVENTIONS/CLIENT EDUCATION
Acute hemolytic reaction (chills, fever, low back pain, tachycardia, tachypnea, hypotension)	• Stop the transfusion immediately if symptoms occur, and notify the provider.
Febrile nonhemolytic reaction, most common (sudden chills); fever (increase in temperature greater than 1° from baseline); headache	• Observe for signs and symptoms of a reaction and stop the transfusion if they occur. • Notify the provider immediately and follow agency policy regarding resumption or discontinuation of transfusion. • Administer acetaminophen for fever.
Anaphylactic reactions (anxiety, urticaria, wheezing, shock, cardiac arrest)	• If symptoms occur, stop the transfusion and notify the provider immediately. • Initiate CPR if necessary. • Have epinephrine ready for IM or IV injection.
Mild allergic reactions (flushing, itching, urticaria)	• If symptoms occur, stop the transfusion and notify the provider immediately. • If symptoms are very mild and there is no respiratory compromise, antihistamines may be prescribed and the transfusion restarted slowly.
Circulatory overload (cough, shortness of breath, crackles, hypertension, tachycardia, distended neck veins)	• Observe clients for signs and symptoms of fluid volume excess. • If symptoms occur, stop the transfusion and notify the provider immediately. • Place the client upright with feet down. • Administer diuretics and oxygen as appropriate. • Monitor I&O. • A slower rate of infusion may be indicated.
Sepsis (rapid onset of chills and fever, vomiting, diarrhea, hypotension, shock)	• Observe clients for signs and symptoms during and following transfusion. • Notify the provider immediately if symptoms occur. • Obtain blood culture, send blood transfusion bag for analysis for possible contaminants, and treat sepsis with antibiotics, IV fluids, vasopressors, and steroids.

Contraindications/Precautions

- Contraindicated in clients with hypersensitivity reactions
- Observe culturally sensitive (religious) issues regarding blood transfusion, such as for clients who are Jehovah's Witnesses. Infusing colloids and other plasma expanders may be acceptable.

Nursing Administration

- Obtain baseline laboratory values: Hgb, Hct, platelet count, total protein, albumin levels, PT, PTT, fibrinogen, potassium, pH, and serum calcium.
- Before starting a transfusion, verify the provider's orders and the client's blood typing, obtain consent for transfusion, and check the client's blood transfusion history.
- Verify identification of donor blood and recipient, blood compatibility, and expiration date with another nurse.
- Obtain baseline vital signs at the start of transfusion. Stay with the client and monitor vital signs every 5 min for 15 min, then monitor according to agency policy.
- Obtain the client's baseline vital signs and assessment of urinary output, and document on the client's medical record. Record the start and completion times of transfusion, total volume of transfusion, and the client's response to the transfusion.
- Assess infusion site for infection or infiltration.
- Assess patency of IV line and prime IV tubing with 0.9% sodium chloride.
- Do not administer blood along with any IV solution other than 0.9% sodium chloride. IV solutions containing dextrose cause hemolysis of red blood cells.
- Administer blood using a 20-gauge or larger intravenous needle (to avoid breakage of cells and blockage of needle lumen, nothing smaller than a 20 gauge should be used due to blood viscosity), a blood filter (to remove particles and possible contaminants within old blood) and a Y tubing connection (so that 0.9% NaCl can be infused by piggyback).
- Observe universal precautions during handling and administration of blood products.
- Do not administer blood products with any other medications.
- Administration of Albumin
    - Identify underlying cause of hypoalbuminemia to completely correct the client's condition.
    - Albumin solutions can be administered piggybacked with saline or glucose solutions.
- Obtain baseline Hgb, Hct, total protein, albumin levels, and continue monitoring the client for the duration of treatment.
- Ensure adequate hydration before and after treatment.
- Obtain and evaluate lab results. Monitor:
    - Whole blood, PRBC: Hemoglobin (Hgb)
    - Platelet concentrate: Platelet count
    - Fresh frozen plasma: Prothrombin time (PT) and partial thromboplastin (PTT) time

   - Pheresed granulocytes: White blood cells
   - Albumin: Albumin level
- Complete transfusion within specified time:
   - Whole blood, packed red blood cells (PRBC), about 250 mL/unit; infuse within 2 to 4 hr.
   - Platelet concentrate, about 300 mL/unit; infuse within 15 to 30 min/unit
   - Fresh frozen plasma (FFP), about 200 mL/unit; infuse within 30 to 60 min/unit
   - Pheresed granulocytes (WBC), about 400 mL/unit; infuse within 45 to 60 min/unit
   - Albumin
      - 5%, 250 to 500 mL bottle; infuse 1 to 10 mL/min
      - 25%, 50 to 100 mL bottle; infuse 4 mL/min
- In the event a blood transfusion reaction is noted:
   - Stop the transfusion and notify the provider immediately.
   - Do not turn on IV fluids that are connected to the Y tubing because the remaining blood in the Y tubing will be infused and aggravate the client's reaction. Administer a new IV solution of 0.9% sodium chloride.
   - Document start and completion times of transfusion, total volume of transfusion, and the client's response to the transfusion.
   - Stay with the client and monitor vital signs and urinary output.
   - Notify the blood bank, recheck the identification tag and numbers on the blood bag, and send the blood bag and IV tubing to the blood bank for analysis.
   - Obtain a urine specimen and send to the laboratory to determine for RBC hemolysis. Insert an indwelling catheter if hemolytic reaction is suspected to monitor urine output.
   - Repeat type and cross match. Obtain CBC and bilirubin to determine hemolysis.
   - Complete a transfusion log sheet, which includes complete record of baseline vital signs, ongoing monitoring, and the client's response to transfusion. Incorporate this in the client's medical record.

- Special Considerations for Older Adult Clients
   - Use caution to prevent overload of fluid. Infuse transfusion more slowly. Space multiple transfusions apart. A diuretic may be needed during transfusions.
   - Administer blood that has been obtained within 1 week. Older RBCs may release potassium and cause hyperkalemia.
   - Monitor older adult clients frequently (every 15 min) during transfusions.
- For massive transfusion (greater than or equal to replacement of total blood volume in 24 hr, about 10 units for an adult or 5 units in 4 hr)
   - Monitor platelets, PT, and aPTT every 5 units and replace as needed.

- Monitor potassium and calcium levels.
- Monitor ECG for changes associated with hypokalemia, hyperkalemia or hypocalcemia.
- Warm blood using blood warmer to prevent hypothermia.

Nursing Evaluation of Medication Effectiveness

- Depending on therapeutic intent, effectiveness may be evidenced by:
    - Whole Blood, Packed RBCs
        - Increase in hemoglobin of 1 to 2 g/dL per unit of blood administered
        - Blood pressure within normal reference range
        - Improved oxygenation as indicated by SaO_2, color and breathing pattern.
    - Platelet Concentrate
        - Reduced bleeding
        - Increase in platelet count
    - Fresh Frozen Plasma
        - Reduced bleeding
        - Prothrombin or activated partial thromboplastin time less than 1.5 times expected reference range
    - Pheresed Granulocytes
        - Increased granulocyte count
    - Albumin
        - Increased serum albumin levels
        - Decreased edema

CHAPTER 27: BLOOD AND BLOOD PRODUCTS

 Application Exercises

1. Prior to initiating a blood transfusion with packed red blood cells, the nurse should do which of the following? (Select all that apply.)

   _____ Insert an IV with a large bore needle, at least 19 gauge when possible and if needed.

   _____ Set up an IV using a Y tubing and flush with D_5W.

   _____ Confirm correct blood, type, expiration date/time with a second qualified nurse.

   _____ Confirm correct client by co-checking the client name and hospital number on the client ID bracelet and comparing to the blood bag tag with a second qualified nurse.

   _____ Take a complete set of vital signs, including a temperature.

   _____ Insert an indwelling urinary catheter.

2. After 15 min of the transfusion, the client begins to have lower back pain and a headache. The nurse suspects a hemolytic transfusion reaction. The nurse should do which of the following? (Select all that apply.)

   _____ Stop the transfusion.

   _____ Flush the IV with 0.9% sodium chloride.

   _____ Slow the transfusion.

   _____ Obtain a urine sample and send to check for hemoglobin.

   _____ Send blood bag and IV tubing to blood bank for analysis.

3. The client has an activated partial thromboplastin time (aPTT) greater than 1.5 times the expected reference range. The nurse should prepare to transfuse which of the following?

   A. Albumin

   B. Platelets

   C. Fresh frozen plasma

   D. Packed red blood cells

CHAPTER 27: BLOOD AND BLOOD PRODUCTS

Application Exercises Answer Key

1. Prior to initiating a blood transfusion with packed red blood cells, the nurse should do which of the following? (Select all that apply.)

 X **Insert an IV with a large bore needle, at least 19 gauge when possible and if needed.**

 ___ Set up an IV using a Y tubing and flush with D_5W.

 X **Confirm correct blood, type, expiration date/time with a second qualified nurse.**

 X **Confirm correct client by co-checking the client name and hospital number on the client ID bracelet and comparing to the blood bag tag with a second qualified nurse.**

 X **Take a complete set of vital signs, including a temperature.**

 ___ Insert an indwelling urinary catheter.

Prior to hanging packed red blood cells, the nurse should establish venous access with a large bore IV. The PRBCs run through a Y type IV tubing that is flushed with 0.9% sodium chloride. Dextrose will cause the RBCs to clot or hemolyze. Always double check the blood, including type and expiration time, and confirm the correct client with a second nurse, using the client's hospital ID number. The insertion of an indwelling urinary catheter is not required prior to a blood transfusion.

NCLEX® Connection: Pharmacological and Parenteral Therapies: Medication Administration

2. After 15 min of the transfusion, the client begins to have lower back pain and a headache. The nurse suspects a hemolytic transfusion reaction. The nurse should do which of the following? (Select all that apply.)

 X **Stop the transfusion.**

 ___ Flush the IV with 0.9% sodium chloride.

 ___ Slow the transfusion.

 X **Obtain a urine sample and send to check for hemoglobin.**

 X **Send blood bag and IV tubing to blood bank for analysis.**

Signs of a transfusion reaction may include headache, low back pain, tachycardia, fever and anxiety. Flushing the line with 0.9% sodium chloride may cause more blood to infuse into the client. The blood transfusion should be stopped and the provider notified.

NCLEX® Connection: Pharmacological and Parenteral Therapies: Adverse Effects/Contraindications/Side Effects/Interactions

3. The client has an activated partial thromboplastin time (aPTT) greater than 1.5 times the expected reference range. The nurse should prepare to transfuse which of the following?

   A. Albumin

   B. Platelets

   C. Fresh frozen plasma

   D. Packed red blood cells

   Fresh frozen plasma is given to correct clotting disorders. It may be given to treat a prothrombin or activated partial thromboplastin time of greater than 1.5 times greater than the expected reference range.

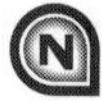

NCLEX® Connection: Pharmacological and Parenteral Therapies: Adverse Effects/Contraindications/Side Effects/Interactions

UNIT 6: MEDICATIONS AFFECTING THE GASTROINTESTINAL SYSTEM AND NUTRITION

- Peptic Ulcer Disease
- Gastrointestinal Disorders
- Vitamins, Minerals, and Supplements

NCLEX® CONNECTIONS

When reviewing the chapters in this unit, keep in mind the relevant sections of the NCLEX® outline, in particular:

CLIENT NEEDS: PHARMACOLOGICAL AND PARENTERAL THERAPIES

Relevant topics/tasks include:

- Adverse Effects/Contraindications/Side Effects/Interactions
  - Document the side effects and adverse effects of medications and parenteral therapy.
- Expected Actions/Outcomes
  - Evaluate the therapeutic effect of medications.
- Parenteral/Intravenous Therapy
  - Evaluate the client's response to intermittent parenteral fluid therapy.

UNIT 6 MEDICATIONS AFFECTING THE GASTROINTESTINAL SYSTEM AND NUTRITION

Chapter 28 Peptic Ulcer Disease

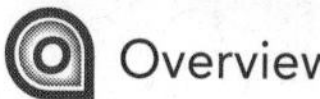

Overview

- Pharmacological management of peptic ulcer disease addresses the imbalance between gastric mucosal defenses and antagonistic factors such as *H. pylori* infection, NSAIDs, and secretions including gastric acid and pepsin.
- Therapeutic management outcomes include:
  - Lessening of symptoms
  - Encouragement of healing
  - Decreased risk of complications
  - Stopping reoccurrence
- The disease process is only altered by the use of antibiotics. All other medications make an environment that is conducive to healing.
- The groups of medications used in the management of peptic ulcer disease include:
  - Antibiotics
  - Antisecretory agents
  - Mucosal protectants
  - Antacids

MEDICATION CLASSIFICATION: ANTIBIOTICS

- Select Prototype Medications:
  - Amoxicillin (Amoxil)
  - Bismuth (Pepto-Bismol)
  - Clarithromycin (Biaxin)
  - Metronidazole (Flagyl)
  - Tetracycline (Achromycin V)

Purpose

- Expected Pharmacological Action
  - Eradication of *H. pylori* bacteria
- Therapy should include:
  - Combination of 2 or 3 antibiotics for 14 days

MEDICATION CLASSIFICATION: HISTAMINE$_2$-RECEPTOR ANTAGONISTS

- Select Prototype Medication: ranitidine hydrochloride (Zantac)
- Other Medications:
  - Cimetidine (Tagamet)
  - Nizatidine (Axid)
  - Famotidine (Pepcid)

Purpose

- Expected Pharmacological Action
  - Histamine$_2$-receptor antagonists suppress the secretion of gastric acid by selectively blocking H_2 receptors in parietal cells lining the stomach.
- Therapeutic Uses
  - Histamine$_2$-receptor antagonists are prescribed for gastric and peptic ulcers, gastroesophageal reflux disease (GERD), and hypersecretory conditions, such as Zollinger-Ellison syndrome.
  - Histamine$_2$-receptor antagonists are used in conjunction with antibiotics to treat ulcers caused by *H. pylori*.

Complications

SIDE/ADVERSE EFFECTS	NURSING INTERVENTIONS/CLIENT EDUCATION
Cimetidine may block androgen receptors, resulting in decreased libido and impotence.	• Inform clients of these possible effects.
Cimetidine may cause CNS effects (lethargy, depression, confusion)	• These effects are seen more often in an older adult with kidney or liver dysfunction. • The use of cimetidine should be avoided in older adults.

- Ranitidine, nizatidine, and famotidine have few adverse effects and interactions.

Contraindications/Precautions

- These medications are Pregnancy Risk Category B.

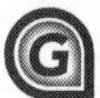

- Use in older adults can cause antiadrenergic effects (e.g., impotence) and CNS effects (e.g., confusion).
- H_2-receptor antagonists decrease gastric acidity, which promotes bacterial colonization of the stomach and the respiratory tract. Use cautiously in clients who are at a high risk for pneumonia, such as clients with chronic obstructive pulmonary disease (COPD).

Interactions

MEDICATION/FOOD INTERACTIONS	NURSING INTERVENTIONS/CLIENT EDUCATION
Cimetidine can inhibit medication-metabolizing enzymes and thus increase the levels of warfarin, phenytoin (Dilantin), theophylline, and lidocaine.	• In clients taking warfarin, monitor for signs of bleeding. • Monitor international normalized ratio (INR) and prothrombin time (PT) levels, and adjust warfarin dosages accordingly. • In clients taking phenytoin, theophylline, and lidocaine, monitor serum levels and adjust dosages accordingly.
Concurrent use of antacids can decrease absorption of histamine$_2$-receptor antagonists	• Advise clients not to take an antacid 1 hr before or after taking a histamine$_2$-receptor antagonist.

Nursing Administration

- Cimetidine, ranitidine, and famotidine can be administered IV for acute situations.
- Advise clients to practice good nutrition. Suggest eating six small meals rather than three large meals a day.
- Inform clients that adequate rest and reduction of stress may promote healing.
- Clients should avoid smoking, because smoking can delay healing.
- Encourage clients to avoid aspirin and other nonsteroidal anti-inflammatory drugs (NSAIDs) unless taking low-dose aspirin therapy for prevention of cardiovascular disease.
- If alcohol exacerbates symptoms, advise clients to stop drinking.
- Availability of these medications OTC may discourage clients from seeking appropriate health care. Encourage clients to see the provider if symptoms persist.
- The medication regimen can be complex, often requiring clients to take two to three different medications for an extended period of time. Encourage clients to adhere to the medication regimen and provide support.
- Ranitidine can be taken with or without food.

- Treatment of peptic ulcer disease is usually started as an oral dose twice a day until the ulcer is healed, followed by a maintenance dose, which is usually taken once a day at bedtime.
- Teach clients to notify the provider for any sign of obvious or occult GI bleeding, such as coffee-ground emesis).

MEDICATION CLASSIFICATION: PROTON PUMP INHIBITOR

- Select Prototype Medication: omeprazole (Prilosec)
- Other Medications:
    - Pantoprazole (Protonix)
    - Lansoprazole (Prevacid)
    - Rabeprazole sodium (AcipHex)
    - Esomeprazole (Nexium)

Purpose

- Expected Pharmacological Action
    - Proton pump inhibitors reduce gastric acid secretion by irreversibly inhibiting the enzyme that produces gastric acid.
    - Proton pump inhibitors reduce basal and stimulated acid production.
- Therapeutic uses
    - Proton pump inhibitors are prescribed for gastric and peptic ulcers, GERD, and hypersecretory conditions such as Zollinger-Ellison syndrome.

Complications

- Insignificant side effects and adverse effects with short-term treatment
- Low incidence of headache, diarrhea, and nausea/vomiting

Contraindications/Precautions

- These medications are Pregnancy Risk Category C.
- Use cautiously with children and women who are breastfeeding.
- Contraindicated for clients hypersensitive to medication
- These medications increase the risk for pneumonia. Omeprazole decreases gastric acid pH, which promotes bacterial colonization of the stomach and the respiratory tract. Use cautiously in clients at high risk for pneumonia, such as clients with COPD.
- Long-term use of proton pump inhibitors increases the risk of gastric cancer and osteoporosis.

Interactions

MEDICATION/FOOD INTERACTIONS	NURSING INTERVENTIONS/CLIENT EDUCATION
Digoxin (Lanoxin) levels may be increased when used concurrently with omeprazole.	• Monitor digoxin levels carefully if prescribed concurrently.
Absorption of ketoconazole (formerly Nizoral), itraconazole (Sporanox), and atazanavir (Reyataz) is extremely decreased when taken concurrently with proton pump inhibitors.	• Concurrent use should be avoided. If necessary to administer concurrently, separate medication administration by 2 to 12 hr.

Nursing Administration

- Do not crush, chew, or break sustained-release capsules.
- Clients may sprinkle the contents of the capsule over food to facilitate swallowing.
- Clients should take omeprazole once a day prior to eating in the morning.
- Encourage clients to avoid alcohol and irritating medications such as NSAIDs.
- Active ulcers should be treated for 4 to 6 weeks.
- Pantoprazole (Protonix) can be administered to clients intravenously. In addition to low incidence of headache and diarrhea, there may be irritation at the injection site leading to thrombophlebitis. Monitor the client's IV site for signs of inflammation (redness, swelling, local pain) and change the IV site if indicated.
- Teach clients to notify the provider for any sign of obvious or occult GI bleeding such as coffee-ground emesis.

MEDICATION CLASSIFICATION: MUCOSAL PROTECTANT

- Select Prototype Medication: sucralfate (Carafate)

Purpose

- Expected Pharmacological Action
  - The acidic environment of the stomach and duodenum changes sucralfate into a thick substance that adheres to an ulcer. This protects the ulcer from further injury that may be caused by acid and pepsin.
  - This viscous substance can stick to the ulcer for up to 6 hr.
- Therapeutic Uses
  - Sucralfate is used for clients with acute duodenal ulcers and those requiring maintenance therapy.
  - Investigational use of sucralfate includes gastric ulcers and gastroesophageal reflux disease.

Complications

- To prevent constipation, encourage clients to increase dietary fiber and drink at least 1,500 mL/day if fluids are not restricted.
- Sucralfate has no systemic effects.

Contraindications/Precautions

- Pregnancy Risk Category B
- Contraindicated in clients who are hypersensitive to the medication

Interactions

MEDICATION/FOOD INTERACTIONS	NURSING INTERVENTIONS/CLIENT EDUCATION
Sucralfate may interfere with the absorption of phenytoin, digoxin, warfarin, and ciprofloxacin.	• Maintain a 2-hr interval between these medications and sucralfate to minimize this interaction.
Antacids interfere with the absorption of sucralfate.	• Antacids should not be administered within 30 min of sucralfate.

Nursing Administration

- Assist clients with the medication regimen.
- Instruct clients that the medication should be taken on an empty stomach.
- Instruct clients that sucralfate should be taken four times a day, 1 hr before meals, and again at bedtime.
- Clients can break or dissolve the medication in water, but should not crush or chew the tablet.
- Encourage clients to complete the course of treatment.

MEDICATION CLASSIFICATION: ANTACIDS

- Select Prototype Medication: aluminum hydroxide (Amphojel)
- Other Medications:
  - Aluminum carbonate
  - Magnesium hydroxide (Milk of Magnesia)
  - Sodium bicarbonate

Purpose

- Expected Pharmacological Action
  - Antacids neutralize gastric acid and inactivate pepsin.
  - Mucosal protection may occur by the antacid's ability to stimulate the production of prostaglandins.
- Therapeutic Uses
  - Antacids are used in clients to treat peptic ulcer disease (PUD) by promoting healing and relieving pain.
  - Antacids provide symptomatic relief for clients with GERD.

Complications

SIDE/ADVERSE EFFECTS	NURSING INTERVENTIONS/CLIENT EDUCATION
Aluminum and calcium compounds cause constipation, whereas magnesium compounds cause diarrhea.	• Advise clients that use of these compounds can be alternated to offset intestinal effects and normalize bowel function. • If a client has difficulty managing bowel function, recommend the use of a combination product. This product contains aluminum hydroxide, magnesium hydroxide, and simethicone.
Antacids containing sodium may result in fluid retention.	• Teach clients with hypertension or heart failure to avoid antacids that contain sodium.
Aluminum hydroxide can lead to hypophosphatemia.	• Monitor the client's phosphate level.
Magnesium compounds can lead to toxicity in clients with renal impairment.	• Teach clients with renal impairment to avoid antacids that contain magnesium.

Contraindications/Precautions

- Antacids are Pregnancy Risk Category C.
- Antacids should be not administered to clients who have GI perforation or obstruction.
- Use cautiously in clients who have abdominal pain.

Interactions

MEDICATION/FOOD INTERACTIONS	NURSING INTERVENTIONS/CLIENT EDUCATION
Aluminum compounds bind to warfarin and tetracycline and interfere with absorption.	• Teach clients to take these medications 1 hr apart.

Nursing Administration

- Clients taking tablets should be instructed to chew the tablets thoroughly and then drink at least 8 oz of water or milk.
- Teach clients to shake liquid formulations to ensure even dispersion of the medication.
- Compliance is difficult for clients because of the frequency of administration. Medication may be administered seven times a day: 1 hr and 3 hr after meals, and again at bedtime. Encourage compliance by reinforcing the intended effect of the antacid (such as relief of pain, healing of ulcer).
- Teach clients to take all medications at least 1 hr before or after taking an antacid.

MEDICATION CLASSIFICATION: PROSTAGLANDIN E ANALOG

- Select Prototype Medication: misoprostol (Cytotec)

Purpose

- Expected Pharmacological Action
  - Prostaglandin E analog acts as an endogenous prostaglandin in the GI tract to decrease acid secretion, increase the secretion of bicarbonate and protective mucus, and promote vasodilation to maintain submucosal blood flow. These actions all serve to prevent gastric ulcers.
- Therapeutic Uses
  - Prostaglandin E analog is used in clients taking long-term NSAIDs to prevent gastric ulcers.
  - Prostaglandin E analog is used in clients who are pregnant to induce labor by causing cervical ripening.

Complications

SIDE/ADVERSE EFFECTS	NURSING INTERVENTIONS/CLIENT EDUCATION
Diarrhea and abdominal pain	• Instruct clients to notify the provider of symptoms of diarrhea or abdominal pain. • Dosage may need to be reduced.
Women may experience dysmenorrhea and spotting.	• Instruct clients to notify the provider if dysmenorrhea and spotting occur. • The provider may discontinue the medication.

Contraindications/Precautions

- Pregnancy Risk Category X

Nursing Administration

- Teach clients to take misoprostol with meals and at bedtime.

Nursing Evaluation of Medication Effectiveness

- Depending on therapeutic intent, effectiveness may be evidenced by:
  - Reduced frequency or absence of GERD symptoms (heartburn, bloating, belching)
  - Absence of GI bleeding
  - Healing of gastric and duodenal ulcers
  - No reoccurrence of ulcer

CHAPTER 28: PEPTIC ULCER DISEASE

Application Exercises

1. A nurse is teaching a client with PUD how to properly self-administer ranitidine (Zantac). Which of the following client statements indicates effective teaching by the nurse?

    A. "I should call my doctor if my stools look black and sticky."

    B. "I will take Zantac regularly until my burning symptoms disappear."

    C. "I need to take Zantac on an empty stomach."

    D. "I can take ibuprofen if I have minor aches and pains."

2. A nurse is caring for a client who is starting omeprazole (Prilosec) PO for management of GERD. The nurse should recognize that this medication works by

    A. improving gastric motility.

    B. decreasing the production of gastric acid.

    C. neutralizing gastric acid.

    D. antagonizing serotonin receptors.

3. A client taking sucralfate (Carafate) PO for peptic ulcer disease has been started on phenytoin (Dilantin) to control seizures. Which of the following should be included in the client's teaching?

    A. Take both of these medications at the same time.

    B. Take sucralfate with a glass of milk.

    C. Allow a 2-hr interval between these medications.

    D. Chew the sucralfate thoroughly before swallowing.

4. For which of the following clients with peptic ulcer disease is misoprostol (Cytotec) contraindicated?

    A. 27-year-old client who is pregnant

    B. 75-year-old client with osteoarthritis

    C. 37-year-old client with a kidney stone

    D. 46-year-old client with a urinary tract infection

CHAPTER 28: PEPTIC ULCER DISEASE

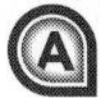

Application Exercises Answer Key

1. A nurse is teaching a client with PUD how to properly self-administer ranitidine (Zantac). Which of the following client statements indicates effective teaching by the nurse?

   A. "I should call my doctor if my stools look black and sticky."

   B. "I will take Zantac regularly until my burning symptoms disappear."

   C. "I need to take Zantac on an empty stomach."

   D. "I can take ibuprofen if I have minor aches and pains."

   Clients need to notify the provider if signs of GI bleeding develop. Symptom relief is not indicative of ulcer healing. Ranitidine can be taken without regard to food, and NSAIDs, such as ibuprofen, should be avoided for clients with PUD due to the risk of bleeding.

NCLEX® Connection: Pharmacological and Parenteral Therapies: Medication Administration

2. A nurse is caring for a client who is starting omeprazole (Prilosec) PO for management of GERD. The nurse should recognize that this medication works by

   A. improving gastric motility.

   B. decreasing the production of gastric acid.

   C. neutralizing gastric acid.

   D. antagonizing serotonin receptors.

   Omeprazole reduces gastric acid secretion by irreversibly inhibiting the enzyme that produces gastric acid. Gastric motility is improved by metoclopramide (Reglan), a prokinetic agent. Gastric acid is neutralized by aluminum hydroxide, an antacid. Ondansetron (Zofran), an antiemetic, antagonizes serotonin receptors, decreasing nausea and vomiting.

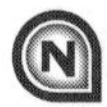

NCLEX® Connection: Pharmacological and Parenteral Therapies: Expected Actions/ Outcomes

3. A client taking sucralfate (Carafate) PO for peptic ulcer disease has been started on phenytoin (Dilantin) to control seizures. Which of the following should be included in the client's teaching?

   A. Take both of these medications at the same time.

   B. Take sucralfate with a glass of milk.

   C. Allow a 2-hr interval between these medications.

   D. Chew the sucralfate thoroughly before swallowing.

   Sucralfate can interfere with the absorption of phenytoin, so the client should allow a 2-hr interval between the sucralfate and phenytoin. Sucralfate should be taken on an empty stomach and it should be swallowed whole.

NCLEX® Connection: Pharmacological and Parenteral Therapies: Expected Actions/ Outcomes

4. For which of the following clients with peptic ulcer disease is misoprostol (Cytotec) contraindicated?

A. 27-year-old client who is pregnant

B. 75-year-old client with osteoarthritis

C. 37-year-old client with a kidney stone

D. 46-year-old client with a urinary tract infection

Misoprostol can induce labor, and therefore is contraindicated in pregnancy. There are no contraindications for use in clients with osteoarthritis, kidney stones, or urinary tract infection.

NCLEX® Connection: Pharmacological and Parenteral Therapies: Adverse Effects/ Contraindications/Side Effects/Interactions

UNIT 6 MEDICATIONS AFFECTING THE GASTROINTESTINAL SYSTEM AND NUTRITION

Chapter 29 Gastrointestinal Disorders

Overview

- The medications in this section affect some aspect of the GI tract to treat or prevent nausea/vomiting, motion sickness, diarrhea, constipation, or to treat GERD by increasing gastric motility.
- Medications include antiemetics, laxatives, antidiarrheals, prokinetic agents, and medications for irritable bowel syndrome.

MEDICATION CLASSIFICATION: ANTIEMETICS

- Select Prototype Medications:
  - Glucocorticoids: dexamethasone (Decadron)
  - Substance P/Neurokinin$_1$ Antagonists: aprepitant (Emend)
  - Serotonin antagonists: ondansetron (Zofran), granisetron (Kytril);
  - Dopamine antagonists: prochlorperazine (Compazine), metoclopramide (Reglan), promethazine (Phenergan)
  - Cannabinoids: dronabinol (Marinol)
  - Anticholinergics: scopolamine (Transderm Scop)
  - Antihistamine: dimenhydrinate (Dramamine), hydroxyzine (Vistaril),
  - Benzodiazepines: lorazepam (Ativan), diazepam (Valium)

Purpose

EXPECTED PHARMACOLOGICAL ACTION	THERAPEUTIC USES
Glucocorticoids: dexamethasone	
The antiemetic mechanism of dexamethasone is unknown.	• Dexamethasone is usually used in combination with other antiemetics to treat chemotherapy-induced nausea and vomiting (CINV). • Administer PO or IV.
Substance P/neurokinin$_1$ antagonists: aprepitant	
Aprepitant inhibits Substance P/neurokinin$_1$ in the brain.	• For best results, it should be used in combination with a glucocorticoid or serotonin antagonist. • Extended duration of action makes it effective for immediate use and delayed response.
Serotonin antagonist: ondansetron	
Ondansetron prevents emesis by blocking the serotonin receptors in the chemoreceptor trigger zone (CTZ), and antagonizing the serotonin receptors on the afferent vagal neurons that travel from the upper GI tract to the CTZ.	• Ondansetron prevents emesis related to chemotherapy, radiation therapy, and postoperative recovery. • Administer PO or IV.
Dopamine antagonists: prochlorperazine (a subset of phenothiazine)	
Antiemetic effects of prochlorperazine result from blockade of dopamine receptors in the CTZ.	• Prochlorperazine prevents emesis related to chemotherapy, opioids, and postoperative recovery. • Administer PO or IV.
Cannabinoids: dronabinol	
Antiemetic mechanism of dronabinol is unknown.	• Dronabinol is used to control CINV and to increase appetite in clients who have AIDS. • Administer PO.
Scopolamine interferes with the transmission of nerve impulses traveling from the vestibular apparatus of the inner ear to the vomiting center (VC) in the brain.	• Scopolamine treats motion sickness. • Administer topical, PO, or subcutaneously.
Muscarinic and histaminergic receptors in nerve pathways that connect the inner ear and VC are blocked by dimenhydrinate.	• Dimenhydrinate treats motion sickness. • Administer PO, IM, or IV.

Complications

SIDE/ADVERSE EFFECTS	NURSING INTERVENTIONS/CLIENT EDUCATION
Substance P/neurokinin antagonist: aprepitant	
Fatigue, diarrhea, dizziness, possible liver damage	• Treat headache with non-opioid analgesics. • Monitor stool pattern.
Serotonin antagonist: ondansetron	
Headache, diarrhea, dizziness	• Treat headache with non-opioid analgesics. • Monitor stool pattern.
Dopamine antagonists: prochlorperazine	
Extrapyramidal symptoms (EPS)	• Inform clients of possible side effects (restlessness, anxiety, spasms of face and neck). • Advise clients to stop the medication and inform the provider if EPS occur. • Administer an anticholinergic medication, such as diphenhydramine (Benadryl), to treat symptoms.
Hypotension	• Monitor clients receiving antihypertensive medications for low blood pressure.
Sedation	• Inform clients of the potential for sedation. • Advise clients to avoid activities that require alertness, such as driving.
Anticholinergic effects (dry mouth, urinary retention, constipation)	• Instruct clients to increase fluid intake. • Instruct clients to increase physical activity by engaging in regular exercise. • Tell clients to suck on hard candy or chew gum to help relieve dry mouth. • Administer a stimulant laxative, such as senna (Senokot) to counteract a decrease in bowel motility, or stool softeners, such as docusate sodium (Colace), to prevent constipation. • Advise clients to void every 4 hr. Monitor I&O and palpate the client's lower abdomen area every 4 to 6 hr to assess the client's bladder.
Cannabinoids: dronabinol	
Potential for dissociation, dysphoria	• Avoid using in clients with mental health disorders.
Hypotension, tachycardia	• Use cautiously in clients with cardiovascular disorders.

SIDE/ADVERSE EFFECTS	NURSING INTERVENTIONS/CLIENT EDUCATION
Anticholinergics: scopolamine and antihistamines: dimenhydrinate	
Sedation	• Inform clients of the potential for sedation. • Advise clients to avoid activities that require alertness, such as driving.
Anticholinergic effects (dry mouth, urinary retention, constipation)	• Instruct clients to increase fluid intake. • Instruct clients to increase physical activity by engaging in regular exercise. • Tell clients to suck on hard candy or chew gum to help relieve dry mouth. • Administer a stimulant laxative, such as senna, to counteract a decrease in bowel motility or stool softeners, such as docusate sodium, to prevent constipation. • Advise clients to void every 4 hr, monitor I&O, and palpate the client's lower abdomen area every 4 to 6 hr to assess the bladder.

Contraindications/Precautions

- Use dopamine antagonists cautiously, if at all, with children and older adults due to the increased risk of extrapyramidal side effects.
- Dopamine antagonists, antihistamines, and anticholinergic antiemetics should be used cautiously in clients with urinary retention or obstruction, asthma, and narrow angle glaucoma.

Interactions

MEDICATION/FOOD INTERACTIONS	NURSING INTERVENTIONS/CLIENT EDUCATION
CNS depressants, such as opioids and alcohol can intensify CNS depression of antiemetics.	• Advise clients that CNS depression is more likely and to avoid activities that require mental alertness.
Concurrent use of antihypertensives can intensify hypotensive effects of antiemetics.	• Advise clients to sit or lie down if symptoms of lightheadedness or dizziness occur. Clients should avoid sudden changes in position by moving slowly from a lying to a sitting or standing position. • Provide assistance with ambulation as needed.
Concurrent use of anticholinergic medications (antihistamines) can intensify anticholinergic effects of antiemetics.	• Provide teaching to reduce anticholinergic effects (sipping on fluids, use of laxatives, voiding on a regular basis).

Nursing Administration

- Antiemetics prevent or treat nausea and vomiting from various causes. Match the medication with the cause.
- When a client is receiving a chemotherapy agent that causes severe nausea, combining three antiemetics and administering them prior to chemotherapy is more effective than treating nausea that is already occurring.

Nursing Evaluation of Medication Effectiveness

- Depending on therapeutic intent, effectiveness may be evidenced by:
  - Absence of nausea and vomiting.

MEDICATION CLASSIFICATION: LAXATIVES

- Select Prototype Medications:
  - Psyllium (Metamucil)
  - Docusate sodium (Colace)
  - Bisacodyl (Dulcolax)
  - Magnesium hydroxide (Milk of Magnesia)
- Other Medications: senna (Senokot), lactulose

Purpose

EXPECTED PHARMACOLOGICAL ACTION	THERAPEUTIC USES
Bulk-forming laxatives: psyllium	
Bulk-forming laxatives soften fecal mass and increase bulk, which is identical to the action of dietary fiber.	• Decrease diarrhea in clients with diverticulosis and irritable bowel syndrome (IBS) • Control stool for clients with an ileostomy or colostomy • Promote defecation in older adults with decrease in peristalsis due to age-related changes in the GI tract
Surfactant laxatives: docusate sodium	
Surfactant laxatives lower surface tension of the stool to allow penetration of water.	• Constipation related to pregnancy or opioid use • Prevention of painful elimination in clients with conditions such as hemorrhoids or following a procedure such as episiotomy • Prevention of straining in clients with conditions such as cerebral aneurysm or post MI • Decrease the risk of fecal impaction in immobile clients and promote defecation in older adults with decreased peristalsis due to age-related changes in the GI tract

EXPECTED PHARMACOLOGICAL ACTION	THERAPEUTIC USES
Stimulant laxatives: bisacodyl	
Stimulant laxatives result in stimulation of intestinal peristalsis.	• Client preparation prior to surgery or diagnostic tests such as a colonoscopy • Short-term treatment of constipation caused by high-dose opioid use
Osmotic laxatives: magnesium hydroxide	
Osmotic laxatives draw water into the intestine to increase the mass of stool, stretching musculature, which results in peristalsis.	• Low dose – Prevent painful elimination (clients with episiotomy or hemorrhoids) • High dose – Client preparation prior to surgery or diagnostic tests such as a colonoscopy • Rapid evacuation of the bowel after ingestion of poisons or following antihelminthic therapy to rid the body of dead parasites

Complications

SIDE/ADVERSE EFFECTS	NURSING INTERVENTIONS/CLIENT EDUCATION
GI irritation	• Instruct clients not to crush or chew enteric-coated tablets.
Rectal burning sensation, leading to proctitis	• Discourage clients from using bisacodyl suppositories on a regular basis.
Laxatives with magnesium salts, such as magnesium hydroxide, can lead to accumulation of toxic levels of magnesium.	• Advise clients with renal dysfunction to read labels carefully and to avoid laxatives that contain magnesium.
Laxatives with sodium salts, such as sodium phosphate, place clients at risk for sodium absorption and fluid retention.	• Advise clients with heart disease to read labels carefully and to avoid laxatives that contain sodium.
Osmotic diuretics may cause dehydration.	• Monitor I&O. • Monitor/assess for signs of dehydration, such as poor skin turgor. • Encourage clients to increase water intake to at least 8 to 10 glasses of water/day.

Contraindications/Precautions

- Laxatives are contraindicated in clients with fecal impaction, bowel obstruction, and acute surgical abdomen to prevent perforation.
- Laxatives are contraindicated in clients with nausea, cramping, and abdominal pain.
- These medications are contraindicated in clients with ulcerative colitis and diverticulitis with the exception of bulk-forming laxatives .
- Use cautiously during pregnancy and lactation.

Interactions

MEDICATION/FOOD INTERACTIONS	NURSING INTERVENTIONS/CLIENT EDUCATION
Milk and antacids can destroy enteric coating of bisacodyl.	• Instruct clients to take bisacodyl at least 1 hr apart from these medications.

Nursing Administration

- Obtain a complete history of laxative use and provide teaching as appropriate.
- Teach clients that chronic laxative use can lead to fluid and electrolyte imbalances.
- To promote defecation and resumption of normal bowel function, instruct clients to increase high-fiber foods in daily diet such as bran, fresh fruits and vegetables and increased amounts of fluids. Recommend at least 2 to 3 L/day from beverages and food sources.
- Encourage clients to maintain a regular exercise regimen to improve bowel function.
- Instruct clients to take bulk-forming and surfactant laxatives with a glass of water.

Nursing Evaluation of Medication Effectiveness

- Depending on therapeutic intent, effectiveness may be evidenced by:
    - Return to regular bowel function.
    - Evacuation of bowel in preparation for surgery or diagnostic tests.

MEDICATION CLASSIFICATION: ANTIDIARRHEALS

- Select Prototype Medication: diphenoxylate plus atropine (Lomotil)
- Other Medications: loperamide (Imodium), difenoxin (Motofen)

Purpose

- Expected Pharmacological Action
    - Antidiarrheals activate opioid receptors in the GI tract to decrease intestinal motility and to increase the absorption of fluid and sodium in the intestine.
- Therapeutic Uses
    - Specific antidiarrheal agents may be used to treat the underlying cause of diarrhea. For example, antibiotics may be used to treat diarrhea caused by a bacterial infection.
    - Nonspecific antidiarrheal agents provide symptomatic treatment of diarrhea (decrease in frequency and fluid content of stool).

Complications

- At recommended doses for diarrhea, diphenoxylate does not affect the CNS system.
- At high doses, clients may experience typical opioid effects, such as euphoria or CNS depression. However, the addition of atropine, which has unpleasant adverse effects (blurred vision, dry mouth, urinary retention, constipation, tachycardia) in diphenoxylate discourages ingestion of doses higher than those prescribed.

Contraindications/Precautions

- There is an increased risk of megacolon in clients with inflammatory bowel disorders. This could lead to a serious complication such as perforation of the bowel.

Interactions

- Alcohol or other CNS depressants may enhance CNS depression.

Nursing Administration

- Administer initial dose of diphenoxylate, 4 mg; follow each loose stool with additional dose of 2 mg, but do not exceed 16 mg/day.
- Loperamide is an analog of the opioid meperidine. This medication is not a controlled substance, and at high doses loperamide does not mimic morphine-like symptoms.
- Advise clients with diarrhea to drink small amounts of clear liquids or a commercial oral electrolyte solution to maintain electrolyte balance for the first 24 hr.
- Advise clients to avoid drinking plain water because it does not contain necessary electrolytes that have been lost in the stool.
- Advise clients to avoid caffeine. Caffeine exacerbates diarrhea by increasing GI motility.
- Clients with severe cases of diarrhea may be hospitalized for management of dehydration.
- Management of dehydration should include monitoring of weight, I&O, and vital signs. A hypotonic solution such as 0.45% sodium chloride may be prescribed.

Nursing Evaluation of Medication Effectiveness

- Depending on therapeutic intent, effectiveness may be evidenced by:
  - Return of normal bowel pattern as evidenced by decrease in frequency and fluid volume of stool.

MEDICATION CLASSIFICATION: PROKINETIC AGENTS

- Select Prototype Medication: metoclopramide (Reglan)

Purpose

- Expected Pharmacological Action
  - Metoclopramide controls nausea and vomiting by blocking dopamine and serotonin receptors in the CTZ.
  - Metoclopramide augments action of acetylcholine, which causes an increase in upper GI motility.
- Therapeutic Uses
  - Control of postoperative and chemotherapy-induced nausea and vomiting
  - Management of GERD and gastroparesis

Complications

SIDE/ADVERSE EFFECTS	NURSING INTERVENTIONS/CLIENT EDUCATION
Extrapyramidal symptoms (EPS)	• Inform clients of the possible side effects, such as restlessness, anxiety, and spasms of face and neck. • Administer an antihistamine, such as diphenhydramine, to minimize extrapyramidal symptoms.
Sedation	• Inform clients of the potential for sedation. • Advise clients to avoid activities that require alertness, such as driving.
Diarrhea	• Monitor the client's bowel function and for signs of dehydration.

Contraindications/Precautions

- Contraindicated in clients with GI perforation, GI bleeding, bowel obstruction, and hemorrhage
- Contraindicated in clients with a seizure disorder due to increased risk of seizures
- Use cautiously in children and older adults due to the increase risk for EPS.

Interactions

MEDICATION/FOOD INTERACTIONS	NURSING INTERVENTIONS/CLIENT EDUCATION
Concurrent use of alcohol and other CNS depressants increases the risk of seizures and sedation.	• Advise clients to avoid the use of alcohol. • Use cautiously with other CNS depressants.
Opioids and anticholinergics decrease the effects of metoclopramide.	• Advise clients to avoid using opioids and medications with anticholinergic effects.

Nursing Administration

- Monitor clients for CNS depression and EPS.
- The medication can be given orally or intravenously. If IV dose is less than or equal to 10 mg, it may be administered IVP undiluted over 2 min. If the dose is greater than 10 mg, it should be diluted and infused over 15 min. Dilute medication in at least 50 mL of dextrose 5% in water or lactated Ringer's solution.

Nursing Evaluation of Medication Effectiveness

- Depending on therapeutic intent, effectiveness may be evidenced by:
  - Absence of nausea and vomiting

MEDICATION CLASSIFICATION: MEDICATIONS FOR IRRITABLE BOWEL SYNDROME WITH DIARRHEA (IBS-D)

- Select Prototype Medication: alosetron (Lotronex)

Purpose

- Expected Pharmacological Action
  - Selective blockade of 5-HT3 receptors, which innervate the viscera and result in increased firmness in stool and decrease in urgency and frequency of defecation
- Therapeutic Uses
  - For female clients who have had irritable bowel syndrome with diarrhea that has lasted more than 6 months and has been resistant to conventional management

Complications

SIDE/ADVERSE EFFECTS	NURSING INTERVENTIONS/CLIENT EDUCATION
Constipation, which may result in GI toxicity such as ischemic colitis, bowel obstruction, impaction or perforation.	• Only clients who meet specific criteria and are willing to sign a treatment agreement may be prescribed medication. • Instruct clients to watch for rectal bleeding, bloody diarrhea, or abdominal pain and report to the provider. Medication should be discontinued.

Contraindications/Precautions

- Contraindicated for clients with chronic constipation, history of bowel obstruction, Crohn's disease, ulcerative colitis, impaired intestinal circulation, or thrombophlebitis

Interactions

MEDICATION/FOOD INTERACTIONS	NURSING INTERVENTIONS/CLIENT EDUCATION
Medications that induce cytochrome P450 enzymes, such as phenobarbital, may decrease levels of alosetron.	Monitor the effectiveness of medication.

Nursing Administration

- Instruct clients that symptoms should resolve within 1 to 4 weeks but will return 1 week after medication is discontinued.
- Dosage will start as once a day and may be increased to BID.

Nursing Evaluation of Medication Effectiveness

- Depending on therapeutic intent, effectiveness may be evidenced by:
    - Relief of diarrhea, decrease in urgency and frequency of defecation.

MEDICATION CLASSIFICATION: MEDICATIONS FOR IRRITABLE BOWEL SYNDROME WITH CONSTIPATION (IBS-C)

- Select Prototype Medication: lubiprostone (Amitiza)

Purpose

- Expected Pharmacological Action
    - Increases fluid secretion in the intestine to promote intestinal motility
- Therapeutic Uses
    - Irritable bowel syndrome with constipation
    - Chronic constipation

Complications

SIDE/ADVERSE EFFECTS	NURSING INTERVENTIONS/CLIENT EDUCATION
Diarrhea	Monitor frequency of stools. Notify provider if severe diarrhea occurs.
Nausea	Instruct clients to take the medication with food.

Contraindications/Precautions

- Pregnancy Risk Category C
- Contraindicated for clients with a history of bowel obstruction, Crohn's disease, ulcerative colitis, or diverticulitis

Interactions

- No significant interactions

Nursing Administration

- Instruct clients to take the medication with food to decrease nausea.
- Oral dosage should be taken BID.

Nursing Evaluation of Medication Effectiveness

- Depending on therapeutic intent, effectiveness may be evidenced by:
  - Relief of constipation

MEDICATION CLASSIFICATION: 5-AMINOSALICYLATES

- Select Prototype Medication: sulfasalazine (Azulfidine)
- Other Medications:
  - 5-aminosalicylates: mesalamine (Asacol, Rowasa)
  - Glucocorticoids, such as hydrocortisone
  - Immunosuppressants, such as azathioprine (Imuran)
  - Immunomodulators such as infliximab (Remicade)
  - Antibiotics, such as metronidazole (Flagyl)

Purpose

- Expected Pharmacological Action
  - Decrease inflammation by inhibiting prostaglandin synthesis
- Therapeutic Uses
  - Inflammatory bowel disease: Crohn's disease, ulcerative colitis

Complications

SIDE/ADVERSE EFFECTS	NURSING INTERVENTIONS/CLIENT EDUCATION
Blood disorders including agranulocytosis, hemolytic and macrocytic anemia	Monitor client's complete blood count

Contraindications/Precautions

- These medications are Pregnancy Risk Category B
- These medications are contraindicated in clients with sensitivity to sulfonamides, salicylates, and/or thiazide diuretics.
- Use cautiously in older adults and in clients with liver or kidney disease or blood dyscrasias.

Interactions

- No significant interactions

Nursing Administration

- Administer in 4 divided oral doses throughout the day.

Nursing Evaluation of Medication Effectiveness

- Depending on therapeutic intent, effectiveness may be evidenced by:
    - Decreased bowel inflammation
    - Return to normal bowel function

CHAPTER 29: GASTROINTESTINAL DISORDERS

Application Exercises

1. For which of the following clients is a laxative indicated? (Select all that apply.)

_____ A young adult female who is postpartum following a vaginal delivery with an episiotomy

_____ A young adult male with constipation and periumbilical pain

_____ A young adult client affected by IBS

_____ An older adult client with limited mobility and minor bowel incontinence

_____ A older adult client preparing for a colonoscopy

2. Children and older adults are usually not administered prochlorperazine (Compazine) for nausea and vomiting due to the increased risk for __________.

3. Laxatives containing sodium are contraindicated for which of the following client conditions?

A. Hypertension
B. Arthritis
C. Depression
D. Seizure disorder

4. A nurse is taking a history for a client who has irritable bowel syndrome with constipation. Which of the following in the client's history is a contraindication to lubiprostone (Amitiza)?

A. Myocardial infarction
B. Ulcerative colitis
C. Diabetes mellitus
D. Rheumatoid arthritis

CHAPTER 29: GASTROINTESTINAL DISORDERS

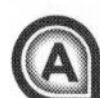

Application Exercises Answer Key

1. For which of the following clients is a laxative indicated? (Select all that apply.)

 X **A young adult female who is postpartum following a vaginal delivery with an episiotomy**

 ___ A young adult male with constipation and periumbilical pain

 X **A young adult client affected by IBS**

 ___ An older adult client with limited mobility and minor bowel incontinence

 X **A older adult client preparing for a colonoscopy**

Laxatives will prevent straining until the episiotomy heals. Bulk-forming laxatives can provide relief of diarrhea for clients with IBS. Laxatives are used for bowel cleansing prior to diagnostic procedures of the GI tract. Appendicitis can begin in the periumbilical area before progressing to the right lower quadrant. The older adult may be experiencing fecal impaction and a laxative could cause perforation.

NCLEX® Connection: Pharmacological and Parenteral Therapies: Expected Actions/ Outcomes

2. Children and older adults are usually not administered prochlorperazine (Compazine) for nausea and vomiting due to the increased risk for ___________.

Extrapyramidal symptoms such as restlessness, anxiety, and spasms of the face and neck are more common in children and older adults.

NCLEX® Connection: Pharmacological and Parenteral Therapies: Adverse Effects/ Contraindications/Side Effects/Interactions

3. Laxatives containing sodium are contraindicated for which of the following client conditions?

A. Hypertension

B. Arthritis

C. Depression

D. Seizure disorder

Laxatives containing sodium can lead to sodium and water retention, which could exacerbate hypertension. Laxatives with sodium are not contraindicated for arthritis, depression, or seizure disorders.

NCLEX® Connection: Pharmacological and Parenteral Therapies: Adverse Effects/ Contraindications/Side Effects/Interactions

4. A nurse is taking a history for a client who has irritable bowel syndrome with constipation. Which of the following in the client's history is a contraindication to lubiprostone (Amitiza)?

   A. Myocardial infarction

   B. Ulcerative colitis

   C. Diabetes mellitus

   D. Rheumatoid arthritis

   A client with ulcerative colitis should not be prescribed lubiprostone. Myocardial infarction, diabetes mellitus, and rheumatoid arthritis are not contraindications to lubiprostone.

NCLEX® Connection: Pharmacological and Parenteral Therapies: Adverse Effects/ Contraindications/Side Effects/Interactions

UNIT 6 MEDICATIONS AFFECTING THE GASTROINTESTINAL SYSTEM AND NUTRITION

Chapter 30 Vitamins, Minerals, and Supplements

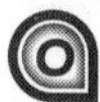 Overview

- The vitamins and minerals described in this section affect production of red blood cells and help prevent various types of anemia.
- Potassium and magnesium regulate body fluid volume. Supplements of these substances prevent multiple serious conditions.
- Categories of medications in this section:
  - Vitamins, including vitamin B_{12} and folic acid
  - Iron supplements
  - Potassium and magnesium supplements
  - Various herbal supplements

MEDICATION CLASSIFICATION: IRON PREPARATIONS

- Select Prototype Medications:
  - Oral: Ferrous sulfate (Feosol)
  - Parenteral: Iron dextran (INFeD)
- Other Medications:
  - Oral: ferrous gluconate (Fergon), ferrous fumarate (Ferro-Sequels)
  - Parenteral: Iron sucrose (Venofer), sodium-ferric gluconate complex (SFGC) (Ferrlecit)

Purpose

- Expected Pharmacological Action
  - Iron preparations provide iron needed for RBC development and oxygen transport to cells. During times of increased growth (in growing children or during pregnancy) or when RBCs are in high demand (after blood loss), the need for iron may be greatly increased. Iron is poorly absorbed by the body, so relatively large amounts must be ingested orally to increase Hgb and Hct levels.

- Therapeutic Uses
  - Iron preparations are used to treat iron-deficiency anemia.
    - Iron sucrose and SFGC are used solely for clients who are undergoing long-term hemodialysis and are deficient in iron.
  - Iron preparations are used to prevent iron deficiency anemia for clients who are at an increased risk, such as pregnant women, infants, and children
  - Parenteral forms should only be used in clients who are unable to take oral medications. IV route is preferred.

Complications

SIDE/ADVERSE EFFECTS	NURSING INTERVENTIONS/CLIENT EDUCATION
GI distress (nausea, constipation, heartburn)	• If intolerable, administer medication with food, but this greatly reduces absorption. • May need to reduce dosage. • Monitor the client's bowel pattern and intervene as appropriate. This side effect usually resolves with continued use.
Teeth staining (liquid form)	• Teach clients to dilute liquid iron with water or juice, drink with a straw, and rinse mouth after swallowing.
Staining of skin and other tissues with IM injections	• Give IM doses deep IM using Z track technique. • Avoid this route if possible.
Anaphylaxis risk with parenteral administration	• IV route is safer. • Administer a test dose and observe the client closely. • Give subsequent doses slowly at no more than 12.4 mg/min. • Be prepared with life-support equipment.
Hypotension, which may progress to circulatory collapse with parenteral administration	• Monitor vital signs when administering parenteral iron.
Fatal iron toxicity in children may occur when an overdose of iron (2-10 g) is ingested.	• Symptoms of toxicity include severe GI symptoms, shock, acidosis, liver and heart failure. A chelating agent, deferoxamine (Desferal), given parenterally, is used to treat toxicity.

Contraindications/Precautions

- Contraindicated for clients with
  - Previous hypersensitivity to iron
  - Hemolytic anemia, peptic ulcer disease, and severe liver disease

Interactions

MEDICATION/FOOD INTERACTIONS	NURSING INTERVENTIONS/CLIENT EDUCATION
Coadministration of antacids or tetracyclines reduces absorption of iron.	• Separate use by at least 2 hr.
Vitamin C increases absorption, but also increases incidence of GI complications.	• Avoid vitamin C intake when taking medication.

Nursing Administration

- Instruct clients to take iron on an empty stomach such as 1 hr before meals to maximize absorption. Stomach acid increases absorption.
- Instruct clients to take with food if GI adverse effects occur. This may increase adherence to therapy even though absorption is also decreased.
- Instruct clients to space doses at approximately equal intervals throughout day to most efficiently increase red blood cell production. Inform clients to anticipate a harmless dark green or black color of stool.
- Teach clients to dilute liquid iron with water or juice, drink with a straw, and rinse the mouth after swallowing.
- Instruct clients to increase water and fiber intake (unless contraindicated), and to maintain an exercise program to counter the constipation effects.
- Advise clients that therapy may last 1 to 2 months. Usually, dietary intake will be sufficient after Hgb levels return to appropriate level.
- Encourage concurrent intake of appropriate quantities of foods high in iron (liver, egg yolks, muscle meats, yeast).

Nursing Evaluation of Medication Effectiveness

- Depending on therapeutic intent, effectiveness may be evidenced by the following:
  - Increase in reticulocyte count is expected by at least 1 week after beginning iron therapy.
  - Increase in hemoglobin of 2 g/dL is expected one month after beginning therapy (Fatigue and pallor subsided or client reports increased energy level, client's skin and mucous membrane color no longer demonstrate pallor).

MEDICATION CLASSIFICATION: VITAMIN B_{12}-CYANOCOBALAMIN

- Select Prototype Medication: vitamin B_{12}
- Other Medications: intranasal cyanocobalamin (Nascobal)

Purpose

- Expected Pharmacological Action
  - Vitamin B_{12} is necessary to convert folic acid from its inactive form to its active form. All cells rely on folic acid for DNA production.
  - Vitamin B_{12} may be administered to prevent or correct a deficiency of this vitamin, which results in megaloblastic anemia (macrocytic) and can cause fatal heart failure if not corrected.
  - Damage to rapidly multiplying cells can affect the skin and mucous membranes, causing GI disturbances. Neurologic damage, which includes numbness and tingling of extremities and CNS damage, may result from deficiency of this vitamin.
  - In addition, a deficiency affects all blood cells and can cause infection and bleeding as well as signs of anemia.
  - Loss of intrinsic factor within the cells of the stomach causes inability to absorb vitamin B_{12}, making it necessary to administer parenteral or intranasal vitamin B_{12} or high doses of oral B_{12} for the rest of the client's life.
- Therapeutic uses
  - Treatment of vitamin B_{12} deficiency
  - Megaloblastic (macrocytic) anemia related to vitamin B_{12} deficiency

Complications

SIDE/ADVERSE EFFECTS	NURSING INTERVENTIONS/CLIENT EDUCATION
Hypokalemia secondary to the increased RBC production effects of vitamin B_{12}	• Monitor the client's potassium levels during the start of treatment. • Observe clients for findings of potassium deficiency (muscle weakness, abnormal cardiac rhythm). • Client may require potassium supplements.

 Contraindications/Precautions

- Vitamin B_{12} deficiency should never be treated only with folic acid. If folic acid is used for a client with vitamin B_{12} deficiency, ensure that dosage is adequate.

Interactions

MEDICATION/FOOD INTERACTIONS	NURSING INTERVENTIONS/CLIENT EDUCATION
Masking of signs of vitamin B_{12} deficiency with concurrent administration of folic acid	• Make sure that clients receive adequate doses of vitamin B_{12} when using folic acid.

Nursing Administration

- Obtain baseline vitamin B_{12}, Hgb, Hct, RBC, and reticulocyte counts. Monitor periodically.
- Monitor clients for signs of vitamin B_{12} deficiency such as beefy red tongue, pallor, neuropathy.
- Cyanocobalamin may be administered intranasally, orally, or by IM or SC injection. Injections are painful and are usually reserved for individuals with significant reduced ability to absorb vitamin B_{12} such as lack of intrinsic factor [pernicious anemia], enteritis, and partial removal of stomach.
- Clients with malabsorption syndrome can use intranasal preparation or parenteral preparation.
- Intranasal cyanocobalamin should be administered 1 hr before or after eating hot foods, which can cause the medication to be removed from nasal passages without being absorbed.
- Clients with irreversible malabsorption syndrome (parietal cell atrophy or total gastrectomy) will need lifelong treatment, usually parenterally. If oral therapy is used, doses must be very high.
    - Encourage concurrent intake of appropriate quantities of foods high in vitamin B_{12}, such as dairy products.
    - Perform Schillings test to determine vitamin B_{12} absorption in the gastrointestinal tract. Measurement of plasma B_{12} levels helps to determine need for therapy.
    - Advise clients to adhere to prescribed laboratory tests. Blood counts and vitamin B_{12} levels should be monitored every 3 to 6 months.

Nursing Evaluation of Medication Effectiveness

- Depending on therapeutic intent, effectiveness may be evidenced by:
    - Improvement of megaloblastic anemia as evidenced by increased reticulocyte count, absence of megaloblast in bone marrow, macrocytes in blood, and normal or increased Hgb and Hct levels.
    - Improvement of neurologic symptoms such as absence of tingling sensation of hands and feet, numbness of extremities. Improvement may take months, and some clients will never attain full recovery.

MEDICATION CLASSIFICATION: FOLIC ACID

- Select Prototype Medication: folic acid

Purpose

- Expected Pharmacological Action
  - Folic acid is essential in the production of DNA and erythropoiesis (RBC, WBC, and platelets).
- Therapeutic Uses
  - Treatment of megaloblastic (macrocytic) anemia secondary to folic acid deficiency
  - Prevention of neural tube defects during pregnancy; therefore it is needed in all women of child-bearing age who may become pregnant
  - Treatment of malabsorption syndrome such as sprue

Contraindications/Precautions

- Indiscriminate use of folic acid is inappropriate because of the risk of masking signs of vitamin B_{12} deficiency.

Interactions

MEDICATION/FOOD INTERACTIONS	NURSING INTERVENTIONS/CLIENT EDUCATION
Decreased folate levels with concurrent use of sulfonamides, sulfasalazine, or methotrexate	• Avoid concurrent use of these medications.

Nursing Administration

- Assess clients for signs and symptoms of megaloblastic anemia (pallor, easy fatigability, palpitations, paresthesias of hands or feet).
- Obtain the client's baseline folic acid levels, RBC and reticulocyte counts, Hgb, and Hct levels. Monitor periodically.
- Advise clients with folic acid deficiency to concurrently increase intake of food sources of folic acid, such as green leafy vegetables and liver. Monitor clients for risk factors indicating that folic acid therapy may be needed, such as heavy alcohol use and child-bearing age.

Nursing Evaluation of Medication Effectiveness

- Depending on therapeutic intent, effectiveness may be evidenced by:
  - Folate level 6 to 15 mcg/mL
  - Return of RBC, reticulocyte count, and Hgb and Hct to levels within expected reference range

- Improvement of anemia findings such as absence of pallor, dyspnea, easy fatigability
- Absence of neural tube defects in newborns

MEDICATION CLASSIFICATION: POTASSIUM SUPPLEMENTS

- Select Prototype Medication: potassium chloride (K-Dur)
- Other Medications:
  - Potassium gluconate
  - Potassium phosphate
  - Potassium bicarbonate

Purpose

- Expected Pharmacological Action
  - Potassium is essential for conducting nerve impulses, maintaining electrical excitability of muscle, and regulation of acid/base balance.
- Therapeutic uses
  - Potassium supplements are used to treat hypokalemia; potassium less than 3.5 mEq/L
  - Potassium supplements are used:
    - For clients receiving diuretics resulting in potassium loss, such as furosemide (Lasix)
    - For clients with potassium loss due to excessive or prolonged vomiting, diarrhea, abuse of laxatives, intestinal drainage, and GI fistulas

Complications

SIDE/ADVERSE EFFECTS	NURSING INTERVENTIONS/CLIENT EDUCATION
GI distress and local GI ulceration, such as nausea, vomiting, diarrhea, abdominal discomfort, and esophagitis with oral administration	• Instruct clients to take the medication with meals or a full glass of water to minimize GI discomfort and prevent ulceration. • Teach clients not to dissolve the tablet in the mouth because oral ulceration will develop.
Hyperkalemia (potassium > 5.0 mEq/L)	• Hyperkalemia rarely occurs with oral administration • Monitor clients receiving IV potassium for signs of hyperkalemia, such as bradycardia, hypotension, ECG changes.

Contraindications/Precautions

- Contraindicated for clients with severe renal disease, hypoaldosteronism

Interactions

MEDICATION/FOOD INTERACTIONS	NURSING INTERVENTIONS/CLIENT EDUCATION
Concurrent use of potassium-sparing diuretics, such as spironolactone, or ACE inhibitors, such as lisinopril, increases the risk of hyperkalemia.	• Concurrent use should be avoided.

Nursing Administration

- Oral formulations
  - Mix powdered formulations in at least 4 oz of liquid.
  - Advise clients to take potassium chloride with a glass of water or with a meal to reduce the risk of adverse GI effects.
  - Instruct clients not to crush extended-release tablets.
  - Instruct clients to notify the provider if they have difficulty swallowing the pills. Medication may be supplied as a powder or sustained-release tablet that is easier to tolerate.
- IV administration
  - Never administer IV bolus. Rapid IV infusion can result in fatal hyperkalemia.
  - Use an IV infusion pump to control the infusion rate.
  - Dilute potassium and give no more than 40 mEq/L of IV solution to prevent vein irritation.
  - Give no faster than 10 mEq/hr.
  - Cardiac monitoring is indicated for serum potassium levels outside of normal parameters.
  - Assess the IV site for local irritation, phlebitis, and infiltration. Discontinue IV immediately if infiltration occurs.
  - Monitor the client's I&O to ensure an adequate urine output of at least 30 mL/hr.

Nursing Evaluation of Medication Effectiveness

- Depending on therapeutic intent, effectiveness may be evidenced by:
  - Serum potassium level within expected reference range: 3.5 to 5.0 mEq/L

MEDICATION CLASSIFICATION: MAGNESIUM SULFATE

- Select Prototype Medication:
  - Parenteral: Magnesium sulfate
  - Oral: Magnesium gluconate, magnesium hydroxide

Purpose

- Expected Pharmacological Action
  - Magnesium activates many intracellular enzymes and plays a role in regulating skeletal muscle contractility and blood coagulation.
- Therapeutic Uses
  - Magnesium supplements are used for clients with hypomagnesemia: magnesium level less than 1.3 mEq/L.
  - Oral preparations are used to prevent low magnesium levels.
  - Parenteral magnesium is used for clients with severe hypomagnesemia.
  - IV magnesium sulfate is used to stop preterm labor.

Complications

SIDE/ADVERSE EFFECTS	NURSING INTERVENTIONS/CLIENT EDUCATION
Neuromuscular blockade and respiratory depression	• IV administration requires careful monitoring of the client's cardiac and neuromuscular status. • Monitor the client's serum magnesium levels.
Diarrhea	• Monitor the client's serum magnesium levels for magnesium loss from diarrhea. • Monitor the client's I&O and observe for signs of dehydration.

Contraindications/Precautions

- Magnesium is Pregnancy Risk Category B.
- Use cautiously with clients who have AV block, rectal bleeding, nausea/vomiting, and abdominal pain.
- Use cautiously with clients who have renal and/or cardiac disease.

Interactions

- Magnesium sulfate may decrease the absorption of tetracyclines.
- Monitor the therapeutic effect to determine if absorption has been affected.

Nursing Administration

  - Monitor serum magnesium, calcium, and phosphorus.
  - Monitor the client's blood pressure, heart rate, and respiratory rate when given intravenously.
  - Assess clients for depressed or absent deep tendon reflexes as a sign of toxicity.
  - Calcium gluconate is given for magnesium sulfate toxicity. Always have an injectable form of calcium gluconate available when administering magnesium sulfate by IV.
  - Teach clients about dietary sources of magnesium (whole grain cereals, nuts, legumes, green leafy vegetables, bananas).

Nursing Evaluation of Medication Effectiveness

- Depending on therapeutic intent, effectiveness may be evidenced by:
  - Serum magnesium levels within expected reference range: 1.3 to 2.1 mEq/L

HERBAL SUPPLEMENTS

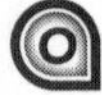
Overview

- Herbal supplements are widely used, but are also frequently less tested and regulated than conventional medications. Dosages are less precise than for more regulated medications. Because different formulations are not standardized, it can be difficult to know which preparations may provide therapeutic effects.

HERBAL SUBSTANCE	ACTION	USES
Aloe, aloe vera (Aloe gel and Aloe latex)	• Antimicrobial, anti-inflammatory, and analgesic actions when applied topically to skin • Cathartic properties when ingested (Aloe latex)	• Soothes pain and heal the inflammation of burns (Aloe gel) • Softens skin • Laxative (Aloe latex)
Black cohosh	• Acts on the female reproductive system as an estrogen substitute; mechanism of action unknown	• Used instead of estrogen therapy for symptoms of menopause

HERBAL SUBSTANCE	ACTION	USES
Echinacea	• Stimulates the immune system, decreases inflammation and can treat viruses through phagocytosis; increases T-lymphocyte, tumor necrosis factor, and interferon production	• Oral form primarily used to prevent and treat the common cold; however research has not proven this • Topical forms used to treat multiple skin disorders, wounds, and burns
Feverfew	• Possibly works by blocking a factor necessary to cause migraine. • Stops release of arachidonic acid in thrombocytes, so can block platelet aggregation.	• Can decrease the number and severity of migraine headaches but has not been found useful in treating an existing migraine
Garlic	• Garlic cells contain an amino acid which, when crushed, forms the enzyme allicin. This enzyme, along with another substance in garlic, has the following actions: ○ Blocks cholesterol synthesis in the liver. ○ Suppresses platelet aggregation and disrupts coagulation. ○ Acts as a vasodilator.	• Lowers total cholesterol, LDL, and triglycerides and slightly increases HDL • Can decrease both systolic (20-30 mm Hg) and diastolic BP (10 to 15 mm Hg)
Ginger root	• By an unknown mechanism, ginger root acts on areas of the CNS that cause nausea • Increases intestinal motility and gastric mucous production. • Decreases GI spasms. • Inhibits prostaglandins and leukotrienes to produce anti-inflammatory effects • Suppresses platelet aggregation	• Used to decrease nausea of morning sickness, motion sickness, and nausea caused by surgery • Can decrease the pain and stiffness of rheumatoid arthritis

HERBAL SUBSTANCE	ACTION	USES
Ginkgo biloba	• Promotes vasodilation throughout the body • Suppresses a substance that can increase platelet aggregation and bronchospasm	• Used to increase recall ability and mental processes by increasing blood flow in the brain; given to people with dementia, including Alzheimer's disease • Used for erectile dysfunction in those who take SSRIs that cause impotence • Can decrease pain in clients with occlusive arterial disorders of the legs • May decrease risk of thrombosis and bronchospasm
Goldenseal	• Suppresses inflammation and may stimulate the immune system; works as an antiseptic; has bactericidal properties • Increases bile secretion	• Used to treat and prevent a wide variety of infections, including bacterial, fungal, and protozoal • Can decrease gall bladder inflammation
Kava (Kava Kava)	• Actual actions unknown, but possibly acts on GABA receptors in CNS	• Used for insomnia, anxiety, and to promote muscle relaxation without decreasing ability to concentrate
Ma Huang (Ephedra sinica)	• May activate all alpha and beta adrenergic receptors to constrict arterioles, increase heart rate, cause bronchodilation, and suppress appetite • Stimulates CNS	• Used to relieve manifestations of colds, influenza, and allergies • Used for weight loss • Has been used to increase athletic abilities
St. John's Wort	• Affects serotonin, NE, dopamine, and GABA uptake to produce antidepressant effects	• Used for mild depression
Saw Palmetto	• Action unknown, but may reduce conversion of testosterone into dihydrotestosterone (DHT) in prostate	• Used to decrease symptoms of BPH
Valerian	• Increases GABA to prevent insomnia • May work in similar way to benzodiazepines	• Promotes sleep, with increased effect over time

HERBAL SUBSTANCE	ADVERSE REACTIONS AND PRECAUTIONS	INTERACTIONS	NURSING ADMINISTRATION
Aloe, Aloe vera (Aloe gel, Aloe Latex)	• Skin preparations: possible hypersensitivity • Laxative: Possible fluid and electrolyte imbalances	• None known	• Teach clients to recognize manifestations of fluid and electrolyte imbalance if using for a laxative.
Black cohosh	• GI distress, lightheadedness, headache, rash, weight gain • Should not be taken during the first two trimesters of pregnancy • Should not be used longer than 6 months due to lack of information regarding long-term effects	• Increases effects of antihypertensive medications • May increase effect of estrogen medications • Increases hypoglycemia in clients taking insulin or other medications for diabetes	• Question clients who take antihypertensives, insulin or hypoglycemic agents, or who may be pregnant, about possible use of black cohosh.
Echinacea	• Bitter taste • Mild GI symptoms or fever may occur. • Allergic reactions, especially in clients who are allergic to plants such as ragweed or others in the daisy family	• With chronic use (more than 6 months), echinacea can decrease positive effects of medications for tuberculosis, HIV, or cancer.	• Echinacea is available in many forms including dried roots or plants, extracts, teas. • Question clients who have tuberculosis, cancer, HIV, lupus erythematosus, and rheumatoid arthritis about concurrent use and advise these clients to talk to their primary care provider.

HERBAL SUBSTANCE	ADVERSE REACTIONS AND PRECAUTIONS	INTERACTIONS	NURSING ADMINISTRATION
Feverfew	• Mild GI symptoms • Post-feverfew syndrome may occur, causing agitation, tiredness, inability to sleep, headache, joint discomfort • May cause allergic reactions in clients allergic to ragweed or echinacea	• May cause increased risk of bleeding in clients taking NSAIDs, heparin, warfarin	• Question clients about concurrent use of NSAIDs, heparin, and warfarin.
Garlic	• GI symptoms	• Due to antiplatelet qualities, can increase risk of bleeding in clients taking NSAIDs, warfarin, and heparin. • Can increase hypoglycemic effects of diabetes medications. • Decreases levels of saquinavir, a medication for HIV treatment.	• Question clients about concurrent use of NSAIDs, heparin, and warfarin. • Have clients taking anti-diabetic medications or saquinavir contact their primary care provider.
Ginger root	• Use cautiously in pregnancy because high doses may cause uterine spasms. • Adverse effects unknown, with potential CNS and cardiac problems with very large overdose.	• Interacts with medications that interfere with coagulation (NSAIDS, warfarin, and heparin)	• Question clients about concurrent use of NSAIDs, heparin, and warfarin.

HERBAL SUBSTANCE	ADVERSE REACTIONS AND PRECAUTIONS	INTERACTIONS	NURSING ADMINISTRATION
Ginkgo biloba	• Mild GI upset, headache, lightheadedness, which may be decreased by reducing dose • Should be taken with caution in those at risk for seizure	• May interact with medications that lower the seizure threshold, such as antihistamines, antidepressants, and antipsychotics • Can interfere with coagulation	• Question clients regarding history of seizures or use of medications that lower seizure threshold. • Question clients about concurrent use of NSAIDs, heparin, and warfarin.
Goldenseal	• None at therapeutic or low doses; can stimulate the CNS and cause death from respiratory failure in large doses • Not advised for use in pregnancy, because it can stimulate the uterus.	• None known	• Question clients who are pregnant regarding use.
Kava (kava kava)	• Chronic use causes dry, flaky skin and jaundice. • Chronic use and large doses can cause liver damage, including severe liver failure.	• Can cause sedation when taken concurrently with CNS depressants.	• Question clients taking any CNS depressant, including alcohol, about use of kava. • Ask clients who have any liver condition about concurrent use.
Ma huang (Ephedra sinica)	• Because it contains ephedrine, ma huang can stimulate the cardiovascular system and, at high doses, can cause death from hypertension and dysrhythmias. • Stimulation of CNS may cause euphoria and, in high doses, psychosis.	• Interacts with any CNS stimulant to potentiate their effect. • May cause severe hypertension when taken with MAOI antidepressants. • Interacts with antihypertensive medications to decrease effect.	• Question clients carefully about other medications. • Products which include more than 10 mg per dose are forbidden to be sold in the U.S.

HERBAL SUBSTANCE	ADVERSE REACTIONS AND PRECAUTIONS	INTERACTIONS	NURSING ADMINISTRATION
St. John's wort	• Mild adverse effects, including dry mouth, lightheadedness, constipation, GI symptoms • Skin rash when exposed to sunlight	• May cause serotonin syndrome when combined with other antidepressants, amphetamine, and cocaine • Decreases effectiveness of oral contraceptives, cyclosporine, warfarin, digoxin, calcium channel blockers, steroids, HIV protease inhibitors, and some cancer chemotherapy medications	• Question clients taking any of the medications with which this substance interacts about concurrent use. • Encourage clients using St. John's wort to prevent prolonged sun exposure and use sunscreen.
Saw palmetto	• Few adverse effects; can cause mild GI effects • Precaution: Can decrease PSA, the marker used to detect prostate cancer	• Possible additive effects with finasteride (Proscar)	• Question male clients about use before they have PSA tests.
Valerian	• Can cause drowsiness, lightheadedness, depression • Risk of physical dependence • Precaution: Clients with mental health disorders should use with caution • Should be avoided by pregnant and lactating women	• Not known if valerian potentiates effects of CNS depressants	• Clients taking valerian should be warned about possibility of drowsiness when operating motor vehicles and other equipment.

CHAPTER 30: VITAMINS, MINERALS, AND SUPPLEMENTS

Application Exercises

1. A client with a hemoglobin of 8 g/dL was started on iron therapy with oral ferrous sulfate. The nurse is now reviewing the client's laboratory values following one month of therapy. The nurse should expect the client's hemoglobin level to be

   A. 8 g/dL.

   B. 10 g/dL.

   C. 11 g/dL.

   D. 12 g/dL.

2. A nurse is caring for a group of clients in a community setting. Which of the following clients should the nurse recognize may benefit from folic acid therapy? (Select all that apply)

   _____ A 12-year-old child with iron deficiency anemia
   _____ A 24-year-old woman with no health problems
   _____ A 44-year-old man with essential hypertension
   _____ A 50-year-old woman with chronic alcohol abuse
   _____ A 55-year-old man with type 2 diabetes mellitus

3. A nurse is reviewing the medication history for a client who has been prescribed potassium chloride (K-Dur). Which of the following medications puts the client at risk for hyperkalemia?

   A. Lisinopril (Zestril)

   B. Furosemide (Lasix)

   C. Digoxin (Lanoxin)

   D. Hydrochlorothiazide (Hydrodiuril)

4. A nurse is admitting a client who has increased liver enzymes and hepatitis. During the nursing assessment, which of the following herbal supplements should the nurse question the client about using?

   A. Ma huang

   B. Saw palmetto

   C. Kava

   D. Feverfew

5. A client asks a nurse about the use of the herbal supplement feverfew. The nurse should reply that feverfew may

   A. treat a variety of microbial infections.

   B. decrease the frequency of migraine headaches.

   C. lessen the nasal congestion of the common cold.

   D. relieve nausea of morning sickness of pregnancy.

6. A nurse is obtaining a medication history for a newly admitted client. The client says she takes gingko biloba to help her memory. The nurse should be concerned about which of the following medications the client also reports taking? (Select all that apply.)

_____ Ibuprofen

_____ Warfarin (Coumadin)

_____ Digoxin (Lanoxin)

_____ Imipramine (Tofranil)

_____ Lisinopril (Zestril)

CHAPTER 30: VITAMINS, MINERALS, AND SUPPLEMENTS

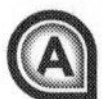

Application Exercises Answer Key

1. A client with a hemoglobin of 8 g/dL was started on iron therapy with oral ferrous sulfate. The nurse is now reviewing the client's laboratory values following one month of therapy. The nurse should expect the client's hemoglobin level to be

   A. 8 g/dL.

   B. 10 g/dL

   C. 11 g/dL

   D. 12 g/dL

   A client's hemoglobin should rise by 2 g/dL after one month of iron therapy. Therefore, this client's hemoglobin should be 10 g/dL at this time.

NCLEX® Connection: Pharmacological and Parenteral Therapies: Expected Actions/ Outcomes

2. A nurse is caring for a group of clients in a community setting. Which of the following clients should the nurse recognize may benefit from folic acid therapy? (Select all that apply)

   _____ A 12-year-old child with iron deficiency anemia

   __X__ **A 24-year-old woman with no health problems**

   _____ A 44-year-old man with essential hypertension

   __X__ **A 50-year-old woman with chronic alcohol abuse**

   _____ A 55-year-old man with type 2 diabetes mellitus

   Women of child-bearing age who may become pregnant benefit from supplemental folic acid (400 mcg/day) to prevent neural tube defects in a developing fetus. Alcoholism is a frequent cause of deficient folic acid in the body; therefore this client is likely to benefit from folic acid therapy until alcohol consumption has decreased. Iron deficiency anemia , hypertension, and diabetes mellitus are not treated by folic acid therapy.

NCLEX® Connection: Pharmacological and Parenteral Therapies: Expected Actions/ Outcomes

3. A nurse is reviewing the medication history for a client who has been prescribed potassium chloride (K-Dur). Which of the following medications puts the client at risk for hyperkalemia?

   A. Lisinopril (Zestril)

   B. Furosemide (Lasix)

   C. Digoxin (Lanoxin)

   D. Hydrochlorothiazide (Hydrodiuril)

   Clients taking lisinopril and other ACE inhibitors are at risk for hyperkalemia and therefore are at greater risk if taking concurrently with a potassium supplement. Digoxin does not interact with potassium supplements to cause hyperkalemia. Both furosemide (a loop diuretic) and hydrochlorothiazide (a thiazide diuretic) can cause hypokalemia when taken concurrently with potassium supplements

NCLEX® Connection: Pharmacological and Parenteral Therapies: Adverse Effects/ Contraindications/Side Effects/Interactions

4. A nurse is admitting a client who has increased liver enzymes and hepatitis. During the nursing assessment, which of the following herbal supplements should the nurse question the client about using?

   A. Ma huang

   B. Saw palmetto

   C. Kava

   D. Feverfew

   Kava can cause liver damage and could aggravate damage to the liver if used concurrently. Ma huang, saw palmetto, and feverfew have no effect on the liver.

NCLEX® Connection: Pharmacological and Parenteral Therapies: Adverse Effects/ Contraindications/ Side Effects/Interactions

5. A client asks a nurse about the use of the herbal supplement feverfew. The nurse should reply that feverfew may

   A. treat a variety of microbial infections.

   B. decrease the frequency of migraine headaches.

   C. lessen the nasal congestion of the common cold.

   D. relieve nausea of morning sickness of pregnancy.

   Feverfew has been found to decrease the frequency of migraine headaches, although it has not been proven to relieve existing headaches. Goldenseal has been used to treat microbial infections. Ma huang has been used to relieve symptoms of the common cold. Ginger root has been used to relieve nausea.

NCLEX® Connection: Pharmacological and Parenteral Therapies: Expected Actions/ Outcomes

6. A nurse is obtaining a medication history for a newly admitted client. The client says she takes gingko biloba to help her memory. The nurse should be concerned about which of the following medications the client also reports taking? (Select all that apply.)

   __X__ **Ibuprofen**
   __X__ **Warfarin (Coumadin)**
   _____ Digoxin (Lanoxin)
   __X__ **Imipramine (Tofranil)**
   _____ Lisinopril (Zestril)

   Concurrent use of ibuprofen and warfarin may lead to bleeding. Concurrent use with imipramine may lead to seizures. There are no known interactions with digoxin or lisinopril.

NCLEX® Connection: Pharmacological and Parenteral Therapies: Adverse Effects/Contraindications/Side Effects/Interactions

UNIT 7: MEDICATIONS AFFECTING THE REPRODUCTIVE SYSTEM

- Medications Affecting the Reproductive Tract
- Medications Affecting Labor and Delivery

NCLEX® CONNECTIONS

When reviewing the chapters in this unit, keep in mind the relevant sections of the NCLEX® outline, in particular:

CLIENT NEEDS: PHARMACOLOGICAL AND PARENTERAL THERAPIES

Relevant topics/tasks include:

- Adverse Effects/Contraindications/Side Effects/Interactions
  - Document the side effects and adverse effects of medications and parenteral therapy.
- Medication Administration
  - Review pertinent data prior to medication administration.

UNIT 7 MEDICATIONS AFFECTING THE REPRODUCTIVE SYSTEM

Chapter 31 Medications Affecting the Reproductive Tract

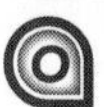

Overview

- Medications that affect the reproductive system include hormones that stimulate puberty, such as estrogen and progesterone in females and testosterone in males. These hormones are also used to replace a hormonal deficiency (male or female) or prevent pregnancy in women (oral contraceptives).
- Medications that are used to treat benign prostatic hyperplasia (BPH) include 5-alpha reductase inhibitors and $alpha_1$-adrenergic antagonists. Medications used to treat erectile dysfunction include the phosphodiesterase type 5 (PDE5) inhibitors.

MEDICATION CLASSIFICATION: ESTROGENS

- Select Prototype Medications: conjugated equine estrogens (Premarin)
- Other Medications: estradiol (Estrace), estradiol hemihydrate (Vagifem)

Purpose

- Expected Pharmacological Action
  - Estrogens are hormones needed for growth and maturation of the female reproductive tract and secondary sex characteristics. Estrogens block bone resorption and reduce low-density lipoprotein (LDL) levels. At high levels, estrogens suppress the release of a follicle-stimulating hormone (FSH) needed for conception.
- Therapeutic Uses
  - Estrogens are used for:
    - Contraception
    - Relief of postmenopausal symptoms, such as hot flashes, mood changes
    - Prevention of postmenopausal osteoporosis
    - Treatment of dysfunctional uterine bleeding and endometriosis
    - Treatment of prostate cancer
- Route of administration: Oral, transdermal, and intravaginal

Complications

SIDE/ADVERSE EFFECTS	NURSING INTERVENTIONS/CLIENT EDUCATION
Endometrial and ovarian cancers when prolonged estrogen is the only postmenopausal therapy	• Give clients progestins along with estrogen. • Instruct clients to report persistent vaginal bleeding. • Advise clients to have an endometrial biopsy every 2 years and yearly pelvic exam.
Potential risk for estrogen-dependent breast cancer	• Rule out estrogen-dependent breast cancer prior to starting therapy. • Encourage regular self-breast examinations and mammograms.
Embolic events such as MI, pulmonary embolism, DVT, cerebrovascular accident)	• Encourage clients to avoid all nicotine products. • Monitor clients for pain, swelling, warmth, or erythema of lower legs.

Contraindications/Precautions

- These medications are Pregnancy Risk Category X.
- These medications are contradicted for clients who have:
  - Client or family history of heart disease
  - Abnormal vaginal bleeding that is undiagnosed
  - Breast or estrogen-dependent cancer
  - History or risk of thromboembolic disease
- Use cautiously during breastfeeding because estrogens decrease quantity and quality of milk and may be excreted in breast milk.
- Use cautiously in prepubescent girls. If administered, monitor bone growth, and check periodically for early epiphyseal plate closure.

Interactions

MEDICATION/FOOD INTERACTIONS	NURSING INTERVENTIONS/CLIENT EDUCATION
Estrogens can reduce the effectiveness of warfarin (Coumadin).	• If used concurrently, monitor client international normalized ratio (INR) and prothrombin time (PT). • Warfarin doses may need to be adjusted.
Concurrent use of phenytoin (Dilantin) can increase the risk of phenytoin toxicity	• Monitor clients for signs of phenytoin toxicity with concurrent use of estrogen and phenytoin.
Corticosteroids may increase effects of estrogen.	• Monitor for increased estrogen effects.
Estrogen may alter effects of tamoxifen.	• Do not use together.
Smoking increases risk for thrombophlebitis.	• Advise clients not to smoke. Use alternative treatment if smoking persists.

Nursing Administration

- Instruct clients to take the medication at the same time each day (e.g., at bedtime).
- Apply estrogen patches to the skin of the trunk.
- Inject IM forms deep in a large muscle mass. Rotate injection sites.
- Instruct clients to report symptoms of menstrual changes, dysmenorrhea, amenorrhea, breakthrough bleeding, and/or breast changes.
- Encourage clients to perform monthly breast self-examinations and schedule annual gynecologic and breast examinations with the primary care provider.
- Advise clients to notify the provider of any swelling or redness in legs, shortness of breath, or chest pain.
- Discontinue prior to knee or hip surgery or any surgical procedures that may cause extensive immobilization.

Nursing Evaluation of Medication Effectiveness

- Depending on therapeutic intent, effectiveness may be evidenced by:
  - No evidence of conception
  - Relief of postmenopausal symptoms (hot flashes, mood changes)
  - No evidence of postmenopausal osteoporosis
  - Reduction in dysfunctional uterine bleeding and endometriosis
  - Decrease in spread of prostate cancer

MEDICATION CLASSIFICATION: PROGESTERONES

- Select Prototype Medications: medroxyprogesterone acetate (Provera)
- Other Medications: norethindrone (Micronor), megestrol acetate (Megace)

Purpose

- Expected Pharmacological Action
  - Progesterones induce favorable conditions for fetal growth and development and maintain pregnancy. A drop in progesterone levels results in menstruation.
- Therapeutic Uses
  - Progesterones counter adverse effects of estrogen in hormone replacement therapy for treatment of:
    - Dysfunctional uterine bleeding due to hormonal imbalance
    - Amenorrhea due to hormonal imbalance
    - Endometriosis
    - Endometrial
- Routes of administration: Oral, IM, subcutaneous, transdermal, and intravaginal

Complications

SIDE/ADVERSE EFFECTS	NURSING INTERVENTIONS/CLIENT EDUCATION
Breast cancer	• Encourage regular self-breast examinations and mammograms.
Thromboembolic events (MI, pulmonary embolism, thrombophlebitis, cerebrovascular accident)	• Discourage clients from smoking. • Monitor clients for pain, swelling, warmth, or erythema of lower legs. • Advise client to notify the provider of chest pain or shortness of breath.
Breakthrough bleeding, amenorrhea, breast tenderness	• Obtain baseline breast exam and Pap smear. • Instruct clients to report abnormal vaginal bleeding.
Edema	• Monitor the client's blood pressure, I&O, and weight gain.
Jaundice	• Monitor for signs of jaundice such as yellowing of the skin and sclera of the eyes. Monitor liver enzymes.
Migraine headaches	• Notify the provider of severe headache.

Contraindications/Precautions

- This medication is Pregnancy Risk Category X.
- This medication is contraindicated in clients who have:
  - Undiagnosed vaginal bleeding
  - History of thromboembolic disease, cardiovascular, or cerebrovascular disease
  - History of breast cancer
- Use cautiously in clients with diabetes, seizures disorders, and migraine headaches.

Interactions

MEDICATION/FOOD INTERACTIONS	NURSING INTERVENTIONS/CLIENT EDUCATION
Use of carbamazepine (Tegretol), Phenobarbital, phenytoin (Dilantin), and rifampin may decrease contraceptive effectiveness.	• Additional contraceptive measures may be needed with concurrent use of these medications.
Bromocriptine (Parlodel) may cause amenorrhea.	• Do not use together.
Smoking increases risk for thrombophlebitis.	• Advise clients not to smoke. Use alternative treatment if smoking persists.

Nursing Administration

- Instruct clients to anticipate withdrawal bleeding 3 to 7 days after stopping the medication.
- Instruct clients to stop taking the medication immediately if pregnancy is suspected. Conception should be delayed for 3 months following use.

Nursing Evaluation of Medication Effectiveness

- Depending on therapeutic intent, effectiveness may be evidenced by:
  - Restoration of hormonal balance with control of uterine bleeding (regular menstrual periods)
  - Restoration of menses
  - Decrease in endometrial hyperplasia in postmenopausal women receiving concurrent estrogen
  - Control of the spread of endometrial cancer

MEDICATION CLASSIFICATION: HORMONAL CONTRACEPTIVES

- Select Prototype Medications:
  - Combination oral contraceptives: Ethinyl estradiol and norethindrone (Ovcon 35, Necon 1/35)
- Other Medications:
  - Transdermal patch: Ethinyl estradiol and norelgestromin (Ortho Evra)
  - Vaginal contraceptive ring: Ethinyl estradiol and etonogestrel (NuvaRing)
  - Parenteral: depot medroxyprogesterone acetate (DMPA) available as Depo-Provera for IM use and Depo-subQ for subcutaneous use

Purpose

- Expected Pharmacological Action
  - Oral contraceptives stop conception by preventing ovulation. They also thicken the cervical mucus and alter the endometrial lining to reduce the chance of fertilization.
- Therapeutic Uses
  - Hormonal contraceptives are used to prevent pregnancy.
- Route of Administration
  - Oral, transdermal, intravaginal, IM, subcutaneous, and subdermal

Complications

SIDE/ADVERSE EFFECTS	NURSING INTERVENTIONS/CLIENT EDUCATION
Thromboembolic events (MI, pulmonary embolism, thrombophlebitis, and cerebrovascular accident)	• Discourage clients from smoking. • Instruct clients to report warmth, edema, tenderness, and/or pain in lower legs.
Hypertension	• Monitor the client's blood pressure and take actions to maintain normal blood pressure.
Breakthrough or abnormal uterine bleeding	• Instruct clients to record duration and frequency of breakthrough bleeding. • Evaluate clients for the possibility of pregnancy if two or more menstrual periods are missed.
Breast cancer	• Oral contraceptives may increase growth of a pre-existing breast cancer. Do not give to women with breast cancer.

Contraindications/Precautions

- These medications are Pregnancy Risk Category X.
- These medications are contraindicated for clients who have:
    - Client history of thrombophlebitis and cardiovascular events
    - Family history or risk factors for breast cancer
- Use cautiously in clients who are obese, who are > 35 years of age and smoke, and who have diabetes mellitus and hypercholesterolemia.

Interactions

MEDICATION/FOOD INTERACTIONS	NURSING INTERVENTIONS/CLIENT EDUCATION
Oral contraceptive effectiveness decreases with use of carbamazepine (Tegretol), phenobarbital, phenytoin (Dilantin), and rifampin.	• Additional contraceptive measures may be needed with concurrent use of these medications.
Oral contraceptives decrease the effects of warfarin (Coumadin) and oral hypoglycemics.	• Monitor the client's INR and PT levels and adjust warfarin dosages accordingly.

Nursing Administration

- Check for pregnancy prior to start of therapy.
- Instruct clients to take pills at the same time each day.
- Instruct clients to take medication for 21 days followed by 7 days of no medication (or inert pill). Begin the sequence on the fifth day after the onset of menses.
- For one missed dose, instruct clients to take two together at the next scheduled dose. For two missed doses, instruct the client to double up for 2 days. For three missed doses, because of an increased risk of ovulation and resulting pregnancy, instruct clients to use an additional form of birth control and to start a new cycle of medications after waiting 7 days.
- Encourage clients who smoke to quit.
- Advise client to report swelling or redness in legs, shortness of breath or severe headache.

Nursing Evaluation of Medication Effectiveness

- Depending on therapeutic intent, effectiveness may be evidenced by:
    - No evidence of conception

MEDICATION CLASSIFICATION: ANDROGENS

- Select Prototype Medications: Testosterone (Andronaq-50, Testred)
- Other Medications: testolactone (Teslac), testosterone pellets (Testopel)

Purpose

- Expected Pharmacological Action
  - Development of sex traits in men and the production and maturation of sperm
  - Increase in skeletal muscle
  - Increase in synthesis of erythropoietin
- Therapeutic Uses
  - Used to treat:
    - Hypogonadism in males
    - Delayed puberty in boys
    - Androgen replacement in testicular failure
    - Post menopausal breast cancer
- Route of administration: IM, transdermal, implantable pellets, buccal tablets

Complications

SIDE/ADVERSE EFFECTS	NURSING INTERVENTIONS/CLIENT EDUCATION
Androgenic effects: • In women these medications may cause irregularity or cessation of menses, hirsutism, weight gain, acne, lowering of voice, growth of clitoris, vaginitis, and baldness. • In boys or men these medications may cause acne, priapism, increased facial and body hair, and penile enlargement.	• Advise clients of possible medication effects. • Advise women to report occurrence of these effects. • Medication may be discontinued to prevent permanent changes.
Epiphyseal closure – Premature closure of epiphysis in boys may reduce mature height.	• Monitor epiphysis with serial X-rays.
Cholestatic hepatitis, jaundice	• Monitor signs of jaundice such as yellowing of the skin and sclera of the eyes. • Monitor liver enzymes.
Hypercholesterolemia – These medications can decrease high-density lipoproteins (HDL) and increase low-density lipoproteins (LDL)	• Monitor cholesterol levels. • Advise clients to adjust diet to reduce cholesterol levels.

SIDE/ADVERSE EFFECTS	NURSING INTERVENTIONS/CLIENT EDUCATION
Increase in growth of prostate cancer.	• Do not give to clients with prostate cancer. • Monitor for prostate cancer.
Polycythemia	• Monitor hemoglobin and hematocrit.
Edema from salt and water retention	• Instruct clients to monitor for weight gain and swelling of extremities and report to the provider. • Medication may be discontinued.
High abuse potential	• Identify high-risk groups and educate regarding abuse potential and potential health risks.

Contraindications/Precautions

- These medications are Pregnancy Risk Category X.

- Androgens are contraindicated in men with prostate or breast cancer, clients who have hypercalcemia, and older adult clients.
- Use cautiously in clients with heart failure, hypertension, and cardiac, renal or liver disease.

Interactions

MEDICATION/FOOD INTERACTIONS	NURSING INTERVENTIONS/CLIENT EDUCATION
Androgens may alter effects of oral anticoagulants.	• Monitor PT and INR.
Androgens may alter effects of insulins and antidiabetic agents.	• Monitor glucose level and adjust dosages.
Concurrent use of androgens and hepatotoxic medications may increase risk for hepatotoxicity.	• Monitor liver enzymes. Assess for jaundice.

Nursing Administration

- Inject into a large muscle and rotate injection sites.
- Monitor women for signs of masculinization (facial hair, baldness, deepened voice, acne).
- Advise clients to use a barrier method of birth control.
- Advise clients to reduce cholesterol in the diet.
- Advise clients at risk about abuse potential

Nursing Evaluation of Medication Effectiveness

- Depending on therapeutic intent, effectiveness may be evidenced by the following:
  - Puberty will be induced in boys and testosterone will be increased in men.
  - There will be a decrease in the progression of breast cancer in women. Medication will produce expected results with minimal side effects.

MEDICATION CLASSIFICATION: 5-ALPHA REDUCTASE INHIBITORS

- Select Prototype Medications: finasteride (Proscar)
- Other Medications: dutasteride (Avodart)

Purpose

- Expected Pharmacological Action
  - Decreases usable testosterone and causes a reduction of the prostate size and increases hair growth
- Therapeutic Uses
  - BPH
  - Male pattern baldness
- Route of administration: Oral

Complications

SIDE/ADVERSE EFFECTS	NURSING INTERVENTIONS/CLIENT EDUCATION
Decreased libido, ejaculate amount	• Advise client to notify the provider if adverse reactions occur.
Gynecomastia	• Advise clients to notify the provider if adverse reactions occur.

Contraindications/Precautions

- These medications are Pregnancy risk category X.
- These medications are contraindicated in clients with medication hypersensitivity.
- Use with caution in clients who have liver disease.

Interactions

- None significant

Nursing Administration

- Advise clients that therapeutic effects may take up to 6 months.

- Pregnant women should not handle crushed or broken medication.
- Advise clients not to donate blood unless medication has been discontinued for at least one month.

Nursing Evaluation of Medication Effectiveness

- Depending on therapeutic intent, effectiveness may be evidenced by the following:
  - Prostate size is decreased and client is able to urinate effectively.
  - Prostate-specific antigen (PSA) levels have decreased from baseline.
  - Client has increased hair growth.

MEDICATION CLASSIFICATION: ALPHA$_1$-ADRENERGIC ANTAGONISTS

- Select Prototype Medication:
  - Selective alpha$_1$ receptor antagonist: tamsulosin (Flomax)
- Other Medications:
  - Selective alpha$_1$ receptor antagonist: silodosin (Rapaflo)
  - Nonselective alpha$_1$ receptor antagonists:
    - Alfuzosin (Uroxatral)
    - Terazosin (Hytrin)
    - Doxazosin (Cardura)

Purpose

- Expected Pharmacological Action
  - These agents decrease mechanical obstruction of the urethra by relaxing smooth muscles of the bladder neck and prostate
  - Nonselective agents also affect blood vessels, resulting in lowered blood pressure. These agents may be used for clients who have BPH and hypertension.
- Therapeutic Uses
  - Benign prostatic hyperplasia (BPH)
- Route of administration: Oral

Complications

SIDE/ADVERSE EFFECTS	NURSING INTERVENTIONS/CLIENT EDUCATION
Hypotension, dizziness, nasal congestion, sleepiness, faintness (more likely with nonselective antagonists)	• Monitor blood pressure. • Advise clients to rise slowly from sitting or lying position. • Advise clients not to drive or operate machinery when starting therapy or with change in dose until response is known.
Problems with ejaculation (failure, decreased volume)	• Advise clients of possible adverse effect.

Contraindications/Precautions

- These agents are contraindicated in clients with medication sensitivity.
- These agents are contraindicated for women.
- Silodosin should be used cautiously in clients who have renal impairment.

Interactions

MEDICATION/FOOD INTERACTIONS	NURSING INTERVENTIONS/CLIENT EDUCATION
Cimetidine may decrease clearance of tamsulosin.	• Use together with caution.
Antihypertensives, PDE5 inhibitors, and nitroglycerin used concurrently with nonselective agents may cause severe hypotension.	• Use with caution. Monitor blood pressure.
Erythromycin and HIV protease inhibitors (Ritonavir) will increase levels of alfuzosin and silodosin when used concurrently.	• Avoid concurrent use.

Nursing Administration

- Monitor blood pressure, especially at the start of therapy and with changes of dose.
- Advise clients to take medication daily as prescribed:
    - Tamsulosin – one half hour after a meal at the same time each day
    - Silodosin – take with same meal each day
    - Alfuzosin – take right after the same meal each day
    - Terazosin – take at bedtime
    - Doxazosin – take at same time each day

Nursing Evaluation of Medication Effectiveness

- Depending on therapeutic intent, effectiveness may be evidenced by:
    - Client has improved urinary flow with minimal adverse effects.

MEDICATION CLASSIFICATION: PHOSPHODIESTERASE TYPE 5 (PDE5) INHIBITORS

- Select Prototype Medications: sildenafil (Viagra)
- Other Medications: tadalafil (Cialis), vardenafil (Levitra)

Purpose

- Expected Pharmacological Action
  - Augments the effects of nitric oxide released during sexual stimulation, resulting in enhanced blood flow to the corpus cavernosum and penile erection
- Therapeutic Uses
  - Erectile dysfunction

Complications

SIDE/ADVERSE EFFECTS	NURSING INTERVENTIONS/CLIENT EDUCATION
MI, sudden death	• Monitor the client's risk factors and history with regard to cardiovascular health.
Priapism	• Instruct clients to notify the provider if erection lasts more than 4 hr.

Contraindications/Precautions

- These medications are contraindicated in clients taking any medications in the nitrate family, such as nitroglycerin.
- Use cautiously in clients who have cardiovascular disease.

Interactions

MEDICATION/FOOD INTERACTIONS	NURSING INTERVENTIONS/CLIENT EDUCATION
Organic nitrates, such as nitroglycerin (Nitrostat) and isosorbide dinitrate (Isordil), can lead to fatal hypotension.	• Discourage concurrent use of organic nitrates.
Ketoconazole, erythromycin, cimetidine, ritonavir, and grapefruit juice inhibit metabolism of sildenafil thereby, increasing plasma levels of medication.	• Use these medications cautiously in clients taking sildenafil.

Nursing Administration

- Administer by oral route.
- Instruct clients to take approximately 1 hr before sexual activity and to limit use to once a day.

Nursing Evaluation of Medication Effectiveness

- Depending on therapeutic intent, effectiveness may be evidenced by:
  - Erection sufficient for sexual intercourse

CHAPTER 31: MEDICATIONS AFFECTING THE REPRODUCTIVE TRACT

Application Exercises

1. Contraindications to estrogen therapy may include which of the following? (Select all that apply.)

   _____ Estrogen-dependent cancer
   _____ Post-menopausal osteoporosis
   _____ Prostate cancer
   _____ Endometriosis
   _____ Thromboembolitic disease

2. Oral contraceptives prevent conception by doing which of the following? (Select all that apply.)

   _____ Thickening the cervical mucus to slow sperm passage
   _____ Inducing maturation of ovarian follicle
   _____ Increasing the development of the corpus luteum
   _____ Altering the endometrial lining to prevent implantation
   _____ Inhibiting ovulation

3. A nurse is providing teaching to a female client who is taking testosterone (Andronaq -50) to treat advanced breast cancer. Which of the following should the nurse instruct the client to watch for and report to the provider?

   _____ Deepening voice
   _____ Male pattern baldness
   _____ Sedation
   _____ Constipation
   _____ Facial hair

4. A nurse is providing teaching to a client who is to start tamsulosin (Flomax) for treatment of benign prostatic hyperplasia. The nurse should monitor the client for which of the following?

   A. Rash
   B. Edema
   C. Hypotension
   D. Jaundice

5. A nurse is taking a medication history from a client who has come to the clinic with reports of erectile dysfunction. Which of the following medications taken by the client for management of angina pain should not be taken concurrently with sildenafil (Viagra)?

   A. Ranolazine (Ranexa)
   B. Isosorbide dinitrate (Isordil)
   C. Clopidogrel (Plavix)
   D. Lisinopril (Zestril)

CHAPTER 31: MEDICATIONS AFFECTING THE REPRODUCTIVE TRACT

Application Exercises Answer Key

1. Contraindications to estrogen therapy may include which of the following? (Select all that apply.)

__X__ **Estrogen-dependent cancer**
_____ Post-menopausal osteoporosis
_____ Prostate cancer
_____ Endometriosis
__X__ **Thromboembolitic disease**

Estrogens are used for contraception, relief of postmenopausal symptoms such as hot flashes, prevention of postmenopausal osteoporosis, treatment of dysfunctional uterine bleeding and endometriosis, and treatment of prostate cancer. They are contraindicated in clients with a history of heart disease, breast- or estrogen-dependent cancer; clients with undiagnosed abnormal vaginal bleeding; or clients with a history of or risk for thromboembolic disease.

NCLEX® Connection: Pharmacological and Parenteral Therapies: Adverse Effects/ Contraindications/ Side Effects/Interactions

2. Oral contraceptives prevent conception by doing which of the following? (Select all that apply.)

__X__ **Thickening the cervical mucus to slow sperm passage**
_____ Inducing maturation of ovarian follicle
_____ Increasing the development of the corpus luteum
__X__ **Altering the endometrial lining to prevent implantation**
__X__ **Inhibiting ovulation**

Oral contraceptives stop conception by preventing ovulation. They also thicken the cervical mucus (which causes a barrier to sperm) and alter the endometrial lining to reduce the chance of fertilization. They do not induce maturation of ovarian follicles or increase the development of the corpus luteum.

NCLEX® Connection: Pharmacological and Parenteral Therapies: Expected Actions/ Outcomes

3. A nurse is providing teaching to a female client who is taking testosterone (Andronaq -50) to treat advanced breast cancer. Which of the following should the nurse instruct the client to watch for and report to the provider?

    __X__ **Deepening voice**
    __X__ **Male pattern baldness**
    _____ Sedation
    _____ Constipation
    __X__ **Facial hair**

    Testosterone may be used in women to treat advanced or metastatic breast cancer. Androgenic effects of testosterone in women may include hirsutism, weight gain, acne, lowering of voice, growth of clitoris, vaginitis, and baldness. Advise women to report occurrence of these effects. Medication may be discontinued to prevent permanent changes. Insomnia and excitation, rather than sedation, are side effects and diarrhea, rather than constipation, is a side effect.

NCLEX® Connection: Pharmacological and Parenteral Therapies: Adverse Effects/Contraindications/Side Effects/Interactions

4. A nurse is providing teaching to a client who is to start tamsulosin (Flomax) for treatment of benign prostatic hyperplasia. The nurse should monitor the client for which of the following?

    A. Rash
    B. Edema
    C. Hypotension
    D. Jaundice

    Tamsulosin relaxes vascular smooth muscle and may cause hypotension. Monitor blood pressure. Advise the client to rise slowly from a sitting or lying position. Tamsulosin may cause additive hypotensive effects when used with other antihypertensives. Rash, edema, and jaundice are not side effects of tamsulosin.

NCLEX® Connection: Pharmacological and Parenteral Therapies: Adverse Effects/Contraindications/Side Effects/Interactions

5. A nurse is taking a medication history from a client has come to the clinic with reports of erectile dysfunction. Which of the following medications taken by the client for management of angina pain should not be taken concurrently with sildenafil (Viagra)?

    A. Ranolazine (Ranexa)
    B. Isosorbide dinitrate (Isordil)
    C. Clopidogrel (Plavix)
    D. Lisinopril (Zestril)

    Isosorbide dinitrate is an organic nitrate that is used to manage angina pain. If taken concurrently with sildenafil it could lead to fatal hypotension. There are no contraindications for concurrent use with ranolazine, clopidogrel, or lisinopril.

NCLEX® Connection: Pharmacological and Parenteral Therapies: Adverse Effects/Contraindications/Side Effects/Interactions

UNIT 7 MEDICATIONS AFFECTING THE REPRODUCTIVE SYSTEM

Chapter 32 Medications Affecting Labor and Delivery

Overview

- Understanding medications affecting labor and delivery is imperative to promote positive maternal and fetal outcomes. This chapter will discuss medications used to induce or augment labor and medication used in the management of preterm labor.

MEDICATION CLASSIFICATION: UTERINE STIMULANTS-OXYTOCICS

- Select Prototype Medication: oxytocin (Pitocin, Syntocinon)
- Other Medication: methylergonovine (Methergine)

Purpose

- Expected Pharmacological Action
  - Uterine stimulants increase the strength, frequency, and length of uterine contractions.
- Therapeutic Uses
  - Oxytocin is used for:
    - Induction of labor (postterm pregnancy, premature rupture of membranes, pre-eclampsia).
    - Enhancement of labor, such as with dysfunctional labor
    - Delivery of placenta (postpartum, miscarriage)
    - Control of postpartum bleeding
    - Fetal stress testing
    - Intranasal: Promotion of milk letdown.
  - Methergine is used for:
    - Emergency intervention for serious postpartum hemorrhage

Complications

SIDE/ADVERSE EFFECTS	NURSING INTERVENTIONS/CLIENT EDUCATION
Oxytocin	
Uterine rupture	• Preassess client risk factors such as multiple deliveries. • Monitor the length, strength, and duration of contractions. • Have magnesium sulfate on standby if needed for relaxation of myometrium.
Methylergonovine	
Hypertensive crisis	• Monitor the client for symptoms of hypertensive crisis (headache, nausea, vomiting, increased blood pressure). • Provide emergency interventions.

Contraindications/Precautions

- Contraindications of Oxytocin
  - Maternal factors include sepsis, labor induction, a cervix that has not ripened, genital herpes, history of multiple births, and/or uterine surgery).
  - Fetal factors include immature lungs, cephalopelvic disproportion, fetal malpresentation, prolapsed umbilical cord, fetal distress, and threatened spontaneous abortion.
- Methergine should not be given to clients with hypertension and used cautiously in clients with organ failure (cardiovascular, renal, or hepatic).

Interactions

MEDICATION/FOOD INTERACTIONS	NURSING INTERVENTIONS/CLIENT EDUCATION
Vasopressors can lead to hypertension.	• Avoid concurrent use of oxytocin and vasopressors. • Monitor maternal blood pressure and report hypertension to the primary care provider.

Nursing Administration

- Use an infusion pump to administer intravenously. Gradually increase the flow rate per prescribed parameters, such as increase by 1 mcg/min every 30 min.
- Carefully monitor uterine contractions. Generally, the goal is contractions that last 1 min or less every 2 to 3 min.

- Continuously monitor the mother's blood pressure, pulse rate, and uterine contractions (frequency and duration).
- Monitor for uterine hyperstimulation (contractions lasting longer than 60 seconds, occurring more frequently than every 2 to 3 min, resting uterine pressure greater than 15 mm Hg). Stop infusion and notify the provider immediately.
- Continuously monitor the fetal heart rate and rhythm. Report signs of fetal distress.

Nursing Evaluation of Medication Effectiveness

- Depending on therapeutic intent, effectiveness may be evidenced by:
  - Effective contractions (lasting less than 60 seconds and occurring every 2 to 3 min)
  - Increase in uterine tone and no evidence of postpartum hemorrhage
  - Effective milk letdown

MEDICATION CLASSIFICATION: TOCOLYTIC MEDICATIONS

- Select Prototype Medication: terbutaline sulfate (Brethine)

Purpose

- Expected Pharmacological Action
  - Terbutaline selectively activates $beta_2$-adrenergic receptors ($beta_2$-adrenergic agonist), resulting in uterine smooth muscle relaxation.
- Therapeutic Uses
  - IV or subcutaneous terbutaline can be used for up to 48 hr to delay preterm labor.

Complications

SIDE/ADVERSE EFFECTS	NURSING INTERVENTIONS/CLIENT EDUCATION
Tachycardia, palpitations, chest pain	• Monitor the client for these $beta_1$ side effects (the medication is not absolutely selective). • Intervene based on tolerance and physiological impact.
Tremors, anxiety, headache	• Monitor the client for these $beta_2$ skeletal muscle stimulant side effects, which will decline with continued use.

 Contraindications/Precautions

- Greater than 34 weeks gestation (the maternal and fetal risks from the tocolytics outweigh the benefits to the fetus of prolonging the pregnancy)
- Acute fetal distress
- Severe pregnancy-induced hypertension or eclampsia
- Vaginal bleeding
- Cervical dilation greater than 6 cm

Interactions

MEDICATION/FOOD INTERACTIONS	NURSING INTERVENTIONS/CLIENT EDUCATION
Concurrent use of adrenergic agonists can cause additive effects.	• Monitor the client for additive adrenergic effects (tachycardia, tremors).
Concurrent use of beta blockers can blunt the effect of terbutaline.	• Monitor the client for negation of effects.

Nursing Administration

- Terbutaline can be administered IV or SC due to high first pass effect with oral administration. Monitor injection site for infection if administered subcutaneously.
- Oral medication is frequently prescribed for clients to take while at home.
- Monitor FHR, uterine contractions, maternal pulse, blood pressure, respiratory rate, lung sounds, and daily weights.
- Withhold/discontinue the medication and contact the provider for reports of chest pain, maternal heart rate greater than 120/min, or presence of cardiac arrhythmias.
- Limit fluid intake to 1,500 to 2,400 mL/24 hr.
- Notify the primary care provider if contractions persist or increase in frequency or duration.

Nursing Evaluation of Medication Effectiveness

- Depending on therapeutic intent, effectiveness may be evidenced by:
  - Cessation of preterm labor (20 to 36 weeks)

MEDICATION CLASSIFICATION: TOCOLYTIC MEDICATIONS

- Select Prototype Medication: magnesium sulfate

Purpose

- Expected Pharmacological Action
    - This central nervous system depressant is commonly used as a tocolytic to relax the smooth muscle of the uterus and causes fewer maternal and fetal side effects than other tocolytics. This medication is also prescribed to treat pregnancy-induced hypertension. It depresses the central nervous system, thus decreasing CNS irritability.
- Therapeutic Uses
    - Magnesium sulfate is administered IV to suppress preterm labor.
    - IV therapy is also used to manage pregnancy-induced hypertension or eclampsia
    - Slow magnesium tablets may be prescribed by the provider once preterm labor has been suppressed.

Complications

SIDE/ADVERSE EFFECTS	NURSING INTERVENTIONS/CLIENT EDUCATION
Lethargy, weakness, blurred vision, headache	• Assess the client's baseline prior to beginning medication. Implement safety measures.
Diarrhea	• Monitor the client's serum magnesium levels due to magnesium loss from diarrhea. • Monitor the client's I&O and observe for signs of dehydration.
Nausea and vomiting	• Provide ice chips and antiemetic medications as prescribed.
Depression of deep tendon reflexes	• Monitor deep tendon reflexes every 2 hr.
Decrease in urinary output	• Monitor urinary output every 2 hr.
Decrease in respiratory rate	• Monitor vital signs per hospital protocol.
Cardiac arrest	• Administer CPR.

 Contraindications/Precautions

- Greater than 34 weeks gestation (the maternal and fetal risks from the tocolytics outweigh the benefits to the fetus of prolonging the pregnancy)
- Acute fetal distress

- Vaginal bleeding
- Cervical dilation greater than 6 cm

Interactions

- No significant interactions

Nursing Administration

- Monitor clients closely. Discontinue medication immediately if pulmonary edema develops and notify the provider.
- Monitor for magnesium sulfate toxicity and discontinue for any of the following adverse effects, which include loss of deep tendon reflexes, urinary output less than 25 to 30 mL/hr, respiratory depression less than 12/min, pulmonary edema, and/or chest pain.
- Calcium gluconate should be available to administer as an antidote for magnesium sulfate toxicity.

Nursing Evaluation of Medication Effectiveness

- Depending on therapeutic intent, effectiveness may be evidenced by:
  - Cessation of preterm labor (20 to 36 weeks)

MEDICATION CLASSIFICATION: OPIOID ANALGESICS

- Select Prototype Medication: meperidine hydrochloride (Demerol)
- Other Medications: butorphanol (Stadol), nalbuphine (Nubain)

Purpose

- Expected Pharmacological Action
  - These medications act in the central nervous system to decrease the perception of pain without the loss of consciousness.
- Therapeutic Uses
  - The client may be given opioid analgesics IM or IV, but the intravenous route is recommended during labor because of its quicker action.
  - Butorphanol and nalbuphine provide pain relief without causing significant respiratory depression in the mother or fetus.

Complications

SIDE/ADVERSE EFFECTS	NURSING INTERVENTIONS/CLIENT EDUCATION
Dry mouth	Provide ice chips.
Nausea and vomiting	Administer antiemetic as prescribed.
Neonatal depression	Have naloxone (Narcan) available at delivery.
Tachycardia, hypotension, decreased fetal heart rate (FHR) variability	Monitor vital signs and fetal heart rate per hospital protocol.
Sedation	Provide safety.

Contraindications/Precautions

- Delivery within 4 hr of administration

Nursing Administration

- Prior to administering analgesic or anesthetic pain relief, the nurse should verify that labor is well established by performing a vaginal exam showing cervical dilation to be at least 4 cm with the fetus engaged.
- Have naloxone (Narcan) available to counteract the effects of respiratory depression in the newborn.
- Administer antiemetics as prescribed.
- Monitor maternal vital signs, uterine contraction pattern, and continuous FHR monitoring.
- Explain to the client that the medication will cause drowsiness.
- Instruct the client to request assistance with ambulation.

Nursing Evaluation of Medication Effectiveness

- Depending on therapeutic intent, effectiveness may be evidenced by:
  - Decreased pain during labor

CHAPTER 32: MEDICATIONS AFFECTING LABOR AND DELIVERY

 Application Exercises

1. A nurse is providing care to a client who is prescribed terbutaline (Brethine) by the provider. The nurse should recognize that terbutaline is administered to

   A. stop uterine contractions.

   B. prevent bleeding.

   C. promotes placental blood flow.

   D. increase prostaglandin production.

2. A labor and delivery nurse is providing care for a client in labor who received meperidine (Demerol) 50 mg IVP 1 hr ago. Assessment reveals imminent delivery. Which of the following medications should the nurse anticipate having available at delivery to reverse neonatal respiratory depression if indicated?

   A. Naloxone (Narcan)

   B. Calcium gluconate

   C. Epinephrine

   D. Sodium bicarbonate

3. Which of the following nursing interventions are indicated for a client in labor receiving oxytocin (Pitocin) to stimulate uterine contractions? (Select all that apply).

   _____ Use an infusion pump to administer medication.

   _____ Provide continuous monitoring of maternal vital signs.

   _____ Stop infusion if uterine contractions occur every 4 min and last 45 seconds.

   _____ Increase medication rapidly to assure adequate contractions.

   _____ Monitor FHR continuously.

4. A nurse is assessing a client with pregnancy-induced hypertension receiving magnesium sulfate. Which of the following findings should the nurse report to the provider?

   A. 2t DTR

   B. 2t pedal edema

   C. 24 mL/hr urinary output

   D. Respirations 12/min

CHAPTER 32: MEDICATIONS AFFECTING LABOR AND DELIVERY

Application Exercises Answer Key

1. A nurse is providing care to a client who is prescribed terbutaline (Brethine) by the provider. The nurse should recognize that terbutaline is administered to

   A. stop uterine contractions.

   B. prevent bleeding.

   C. promotes placental blood flow.

   D. increase prostaglandin production.

   Terbutaline blocks beta$_2$ adrenergic receptors, which causes uterine smooth muscle relaxation. Terbutaline does not have the other actions.

NCLEX® Connection: Pharmacological and Parenteral Therapies: Expected Actions/Outcomes

2. A labor and delivery nurse is providing care for a client in labor who received meperidine (Demerol) 50 mg IVP 1 hr ago. Assessment reveals imminent delivery. Which of the following medications should the nurse anticipate having available at delivery to reverse neonatal respiratory depression if indicated?

   A. Naloxone (Narcan)

   B. Calcium gluconate

   C. Epinephrine

   D. Sodium bicarbonate

   Opioid administration may cause respiratory depression the newborn. Therefore, the nurse should have naloxone (Narcan) available at delivery. The other medications do not affect neonatal depression.

NCLEX® Connection: Pharmacological and Parenteral Therapies: Adverse Effects/ Contraindications/Side Effects/Interactions

3. Which of the following nursing interventions are indicated for a client in labor receiving oxytocin (Pitocin) to stimulate uterine contractions? (Select all that apply).

   __X__ **Use an infusion pump to administer medication.**

   __X__ **Provide continuous monitoring of maternal vital signs.**

   _____ Stop infusion if uterine contractions occur every 4 min and last 45 seconds.

   _____ Increase medication rapidly to assure adequate contractions.

   __X__ **Monitor FHR continuously.**

   Oxytocin must be administered by an infusion pump to ensure precise dosage. Continuous maternal and fetal monitoring is required to assess for therapeutic effects and development of adverse effects of oxytocin. Infusion should not be stopped because therapeutic effect has not been achieved. Oxytocin rate is increased gradually to prevent hypertonic uterine contractions.

NCLEX® Connection: Pharmacological and Parenteral Therapies: Medication Administration

4. A nurse is assessing a client with pregnancy-induced hypertension receiving magnesium sulfate. Which of the following findings should the nurse report to the provider?

    A. 2t DTR

    B. 2t pedal edema

    C. 24 mL/hr urinary output

    D. Respirations 12/min

    Signs of magnesium sulfate toxicity include loss of deep tendon reflexes, urinary output less than 25 to 30 mL/hr, respiratory depression less than 12/min, pulmonary edema, and/or chest pain. Any of these findings requires immediate notification of the provider.

NCLEX® Connection: Pharmacological and Parenteral Therapies: Adverse Effects/ Contraindications/Side Effects/Interactions

UNIT 8: MEDICATIONS FOR JOINT AND BONE CONDITIONS

- Rheumatoid Arthritis
- Bone Disorders

NCLEX® CONNECTIONS

When reviewing the chapters in this unit, keep in mind the relevant sections of the NCLEX® outline, in particular:

CLIENT NEEDS: PHARMACOLOGICAL AND PARENTERAL THERAPIES

Relevant topics/tasks include:

- Adverse Effects/Contraindications/Side Effects/Interactions
  - Monitor for anticipated interactions among the client's prescribed medications and fluids.
- Expected Actions/Outcomes
  - Evaluate the client's use of medications over time.
- Medication Administration
  - Administer and document medications given by common routes.

UNIT 8 MEDICATIONS FOR JOINT AND BONE CONDITIONS

Chapter 33 Rheumatoid Arthritis

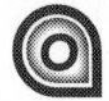

Overview

- Rheumatoid arthritis (RA) is a chronic disorder with autoimmune and inflammatory components. Pharmacological management provides symptomatic relief and some delay in progression of the disorder without resulting in cure. Disease-modifying antirheumatic drugs (DMARDs), glucocorticoids, and nonsteroidal antiinflammatory drugs (NSAIDs) may be used individually or in combination to manage this chronic disorder.
- The American College of Rheumatology (ACR) provides recommendations for management of rheumatoid arthritis. These guidelines can be found at http://www.rheumatology.org/
- Categories of medications in this section include disease-modifying antirheumatic medications (DMARDs), glucocorticoids, immunosuppressants, and NSAIDs.

MEDICATION CLASSIFICATION: DISEASE MODIFYING ANTIRHEUMATIC DRUGS (DMARDs)

- DMARDs I – Major Nonbiologic DMARDs
  - Cytotoxic medications: Methotrexate (Rheumatrex), leflunomide (Arava)
  - Antimalarial agents: Hydroxychloroquine (Plaquenil)
  - Antiinflammatory medication: Sulfasalazine (Azulfidine)
  - Tetracycline antibiotic: Minocycline (Minocin)
- DMARDs II – Major Biologic DMARDs
  - Biologic response modifiers:
    - Etanercept (Enbrel)
    - Infliximab (Remicade)
    - Adalimumab (Humira)
    - Rituximab (Rituxan)
    - Abatacept (Orencia)

- DMARDs III – Minor nonbiologic and biologic DMARDs
  - Gold salts: Aurothioglucose (Solganal)
  - Penicillamine (Cuprimine, Depen)
  - Cytotoxic medications: azathioprine (Imuran), cyclosporine (Sandimmune, Gengraf, Neoral)
- Glucocorticoids:
  - Prednisone (Deltasone), prednisolone (Prelone)
- NSAIDs:
  - Aspirin
  - Ibuprofen
  - Diclofenac (Voltaren)
  - Indomethacin (Indocin)
  - Meloxicam (Mobic)
  - Naproxen (Naprosyn)
  - Celecoxib (Celebrex)

Purpose

- Expected Pharmacological Action
  - DMARDs slow joint degeneration and progression of rheumatoid arthritis.
  - Glucocorticoids provide symptomatic relief of inflammation and pain.
  - NSAIDs provide rapid, symptomatic relief of inflammation and pain.
- Therapeutic Uses
  - Analgesia for pain, swelling, and joint stiffness
  - Maintenance of joint function
  - Slow/delay the worsening of the disease (DMARDs, glucocorticoids)
  - Short-term therapy until long-acting DMARDs take effect (NSAIDs, glucocorticoids)
  - Prevention of organ rejection in transplant clients such as kidney, liver, and heart transplants (cytotoxic agents, glucocorticoids, immunosuppressants).
  - Management of inflammatory bowel disease (glucocorticoids, immunosuppressants, DMARDs)

Complications

SIDE/ADVERSE EFFECTS	NURSING INTERVENTIONS/CLIENT EDUCATION
Cytotoxic agents: Methotrexate	
Increased risk of infection (fever and/or sore throat)	• Advise clients to notify the provider immediately if symptoms occur.
Hepatic fibrosis	• Monitor liver function test. • Advise clients to observe for anorexia, abdominal fullness, and jaundice and to notify the provider if symptoms occur.
Bone marrow suppression	• Obtain the client's baseline CBC and platelet counts. Repeat every 3 to 6 months.
GI ulceration	• Advise clients to take the medication with food or a full glass of water. • Stop the medication if symptoms occur. • H_2 antagonists, such as ranitidine (Zantac), can be used prophylactically.
Fetal death/congenital abnormalities	• Avoid use during pregnancy. • Use adequate contraception during therapy.
Antimalarial agents: Hydroxychloroquine	
Retinal damage (blindness)	• Advise clients to have baseline eye examination and follow-up eye exams every 6 months with an ophthalmologist. • Stop the medication and notify the provider if blurred vision occurs.
Sulfasalazine	
Gastrointestinal discomfort (nausea, vomiting, diarrhea, abdominal pain)	• Use an enteric-coated preparation and divide dosage daily.
Hepatic dysfunction	• Monitor liver function tests.
Bone marrow suppression	• Monitor CBC and platelet counts.

SIDE/ADVERSE EFFECTS	NURSING INTERVENTIONS/CLIENT EDUCATION
Biologic response modifiers: Etanercept, infliximab	
Subcutaneous injection-site irritation (redness, swelling, pain, itching)	• Monitor the client's injection site, and stop the medication if signs of irritation occur.
Risk of infection, especially TB	• Instruct client to monitor for infection (fever, sore throat, inflammation) and notify the provider if symptoms occur. Medication should be discontinued. • Perform TB testing.
Severe skin reactions	• Instruct clients to monitor for adverse skin reactions and notify the provider if symptoms occur. Medication should be discontinued.
Heart failure	• Monitor for development or worsening of heart failure (distended neck veins, crackles in lungs, dyspnea). Medication should be discontinued.
Blood dyscrasias	• Monitor for signs of bleeding, bruising or fever. Medication should be discontinued.
Gold salts: Aurothioglucose	
Toxicity (severe pruritus, rashes, stomatitis)	• Stop medication. • Notify the provider if symptoms occur.
Renal toxicity such as proteinuria	• Stop the medication. • Monitor I&O, BUN, creatinine, and UA.
Blood dyscrasias (thrombocytopenia, leukopenia, agranulocytosis, aplastic anemia)	• Monitor CBC, WBC, and platelet counts periodically. • Advise clients to observe for bruising and gum bleeding and to notify the provider if these occur.
Hepatitis	• Monitor liver function tests.
GI discomfort (nausea, vomiting, abdominal pain)	• Observe for symptoms and notify the provider if they occur.
Penicillamine	
Bone marrow suppression	• Obtain the client's baseline CBC and platelet counts, and repeat every 3 to 6 months.
Toxicity (severe pruritus, rashes)	• Stop the medication. • Notify the provider if symptoms occur.

SIDE/ADVERSE EFFECTS	NURSING INTERVENTIONS/CLIENT EDUCATION
	Cyclosporine
Risk of infection (fever and/or sore throat)	• Advise clients to notify the provider immediately if symptoms occur.
Hepatotoxicity (jaundice)	• Monitor liver function and adjust dosage.
Nephrotoxicity	• Monitor BUN and creatinine. • Measure I&O.
Hirsutism	• This effect is reversible with discontinuation of the medication.
	Glucocorticoids: Prednisone
Risk of infection (fever and/or sore throat)	• Advise clients to notify the provider immediately if symptoms occur.
Osteoporosis	• Advise clients to take calcium supplements, vitamin D, and/or bisphosphonate (etidronate).
Adrenal suppression	• Advise clients to observe for symptoms, and to notify the provider if symptoms occur. • Administer fluids such as normal saline, salt, and hydrocortisone IV. Advise clients not to discontinue the medication suddenly.
Fluid retention	• Monitor for signs of fluid excess such as crackles, weight gain, edema.
GI discomfort	• Advise clients to observe for symptoms, and to notify the provider if symptoms occur. • H_2 antagonists can be used prophylactically. • Advise client to report symptoms of GI bleeding (coffee-ground emesis or black, tarry stools).
Hyperglycemia	• Monitor blood glucose level. Clients with diabetes mellitus may need to adjust hypoglycemic agent.
Hypokalemia	• Monitor serum potassium levels. • Advise clients to eat potassium-rich foods. • Administer potassium supplements.

 Contraindications/Precautions:

- Methotrexate
  - This medication is Pregnancy Risk Category X.
  - Methotrexate is contraindicated in clients with psoriasis, renal or liver failure, alcoholism, or blood dyscrasias.

- Use with caution in clients who have liver or kidney dysfunction, cancer and suppressed bone marrow function, peptic ulcer disease, ulcerative colitis, impaired nutritional status, or infections.

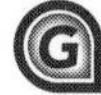

- Use cautiously with children or older adult clients.

- Etanercept (Enbrel)
  - Use caution in clients with heart failure, CNS demyelinating disorders such as multiple sclerosis, or blood dyscrasias.
- Cyclosporine is contraindicated in pregnancy, recent vaccination with live virus vaccines, and recent contact with or active infection of chickenpox or herpes zoster.
- Glucocorticoids are contraindicated in systemic fungal infections and live virus vaccines.

Interactions

MEDICATION/FOOD INTERACTIONS	NURSING INTERVENTIONS/CLIENT EDUCATION
Methotrexate	
Concurrent use may reduce digoxin level.	Monitor digoxin level. Monitor ECG.
NSAIDs, salicylates, and sulfonamides may cause methotrexate toxicity.	Monitor methotrexate levels.
Methotrexate may reduce levels of phenytoin (Dilantin).	Monitor phenytoin level.
Food may decrease absorption.	Take on an empty stomach.
Methotrexate may decrease vaccine strength.	Use precautions against illness.
Alcohol use may increase risk of hepatotoxicity.	Do not use together.
Etanercept	
Concurrent use of etanercept with a live vaccine increases the risk of getting or transmitting infection.	Avoid live vaccines
Cyclosporine	
Concurrent use of phenytoin, phenobarbital, rifampin, carbamazepine, and trimethoprim-sulfamethoxazole decreases cyclosporine level, which can lead to organ rejection.	Monitor the client's cyclosporine levels and adjust dosage accordingly.
Concurrent use of ketoconazole, erythromycin, and amphotericin B may increase cyclosporine level, leading to toxicity.	Monitor cyclosporine dosage and adjust accordingly to prevent toxicity.
Amphotericin B, aminoglycoside, and NSAIDs are nephrotoxic, and concurrent use with cyclosporine increases the risk for renal dysfunction.	Monitor BUN, creatinine, and I&O.
Consumption of grapefruit juice increases cyclosporine levels by 50%, which poses an increased risk of toxicity.	Advise clients to avoid drinking grapefruit juice.

MEDICATION/FOOD INTERACTIONS	NURSING INTERVENTIONS/CLIENT EDUCATION
Glucocorticoids	
Diuretics that promote potassium loss increase the risk of hypokalemia.	Monitor the client's potassium level and administer supplements as needed.
Because of the risk for hypokalemia, concurrent use of glucocorticoids with digoxin increases the risk of digoxin-induced dysrthymias.	Monitor digoxin and potassium levels.
NSAIDs increase the risk of GI ulceration.	Advise clients to avoid use of NSAIDs. If GI distress occurs, instruct clients to notify the provider.
Glucocorticoids promote hyperglycemia, thereby counteracting the effects of insulin and oral hypoglycemics.	The dose of hypoglycemic medications may need to be increased.

Nursing Administration

- Advise clients that effects of DMARDs are delayed and may take 3 to 6 weeks with full therapeutic effect taking several months.
- Administer etanercept by subcutaneous injection two times a week. Ensure solution is clear without particles present.
- Glucocorticoids may be used as oral agents or as intra-articular injections. Short-term therapy may be used to control exacerbations of symptoms and also may be used while waiting for the effects of DMARDs to develop.
- Cyclosporine:
    - Administer the initial IV dose of cyclosporine over 2 to 6 hr.
    - Monitor clients for hypersensitivity reactions. Stay with clients for 30 min after administration of cyclosporine.
    - Mix oral cyclosporine with milk or orange juice right before ingestion to increase palatability.
    - Instruct clients regarding the importance of lifelong therapy if used to prevent organ rejection.

Nursing Evaluation of Medication Effectiveness

- Depending on the therapeutic intent, effectiveness may be evidenced by:
    - Improvement of symptoms of rheumatoid arthritis, (reduced swelling of joints, absence of joint stiffness, ability to maintain joint function, and absence of pain)
    - Decrease in systemic complications such as weight loss and fatigue
    - Prevention of organ rejection

CHAPTER 33: RHEUMATOID ARTHRITIS

Application Exercises

1. A nurse is preparing to administer a regular intramuscular dose of aurothioglucose (Solganal) for a client who has rheumatoid arthritis. For which of the following reported adverse effects should the nurse hold the medication and notify the provider? (Select all that apply)

    _____ Insomnia

    _____ Stomatitis

    _____ Visual changes

    _____ Bruising

    _____ Pruritus

2. A nurse is evaluating teaching for a client who is diagnosed with rheumatoid arthritis and has a new prescription for methotrexate (Rheumatrex). Which of the following statements by the client indicates a need for further teaching?

    A. "If I get pregnant, I will need to stop taking this medication before giving birth."

    B. "I'll stop taking this medication and let my doctor know if I have stomach pain."

    C. "I will need several blood tests every few months while I take this medication."

    D. "I should give up my daily glass of wine while I take this medication."

3. A nurse is caring for a client who is beginning a new prescription for etanercept (Enbrel) for rheumatoid arthritis. Based on the route of administration of etanercept, which of the following should the nurse plan to monitor?

    A. The client's vein for thrombophlebitis during IV administration

    B. The client's subcutaneous site for redness following injection

    C. The client's oral mucosa for ulceration after oral administration

    D. The client's skin for irritation following removal of transdermal patch

4. A nurse is caring for a client with a prescription for cyclosporine (Sandimmune) to treat rheumatoid arthritis. Which of the following medications, if taken concurrently with cyclosporine, should the nurse anticipate causing a risk for cyclosporine toxicity?

    A. Phenytoin (Dilantin)

    B. Trimethoprim/sulfamethoxazole (Septra)

    C. Carbamazepine (Tegretol)

    D. Erythromycin (E-Mycin)

CHAPTER 33: RHEUMATOID ARTHRITIS

Application Exercises Answer Key

1. A nurse is preparing to administer a regular intramuscular dose of aurothioglucose (Solganal) for a client who has rheumatoid arthritis. For which of the following reported adverse effects should the nurse hold the medication and notify the provider? (Select all that apply)

    ____ Insomnia

    _X_ **Stomatitis**

    ____ Visual changes

    _X_ **Bruising**

    _X_ **Pruritus**

    The nurse should hold the medication and notify the provider for stomatitis, bruising (possible thrombocytopenia), and pruritus. Insomnia and visual changes are not manifestations of aurothioglucose therapy and should not require holding the medication.

NCLEX® Connection: Pharmacological and Parenteral Therapies: Adverse Effects/ Contraindications/Side Effects/Interactions

2. A nurse is evaluating teaching for a client who is diagnosed with rheumatoid arthritis and has a new prescription for methotrexate (Rheumatrex). Which of the following statements by the client indicates a need for further teaching?

    A. "If I get pregnant, I will need to stop taking this medication before giving birth."

    B. "I'll stop taking this medication and let my doctor know if I have stomach pain."

    C. "I will need several blood tests every few months while I take this medication."

    D. "I should give up my daily glass of wine while I take this medication."

    Methotrexate is rated Pregnancy Risk Category X and may cause fetal malformation or death if taken while pregnant. The client will be given a pregnancy test before beginning the medication and will be advised to use birth control during treatment. If the client becomes pregnant while taking this medication it will need to be discontinued. Methotrexate may cause GI ulceration; therefore the client should stop taking the medication and notify the provider if abdominal pain occurs. The client's CBC and renal and hepatic function will be carefully monitored while she is taking methotrexate. Clients taking this medication should avoid alcohol due to the risk for hepatic dysfunction.

NCLEX® Connection: Pharmacological and Parenteral Therapies: Adverse Effects/ Contraindications/Side Effects/Interactions

3. A nurse is caring for a client who is beginning a new prescription for etanercept (Enbrel) for rheumatoid arthritis. Based on the route of administration of etanercept, which of the following should the nurse plan to monitor?

    A. The client's vein for thrombophlebitis during IV administration.

    B. The client's subcutaneous site for redness following injection.

    C. The client's oral mucosa for ulceration after oral administration.

    D. The client's skin for irritation following removal of transdermal patch.

    Etanercept is administered subcutaneously; therefore the site of injection should be monitored for redness. None of the other administration routes should be prescribed for this medication.

NCLEX® Connection: Pharmacological and Parenteral Therapies: Adverse Effects/ Contraindications/Side Effects/Interactions

4. A nurse is caring for a client with a prescription for cyclosporine (Sandimmune) to treat rheumatoid arthritis. Which of the following medications, if taken concurrently with cyclosporine, should the nurse anticipate causing a risk for cyclosporine toxicity?

    A. Phenytoin (Dilantin)

    B. Trimethoprim/sulfamethoxazole (Septra)

    C. Carbamazepine (Tegretol)

    D. Erythromycin (E-Mycin)

    Erythromycin can increase levels of cyclosporine and increase risk for toxicity. Phenytoin, carbamazepine, and trimethoprim/sulfamethoxazole can decrease cyclosporine levels, and do not increase the risk of toxicity.

NCLEX® Connection: Pharmacological and Parenteral Therapies: Adverse Effects/ Contraindications/Side Effects/Interactions

UNIT 8 MEDICATIONS FOR JOINT AND BONE CONDITIONS

Chapter 34 Bone Disorders

Overview

- Calcium is necessary for the proper functioning of bones, nerves, muscles, the heart and blood coagulation.
- Calcium may be given as a supplement when dietary intake is insufficient. Uses for other medications that affect the bones include prevention and treatment of osteoporosis and prevention of fractures.
- Medication classifications include calcium supplements, selective estrogen receptor modulators, bisphosphonates, and calcitonin.

MEDICATION CLASSIFICATION: CALCIUM SUPPLEMENTS

- Select Prototype Medication: calcium citrate (Citracal)
- Other Medications:
  - Calcium carbonate (Tums, Rolaids)
  - Calcium acetate (PhosLo)
  - For IV administration:
    - Calcium chloride
    - Calcium gluconate

Purpose

- Expected Pharmacological Action
  - Maintenance of normal musculoskeletal, neurological, and cardiovascular function.
- Therapeutic Uses
  - Oral calcium supplements are used for clients with hypocalcemia, or deficiencies of parathyroid hormone, vitamin D, or dietary calcium.
  - Oral dietary supplements are used for adolescents, older adults, and women who are postmenopausal, pregnant or breastfeeding.
  - Intravenous medications are used for clients with critically low levels of calcium.

Complications

SIDE/ADVERSE EFFECTS	NURSING INTERVENTIONS/CLIENT EDUCATION
Hypercalcemia (Calcium level greater than 10.5 mg/dL) • Findings include tachycardia and elevated blood pressure leading to bradycardia and hypotension, muscle weakness and hypotonia, constipation, nausea, vomiting and abdominal pain, lethargy, and confusion.	• Instruct clients to monitor for symptoms and report to the provider. • Monitor serum calcium levels to maintain between 9.0 to 10.5 mg/dL.

Contraindications/Precautions

- Calcium supplements are contraindicated in clients who have hypercalcemia, bone tumors, and hyperparathyroidism.
- Use cautiously in clients with kidney disease or a decrease in GI function.

Interactions

MEDICATION/FOOD INTERACTIONS	NURSING INTERVENTIONS/CLIENT EDUCATION
Concurrent use of glucocorticoids reduces absorption of calcium.	• Give medications at least 1 hr apart.
Concurrent use of calcium decreases absorption of tetracyclines and thyroid hormone.	• Ensure 1 hr between administration of medications.
Concurrent administration of thiazide diuretics increases risk of hypercalcemia.	• Assess clients for hypercalcemia. • Avoid concurrent use.
Spinach, rhubarb, bran, and whole grains may decrease calcium absorption.	• Do not administer calcium with foods that decrease absorption. • Instruct clients to avoid consuming these foods at the same time as taking calcium.
IV calcium precipitates with phosphates, carbonates, sulfates, and tartrates.	• Do not mix parenteral calcium with compounds that cause precipitation.
Concurrent use of digoxin and parenteral calcium can lead to severe bradycardia.	• IV injection of calcium must be given slowly with careful monitoring of client status.

Nursing Administration

- Instruct clients to take a calcium supplement at least 1 hr apart from glucocorticoids, tetracyclines, and/or thyroid hormone.
- Chewable tablets provide more consistent bioavailability.

- Recommended doses of oral calcium vary widely depending on the specific calcium preparation. Instruct client to follow provider prescription.
- Prior to administration, warm IV infusions of calcium to body temperature.
- Administer IV injections at 0.5 to 2 mL/min.

Nursing Evaluation of Medication Effectiveness

- Depending on therapeutic intent, effectiveness may be evidenced by:
  - Serum calcium level within expected reference range: 9.0 to 10.5 mg/dL.

MEDICATION CLASSIFICATION: SELECTIVE ESTROGEN RECEPTOR MODULATORS/SERMS

- Select Prototype Medication: raloxifene (Evista)

Purpose

- Expected Pharmacological Action
  - Works as endogenous estrogen in bone, lipid metabolism, and blood coagulation
  - Decreases bone resorption, which results in slowing down of bone loss and preservation of bone mineral density
  - Works as an antagonist to estrogen on breast and endometrial tissue
  - Can decrease plasma levels of cholesterol
- Therapeutic Uses
  - Used in female clients to prevent and treat postmenopausal osteoporosis and to prevent spinal fractures
  - Used to protect against breast cancer

Complications

SIDE/ADVERSE EFFECTS	NURSING INTERVENTIONS/CLIENT EDUCATION
Increases the risk for pulmonary embolism and deep vein thrombosis (DVT)	• Medication should be stopped prior to scheduled immobilization such as surgery. Medication can be resumed when the client is fully mobile. • Discourage long periods of sitting and inactivity.
Hot flashes	• Inform clients that the medication may exacerbate, rather than reduce, hot flashes.

Contraindications/Precautions

- Raloxifene is Pregnancy Risk Category X.
- This medication is contraindicated in clients with a history of venous thrombosis. The medication should be stopped three days before periods in which risk of DVT is high (such as before surgical procedures).

Interactions

- No significant interactions

Nursing Administration

- For maximum benefit of the medication, encourage clients to consume adequate amounts of calcium (such as from dairy products) and vitamin D (such as from egg yolks). Inadequate amounts of dietary calcium and vitamin D cause release of parathyroid hormone, which stimulates calcium release from the bone.
- Medication may be taken with or without food once a day.
- Monitor the client's bone density; clients should undergo a bone density scan every 12 to 18 months.
- Monitor the client's serum calcium. Expected reference range is 9.0 to 10.5 mg/dL.
- Monitor liver function tests. Raloxifene levels may be increased in clients with hepatic impairment.
- Encourage clients to perform weight-bearing exercises daily, such as walking 30 to 40 min each day.

Nursing Evaluation of Medication Effectiveness

- Depending on therapeutic intent, effectiveness may be evidenced by:
  - Increase in bone density
  - No fractures

MEDICATION CLASSIFICATION: BISPHOSPHONATES

- Select Prototype Medications: alendronate sodium (Fosamax)
- Other Medications:
  - Ibandronate sodium (Boniva)
  - Risedronate (Actonel)
  - For IV infusion – Zoledronate (Reclast, Zometa)

Purpose

- Expected Pharmacological Action
  - Bisphosphonates decrease the number and action of osteoclasts, which thereby inhibits bone resorption.
- Therapeutic Uses
  - As prophylaxis and treatment of postmenopausal osteoporosis
  - In male clients who have osteoporosis
  - As prophylaxis and treatment of osteoporosis produced by long-term glucocorticoid use
  - For clients who have Paget's disease of the bone and hypercalcemia of malignancy

Complications

SIDE/ADVERSE EFFECTS	NURSING INTERVENTIONS/CLIENT EDUCATION
Esophagitis, other GI disturbances including nausea, diarrhea, constipation, dyspepsia	• Instruct client to sit upright or ambulate for 30 minutes after taking this medication orally. • Instruct client to take tablets with at least 8 oz of water and liquid formulation with at least 2 oz.
Musculoskeletal pain	• Advise client to take mild analgesic. • Instruct client to notify provider if pain persists. Alternate medication may be prescribed.
Visual disturbances such as blurred vision, eye pain	• Instruct clients to watch for symptoms and report to the provider. Medication should be discontinued.
Bisphosphonate-related osteonecrosis of the jaw with IV infusion	• Avoid dental work during administration of medication.
Risk for hyperparathyroidism at higher dose used for Paget's disease	• Monitor the client's parathyroid hormone (PTH) levels.

Contraindications/Precautions

- Bisphosphonates are Pregnancy Risk Category C.
- These medications are contraindicated for women who are lactating.
- These medications are contraindicated in clients who have esophageal stricture or difficulty swallowing, esophageal disorders, serious renal impairment, and hypocalcemia.
- Use cautiously in clients with upper GI disorders, infection, and liver impairment.

Interactions

MEDICATION/FOOD INTERACTIONS	NURSING INTERVENTIONS/CLIENT EDUCATION
Alendronate absorption decreases when taken with calcium supplements, antacids, orange juice, and caffeine.	• Advise clients to take the medication on an empty stomach with at least 8 oz of water. • Wait 2 hr after administration to take antacids or calcium.

Nursing Administration

- Instructions for clients should include:
  - Take the medication first thing in the morning after getting out of bed.
  - Take oral medication on an empty stomach, drinking at least 8 oz of water with tablets and at least 2 oz of water with liquid formulation.
  - Sit or ambulate for 30 min after taking the medication.
  - Avoid all calcium-containing foods and liquids or any medications within 2 hr of taking alendronate.
  - Avoid chewing or sucking on the tablet.
  - Perform weight-bearing exercises daily, such as walking 30 to 40 min each day.
  - Notify the provider of difficulty swallowing, painful swallowing, and/or new or worsening heartburn.
  - If a dose is skipped, wait until the next day to take the next dose. Clients should not take the skipped dose.
  - For maximum benefit of the medication, consume adequate amounts of calcium and vitamin D.
- Tablets are prescribed once daily or once a week. Liquid form is prescribed for once a week.
- Monitor the client's bone density; clients should have a bone density scan every 12 to 18 months.
- Monitor the client's serum calcium: expected reference range 9.0 to 10.5 mg/dL.

Nursing Evaluation of Medication Effectiveness

- Depending on therapeutic intent, effectiveness may be evidenced by:
  - Increase in bone density
  - No fractures

MEDICATION CLASSIFICATION: CALCITONIN

- Select Prototype Medication: calcitonin-salmon (Fortical, Miacalcin)

Purpose

- Expected Pharmacological Action
    - Decreases bone resorption by inhibiting the activity of osteoclasts in osteoporosis
    - Increases renal calcium excretion by inhibiting tubular resorption
- Therapeutic Uses
    - Postmenopausal osteoporosis and moderate to severe Paget's disease
    - Hypercalcemia caused by hyperparathyroidism and cancer

Complications

SIDE/ADVERSE EFFECTS	NURSING INTERVENTIONS/CLIENT EDUCATION
Nausea	• Advise clients that nausea is usually self-limiting.
With intranasal route, nasal dryness and irritation can occur.	• Instruct clients to alternate nostrils daily. • Inspect nasal mucosa periodically for ulceration.

Contraindications/Precautions

- This medication is Pregnancy Risk Category C.
- The medication is contraindicated in clients with hypersensitivity to the medication and fish protein. Perform an allergy skin test prior to administration if the client is at risk.
- Use cautiously with women who are lactating, children, and clients diagnosed with kidney disease.

Interactions

- Concurrent use with lithium may decrease serum lithium levels. Monitor lithium levels closely.

Nursing Administration

- Calcitonin-salmon is most commonly given by nasal spray. It can also be given IM or SC. Rotate injection sites to prevent inflammation
- Keep the container in an upright position.
- Teach clients to alternate nostrils daily.

- Check for Chvostek's or Trousseau's signs to monitor for hypocalcemia.
- Monitor the client's bone density scans periodically.
- Encourage clients to consume a diet high in calcium and vitamin D

Nursing Evaluation of Medication Effectiveness

- Depending on therapeutic intent, effectiveness may be evidenced by:
  - Increase in bone density
  - Serum calcium level within expected reference range of 9.0 to 10.5 mg/dL

CHAPTER 34: BONE DISORDERS

Application Exercises

1. A nurse is providing teaching to a client who is taking raloxifene (Evista) to prevent post-menopausal osteoporosis. The nurse should advise the client to monitor for which of the following possible adverse reactions? (Select all that apply.)

    _____ Hot flashes
    _____ Lump in breast
    _____ Swelling or redness in calf
    _____ Shortness of breath
    _____ Difficulty swallowing

2. A client with osteoporosis is started on alendronate sodium (Fosamax). The client should be instructed to do which of the following? (Select all that apply.)

    _____ Take medication in the morning after arising and before eating.
    _____ Chew tablets to increase bioavailability.
    _____ Drink a full glass of water with each tablet.
    _____ Take Fosamax with an antacid if heartburn occurs.
    _____ Avoid lying down after taking this medication.

3. The nurse recognizes that calcitonin-salmon (Miacalcin) may be given to a client with hypercalcemia to:

    A. Increase renal reabsorption of calcium.
    B. Decrease intestinal absorption of calcium.
    C. Increase parathyroid response to hypercalcemia.
    D. Decrease bone resorption of calcium.

CHAPTER 34: BONE DISORDERS

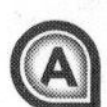

Application Exercises Answer Key

1. A nurse is providing teaching to a client who is taking raloxifene (Evista) to prevent post-menopausal osteoporosis. The nurse should advise the client to monitor for which of the following possible adverse reactions? (Select all that apply.)

 ___X___ **Hot flashes**
 _______ Lump in breast
 ___X___ **Swelling or redness in calf**
 ___X___ **Shortness of breath**
 _______ Difficulty swallowing

Raloxifene is given to treat or prevent postmenopausal osteoporosis. It may cause increased hot flashes or thromboembolism as evidenced by swelling or redness in the calf or shortness of breath. Raloxifene may be used to prevent breast cancer. It does not cause difficulty swallowing.

NCLEX® Connection: Pharmacological and Parenteral Therapies, Adverse Effects/Contraindications/Side Effects/Interactions

2. A client with osteoporosis is started on alendronate sodium (Fosamax). The client should be instructed to do which of the following? (Select all that apply.)

 ___X___ **Take medication in the morning after arising and before eating.**
 _______ Chew tablets to increase bioavailability.
 ___X___ **Drink a full glass of water with each tablet.**
 _______ Take Fosamax with an antacid if heartburn occurs.
 ___X___ **Avoid lying down after taking this medication.**

To prevent esophagitis, alendronate sodium should be taken first thing in the morning before eating; the client should swallow the tablet with at least a full 8 oz glass of water, and should avoid lying down after taking the medication. Tablets should not be chewed, because this could cause esophagitis. To optimize absorption, alendronate sodium should not be taken within 2 hr of an antacid or calcium.

NCLEX® Connection: Pharmacological and Parenteral Therapies, Medication Administration

3. The nurse recognizes that calcitonin-salmon (Miacalcin) may be given to a client with hypercalcemia to

   A. increase renal reabsorption of calcium.

   B. decrease intestinal absorption of calcium.

   C. increase parathyroid response to hypercalcemia.

   D. decrease bone resorption of calcium.

   High calcium blood levels cause the parathyroid hormone to release calcitonin. Calcitonin-salmon is a synthetic calcitonin hormone that decreases bone resorption of calcium. It decreases the renal reabsorption of calcium, increases intestinal absorption of calcium, and does not increase the parathyroid response to hypercalcemia.

NCLEX® Connection: Pharmacological and Parenteral Therapies, Expected Actions/ Outcomes

UNIT 9: MEDICATIONS FOR PAIN AND INFLAMMATION

- Nonopioid Analgesics
- Opioid Agonists and Antagonists
- Adjuvant Medications for Pain
- Miscellaneous Pain Medications

NCLEX® CONNECTIONS

When reviewing the chapters in this unit, keep in mind the relevant sections of the NCLEX® outline, in particular:

CLIENT NEEDS: PHARMACOLOGICAL AND PARENTERAL THERAPIES

Relevant topics/tasks include:

- Medication Administration
  - Evaluate the appropriateness/accuracy of a medication order for the client per institution policy, including reconciling orders.
- Parenteral/Intravenous Therapy
  - Monitor the use of an infusion pump.
- Pharmacological Pain Management
  - Use pharmacological measures for pain management, as needed.

UNIT 9 MEDICATIONS FOR PAIN AND INFLAMMATION

Chapter 35 Nonopioid Analgesics

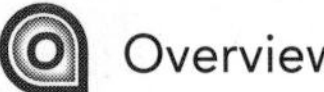

Overview

- Nonopioid analgesics may have anti-inflammatory, antipyretic, and analgesic action. These medications include nonsteroidal anti-inflammatory drugs and acetaminophen.

MEDICATION CLASSIFICATION: NONSTEROIDAL ANTI-INFLAMMATORY DRUGS

- 1st generation NSAIDs (COX-1 and COX-2 inhibitors):
  - Aspirin
  - Ibuprofen (Motrin, Advil)
  - Naproxen (Naprosyn)
  - Indomethacin (Indocin)
  - Diclofenac (Voltaren)
  - Ketorolac (Toradol)
  - Meloxicam (Mobic)
- 2nd generation NSAIDs (selective COX-2 Inhibitor):
  - Celecoxib (Celebrex)

Purpose

- Expected Pharmacological Action
  - Inhibition of cyclooxygenase — Inhibition of COX-1 can result in decreased platelet aggregation and kidney damage. Inhibition of COX-2 results in decreased inflammation, fever, and pain.
- Therapeutic Uses
  - Inflammation suppression
  - Analgesia for mild to moderate pain, such as with osteoarthritis and rheumatoid arthritis
  - Fever reduction
  - Dysmenorrhea
  - Inhibition of platelet aggregation, which protects against stroke and myocardial infarction (aspirin)

Complications

SIDE/ADVERSE EFFECTS	NURSING INTERVENTIONS/CLIENT EDUCATION
• Gastrointestinal discomfort (dyspepsia, abdominal pain, heartburn, nausea) • Damage to gastric mucosa may lead to GI bleeding and perforation, especially with long-term use.	• Advise clients to take medication with food or with a full glass of water or milk. • Advise clients to avoid alcohol. • Observe for signs of bleeding (passage of black or dark-colored stools, severe abdominal pain, nausea, vomiting). • Administer a proton pump inhibitor, such as omeprazole (Prilosec), or an H_2 receptor antagonist, such as ranitidine (Zantac) to decrease the risk of ulcer formation. • Use prophylaxis agents such as misoprostol (Cytotec).
• Renal dysfunction (decreased urine output, weight gain from fluid retention, increased BUN and creatinine levels)	• Use cautiously with older adults and clients who have heart failure. • Monitor I&O and kidney function (BUN, creatinine).
• Increased risk of heart attack and stroke (nonaspirin NSAIDs)	• Use the smallest effective dose for clients with known cardiovascular disease.
• Salicylism may occur with aspirin. Signs and symptoms include tinnitus, sweating, headache and dizziness, and respiratory alkalosis.	• Advise clients to notify the provider and to stop taking aspirin if symptoms occur.
• Reye syndrome is rare, but serious in childhood. This occurs when aspirin is used for fever reduction in children who have a viral illness, such as chickenpox or influenza	• Advise clients to avoid giving aspirin when a child has a viral illness, such as chickenpox or influenza.
• Aspirin toxicity	• Aspirin toxicity should be managed as a medical emergency in the hospital. • Therapy includes: ○ Cooling with tepid water ○ Correction of dehydration and electrolyte imbalance with IV fluids ○ Reversal of acidosis and promotion of salicylate excretion with bicarbonate ○ Gastric lavage • Activated charcoal may also be given to decrease absorption. • Hemodialysis may be indicated.

Contraindications/Precautions

- Contraindications for aspirin and other 1st generation NSAIDs include:
    - Pregnancy (Pregnancy Risk Category D)
    - Peptic ulcer disease
    - Bleeding disorders such as hemophilia, vitamin K deficiency
    - Hypersensitivity to aspirin and other NSAIDs
    - Children with chickenpox or influenza (aspirin)

- Use NSAIDs cautiously in older adults, clients who smoke cigarettes, and in clients with *H. pylori* infection, hypovolemia, asthma, chronic urticaria, and/or a history of alcoholism.
- Celecoxib is contraindicated in clients with allergy to sulfonamides.
- Ketorolac is contraindicated in clients with advanced renal dysfunction. Use should be no longer than five days because of the risk for kidney damage.
- 2nd generation NSAIDs should be used cautiously in clients who have known cardiovascular disease.

Interactions

MEDICATION/FOOD INTERACTIONS	NURSING INTERVENTIONS/CLIENT EDUCATION
Anticoagulants, such as heparin and warfarin, increase the risk of bleeding.	• Monitor the client's PTT, PT, and INR. • Advise clients about the potential risk of bleeding when a NSAID is combined with an anticoagulant. Instruct clients to report signs of bleeding.
Glucocorticoids increase the risk of gastric bleeding.	• Advise clients to take antiulcer prophylaxis, such as misoprostol (Cytotec), to decrease the risk for gastric ulcer.
Alcohol increases the risk of bleeding.	• Advise clients to avoid consuming alcoholic beverages to decrease the risk of GI bleeding.
Ibuprofen decreases the antiplatelet effects of low-dose aspirin used to prevent MI.	• Advise clients not to take ibuprofen.
Ketorolac and concurrent use of other NSAIDs increase the risk of known side effects.	• Ketorolac should not be used concurrently with other NSAIDs.

Nursing Administration

- Advise clients to stop aspirin 1 week before an elective surgery or expected date of childbirth.
- Advise clients to take NSAIDs with food, milk, or a full glass of water to reduce gastric discomfort.
- Instruct clients not to chew or crush enteric-coated or sustained-release aspirin tablets.
- Advise clients to notify the provider if signs and symptoms of gastric discomfort or ulceration occur.
- Advise clients to notify the provider if symptoms of salicylism occur. Medication should be discontinued until symptoms are resolved. Medication can be restarted at a lower dose.
- Ketorolac may be used for short-term treatment of moderate to severe pain such as that associated with postoperative recovery.
    - Concurrent use with opioids allows for lower dosages of opioids and thus minimizes adverse effects such as constipation and respiratory depression.
    - Ketorolac is usually first administered parenterally and then switched to oral doses. Use should not be longer than 5 days because of the risk for kidney damage.

Nursing Evaluation of Medication Effectiveness

- Depending on therapeutic intent, effectiveness may be evidenced by:
    - Reduction in inflammation
    - Reduction of fever
    - Relief from mild to moderate pain
    - Absence of injury

MEDICATION CLASSIFICATION: ACETAMINOPHEN

- Select Prototype Medication: acetaminophen (Tylenol)

Purpose

- Expected Pharmacological Action
    - Acetaminophen slows the production of prostaglandins in the central nervous system.
- Therapeutic Uses
    - Analgesic (relief of pain) effect
    - Antipyretic (reduction of fever) effects

Complications

SIDE/ADVERSE EFFECTS	NURSING INTERVENTIONS/CLIENT EDUCATION
Acute toxicity that results in liver damage with early symptoms of nausea, vomiting, diarrhea, sweating, and abdominal discomfort progressing to hepatic failure, coma, and death	• Advise clients to take acetaminophen as prescribed and not to exceed 4 g/day. • Administer the antidote, acetylcysteine (Mucomyst).

Contraindications/Precautions

- Use cautiously in clients who consume three or more alcoholic drinks/day and those taking warfarin (interferes with metabolism).

Interactions

MEDICATION/FOOD INTERACTIONS	NURSING INTERVENTIONS/CLIENT EDUCATION
• Alcohol increases the risk of liver damage.	• Advise clients about the potential risk of liver damage with consumption of alcohol.
• Acetaminophen slows the metabolism of warfarin (Coumadin) leading to increased levels of warfarin. This places clients at risk for bleeding.	• Instruct clients to observe for signs of bleeding (bruising, petechiae, hematuria). • Monitor prothrombin time and INR levels and adjust dosages of warfarin accordingly.

Nursing Administration

- Acetaminophen is a component of multiple prescribed and over-the-counter medications. Keep a running total of daily acetaminophen intake and follow recommended dosages as prescribed by the provider to prevent toxicity, not to exceed 4 g/day.
- In the event of an overdose, administer acetylcysteine (Mucomyst), the antidote for acetaminophen, to prevent liver damage. Administer via an oroduodenal tube to prevent emesis and subsequent aspiration.

Nursing Evaluation of Medication Effectiveness

- Depending on therapeutic intent, effectiveness may be evidenced by:
  - Relief of pain
  - Reduction of fever

CHAPTER 35: NONOPIOID ANALGESICS

Application Exercises

1. Which of the following are potential adverse effects of aspirin? (Select all that apply.)

    _____ Tinnitus
    _____ GI distress
    _____ Hepatoxicity
    _____ Platelet interference
    _____ Reye syndrome

2. A nurse is admitting a toddler to the hospital after an acetaminophen overdose. Which of the following medications should the nurse anticipate administering to this client?

    A. Acetylcysteine (Mucomyst)
    B. Pegfilgrastim (Neulasta)
    C. Misoprostol (Cytotec)
    D. Naltrexone (ReVia)

3. A nurse is caring for a postoperative client who is prescribed ketorolac (Toradol) for pain management. When reviewing the client's medication administration record, which of the following medications should the nurse expect the client will also be receiving for pain management?

    A. Naproxen (Naprosyn)
    B. Indomethacin (Indocin)
    C. Morphine sulfate
    D. Meloxicam (Mobic)

CHAPTER 35: NONOPIOID ANALGESICS

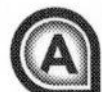

Application Exercises Answer Key

1. Which of the following are potential adverse effects of aspirin? (Select all that apply.)

   __X__ **Tinnitus**

   __X__ **GI distress**

   _____ Hepatoxicity

   __X__ **Platelet interference**

   __X__ **Reye syndrome**

   Tinnitus, GI distress, platelet interference and Reye syndrome are all potential adverse effects of aspirin. Hepatotoxicity is a potential adverse effect of acetaminophen overdoses.

NCLEX® Connection: Pharmacological and Parenteral Therapies, Adverse Effects/ Contraindications/Side Effects/Interactions

2. A nurse is admitting a toddler to the hospital after an acetaminophen overdose. Which of the following medications should the nurse anticipate administering to this client?

   A. Acetylcysteine (Mucomyst)

   B. Pegfilgrastim (Neulasta)

   C. Misoprostol (Cytotec)

   D. Naltrexone (ReVia)

   Acetylcysteine is the antidote for acetaminophen overdose. Pegfilgrastim is a long-acting medication used to increase the body's production of neutrophils. Misoprostol is a prostaglandin hormone and is often used to prevent the formation of gastric ulcers. Naltrexone is an opioid antagonist used to prevent alcohol craving.

NCLEX® Connection: Pharmacological and Parenteral Therapies, Expected Actions/Outcomes

3. A nurse is caring for a postoperative client who is prescribed ketorolac (Toradol) for pain management. When reviewing the client's medication administration record, which of the following medications should the nurse expect the client will also be receiving for pain management?

   A. Naproxen (Naprosyn)

   B. Indomethacin (Indocin)

   C. Morphine sulfate

   D. Meloxicam (Mobic)

   Ketorolac is an effective postoperative pain medication. Concurrent use with morphine sulfate will increase analgesia without increasing risk of opioid side effects. Use is short term, no longer than 5 days. Concurrent use with other NSAIDs such as naproxen, indomethacin, and meloxicam is contraindicated because of the increased risk of side effects.

NCLEX® Connection: Pharmacological and Parenteral Therapies, Pharmacological Pain Management

UNIT 9 MEDICATIONS FOR PAIN AND INFLAMMATION

Chapter 36 Opioid Agonists and Antagonists

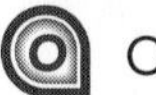

Overview

- Opioid analgesics are medications used to treat moderate to severe pain. Most opioid analgesics reduce pain by attaching to a receptor in the central nervous system, altering perception and response to pain.
- Opioids are classified as agonists, agonist-antagonists, and antagonists.
- An agonists attaches to a receptor and produces a response.
  - An agonist-antagonist binds to one receptor, causing a response, and binds to another receptor, which prevents a response.
  - An antagonist attaches to a receptor site and prevents a response.
- The desired outcome is to reduce pain and increase activity with few adverse effects.

OPIOID AGONISTS

- Select Prototype Medication: morphine sulfate
- Other Medications:
  - Fentanyl (Sublimaze, Duragesic)
  - Meperidine (Demerol)
  - Methadone (Dolophine)
  - Codeine, oxycodone (OxyContin)

Purpose

- Expected Pharmacological Action
  - Opioid agonists, such as morphine, codeine, meperidine, and other morphine-like medications (fentanyl), act on the mu receptors, and to a lesser degree on kappa receptors. Activation of mu receptors produces analgesia, respiratory depression, euphoria, and sedation, whereas kappa receptor activation produces analgesia, sedation, and decreased GI motility.

- Therapeutic Uses
  - Relief of moderate to severe pain (postoperative, myocardial infarction, cancer)
  - Sedation
  - Reduction of bowel motility
  - Codeine: cough suppression
- Route of administration:
  - Morphine sulfate – Oral, subcutaneous, IM, rectal, IV, epidural, and intrathecal
  - Other Medications:
    - Fentanyl (Sublimaze, Duragesic) – IV, IM, transmucosal and transdermal
    - Meperidine (Demerol) – Oral, subcutaneous IM, and IV
    - Codeine – Oral, subcutaneous IM, and IV
    - Methadone (Dolophine) – Oral, subcutaneous, and IM
    - Oxycodone (OxyContin) – Oral, rectal
    - Hydromorphone (Dilaudid) – Oral, subcutaneous, IM, IV

Complications

SIDE/ADVERSE EFFECTS	NURSING INTERVENTIONS/CLIENT EDUCATION
Respiratory depression	• Monitor the client's vital signs. • Stop opioids if the client's respiratory rate is less than 12/min, and then notify the provider. • Have naloxone (Narcan) and resuscitation equipment available. • Avoid the use of opioids with CNS depressant medications (barbiturates, benzodiazepines, and consumption of alcohol).
Constipation	• Increased fluid intake and physical activity. • Administer a stimulant laxative, such as bisacodyl (Dulcolax), to counteract decreased bowel motility, or a stool softener, such as docusate sodium (Colace), to prevent constipation.
Orthostatic hypotension	• Advise clients to sit or lie down if symptoms of lightheadedness or dizziness occur. • Avoid sudden changes in position by slowly moving clients from a lying to a sitting or standing position. • Provide assistance with ambulation as needed.
Urinary retention	• Advise clients to void every 4 hr. • Monitor I&O. • Assess the client's bladder for distention by palpating the lower abdomen area every 4 to 6 hr.

SIDE/ADVERSE EFFECTS	NURSING INTERVENTIONS/CLIENT EDUCATION
Cough suppression	• Advise clients to cough at regular intervals to prevent accumulation of secretions in the airway. • Auscultate the client's lungs for crackles, and instruct clients to increase intake of fluid to liquefy secretions.
Sedation	• Advise clients to avoid hazardous activities such as driving or operating heavy machinery.
Biliary colic	• Avoid giving morphine to clients who have a history of biliary colic. Use meperidine as an alternative.
Emesis	• Administer an antiemetic such as promethazine (Phenergan).
Opioid overdose triad of coma, respiratory depression, and pinpoint pupils	• Monitor the client's vital signs. • Provide mechanical ventilation. • Administer opioid antagonists, such as naloxone (Narcan) or nalmefene (Revex).

Contraindications/Precautions

- Morphine is contraindicated after biliary tract surgery.
- Morphine is contraindicated for premature infants during and after delivery because of respiratory depressant effects.
- Meperidine is contraindicated for clients with renal failure because of the accumulation of normeperidine, which can result in seizures and neurotoxicity.
- Use cautiously with:

  - Clients who have asthma, emphysema, and/or head injuries; infants, and older adult clients (risk of respiratory depression)
  - Clients who are pregnant (risk of physical dependence of the fetus)
  - Clients in labor (risk of respiratory depression in the newborn and inhibition of labor by decreasing uterine contractions)
  - Clients who are extremely obese (greater risk for prolonged side effects because of the accumulation of medication that is metabolized at a slower rate)
  - Clients with inflammatory bowel disease (risk of megacolon or paralytic ileus)
  - Clients with an enlarged prostate (risk of acute urinary retention)
  - Clients with hepatic or renal disease

Interactions

MEDICATION/FOOD INTERACTIONS	NURSING INTERVENTIONS/CLIENT EDUCATION
CNS depressants (barbiturates, phenobarbital, benzodiazepines, alcohol) have additive CNS depression action.	• Warn clients about the use of these medications in conjunction with opioid agonists • Advise clients to avoid consumption of alcohol.
Anticholinergic agents (atropine sulfate or scopolamine), antihistamines (diphenhydramine [Benadryl]), and tricyclic antidepressants (amitriptyline [Elavil]) have additive anticholinergic effects (constipation, urinary retention).	• Advise clients to increase fluids and dietary fiber to prevent constipation.
Monoamine oxidase inhibitors (MAOIs) may cause hyperpyrexic coma, characterized by excitation, seizures, and respiratory depression.	• Avoid the use of meperidine with MAOIs to prevent occurrence of this syndrome.
Antihypertensives have additive hypotensive effects	• Warn clients to refrain from using opioids with antihypertensive agents.

Nursing Administration

- Assess the client's pain level on a regular basis. Document the client's response.
- Take the client's baseline vital signs. If the respiratory rate is less than 12/min, notify the provider and withhold the medication.
- Follow controlled substance procedures.
- Double check opioid doses with another nurse prior to administration.
- Administer opioids intravenously slowly over a period of 4 to 5 min; have naloxone (Narcan) and resuscitation equipment available.
- Warn clients not to increase dosage without consulting the provider.
- For clients who have cancer, administer opioids on a fixed schedule around the clock. Administer supplemental doses as needed.
- Advise clients with physical dependence not to discontinue opioids abruptly. Opioids should be withdrawn slowly, and the dosage should be tapered over a period of 3 days.
- Closely monitor patient-controlled analgesia pump (PCA) settings (dose, lockout interval, and 4-hr limit). Reassure clients regarding safety measures that safeguard against self-administration of excessive doses. Encourage clients to use PCA prophylactically prior to activities likely to augment pain levels.
- When switching clients from PCA to oral doses of opioids, make sure the client receives adequate PCA dosing until the onset of oral medication takes place.
- The first administration of a transdermal fentanyl patch will take several hours to achieve the desired therapeutic effect. Administer short-acting opioids prior to onset of therapeutic effects and for breakthrough pain.

Nursing Evaluation of Medication Effectiveness

- Depending on the therapeutic intent, effectiveness may be evidenced by:
  - Relief of moderate to severe pain (postoperative pain, cancer pain, myocardial pain)
  - Cough suppression
  - Resolution of diarrhea

MEDICATION CLASSIFICATION: AGONIST-ANTAGONIST OPIOIDS

- Select Prototype Medication: butorphanol (Stadol)
- Other Medications:
  - Nalbuphine hydrochloride (Nubain)
  - Buprenorphine hydrochloride (Buprenex)

Purpose

- Expected Pharmacological Action
  - These medications act as antagonists on mu receptors and agonists on kappa receptors.
  - Compared to pure opioid agonists, agonist-antagonists have:
    - A low potential for abuse causing little euphoria. In fact, high doses can cause adverse effects (anxiety, restlessness, mental confusion).
    - Less respiratory depression.
    - Less analgesic effect.
- Therapeutic Uses
  - Relief of moderate to severe pain
  - Treatment of opioid dependence (buprenorphine)
  - Adjunct to balanced anesthesia
  - Relief of labor pain (butorphanol)
- Route of administration:
  - Butorphanol – IV, IM, intranasal
  - Nalbuphine – IV, IM, subcutaneous
  - Buprenorphine – IV, sublingual, epidural

Complications

SIDE/ADVERSE EFFECTS	NURSING INTERVENTIONS/CLIENT EDUCATION
Abstinence syndrome (cramping, hypertension, vomiting)	• This syndrome may be precipitated when these medications are given to clients who are physically dependent on opioid agonists. • Advise clients to stop opioid agonists, such as morphine sulfate, before using agonist-antagonist medications, such as pentazocine. • Avoid giving to clients if undisclosed opioid use is suspected.
Sedation, respiratory depression	• Have naloxone (Narcan) and resuscitation equipment available. Monitor for respiratory depression.
Dizziness	• Use caution in standing up. Avoid driving or using heavy machinery.
Increased intracranial pressure, headache	• Monitor for headache. Assess level of consciousness.
Increased cardiac workload	• Do not use for angina, myocardial infarction.

Contraindications/Precautions

- Use cautiously in clients who have a history of myocardial infarction, renal or liver disease, respiratory depression, or head injury, and clients who are physically dependent on opioids.

Interactions

MEDICATION/FOOD INTERACTIONS	NURSING INTERVENTIONS/CLIENT EDUCATION
CNS depressants and alcohol may cause additive effects.	• Use together cautiously. Monitor respirations.
Opioid agonists may antagonize and reduce analgesic effects of the opioid.	• Do not use concurrently.

Nursing Administration

- Take the client's baseline vital signs. If the respiratory rate is less than 12/min, withhold the medication and notify the provider.
- Have naloxone and resuscitation equipment available.
- Assess clients for opioid dependence prior to administration. Agonist-antagonists may trigger withdrawal symptoms.
- Warn clients not to increase dosage without consulting the provider.
- Advise clients to use caution when getting out of bed or standing. Clients should not operate heavy machinery or drive until CNS effects are known.
- Warn clients not to increase dosage without consulting the provider.

Nursing Evaluation of Medication Effectiveness

- Monitor for improvement of symptoms, such as relief of pain.

MEDICATION CLASSIFICATION: OPIOID ANTAGONISTS

- Select Prototype Medication: Naloxone (Narcan)
- Other Medications: Naltrexone (Re Via, Depade), nalmefene (Revex)

Purpose

- Expected Pharmacological Action
  - Opioid antagonists interfere with the action of opioids by competing for opioid receptors. Opioid antagonists have no effect in the absence of opioids.
- Therapeutic Uses
  - Treatment of opioid overdose
  - Reversal of effects of opioids, such as respiratory depression
  - Reversal of respiratory depression in an infant
- Route of administration:
  - Naloxone, nalmefene – IV, IM, subcutaneous
  - Naltrexone – Oral

Complications

SIDE/ADVERSE EFFECTS	NURSING INTERVENTIONS/CLIENT EDUCATION
Tachycardia and tachypnea	• Monitor the client's heart rhythm (risk of ventricular tachycardia) and respiratory function. • Have resuscitative equipment, including oxygen, on standby during administration.
Abstinence syndrome (cramping, hypertension, vomiting)	• These symptoms may occur when given to clients physically dependent on opioid agonists.
Pulmonary edema	• Monitor for pulmonary edema (rales). • Use with caution in clients with history of pulmonary edema.

Contraindications/Precautions

- Opioid antagonists are Pregnancy Risk Category B.
- These medications are contraindicated in clients with opioid dependency.

Interactions

- None noted

Nursing Administration

- Naloxone has rapid first-pass inactivation and should be administered IV, IM, or SC. Do not administer orally.
- Observe clients for withdrawal symptoms and/or abrupt onset of pain. Be prepared to address the client's need for analgesia (if given for postoperative opioid-related respiratory depression).
- Titrate dosage to achieve reversal of respiratory depression without full reversal of pain management effects.
- Rapid infusion of naloxone may cause hypertension, tachycardia, nausea, and vomiting.
- Half-life of opioid analgesic may exceed the half-life of naloxone (60 to 90 min).
- Monitor respirations for up to 2 hr after use to assess for reoccurrence of respiratory depression and the need for repeat dosage of naloxone.

Nursing Evaluation of Medication Effectiveness

- Reversal of respiratory depression (respirations are regular, client is without shortness of breath, respiratory rate is 16 to 20/min in adults and 40 to 60/min in newborns)

CHAPTER 36: OPIOID AGONISTS AND ANTAGONISTS

Application Exercises

1. Which of the following opioids can result in the buildup of a toxic metabolite with repetitive dosing and should not be used for more than 48 hr?

   A. Dolophine (Methadone)

   B. Hydromorphone (Dilaudid)

   C. Meperidine (Demerol)

   D. Morphine sulfate

2. Which of the following opioids is available as a transdermal patch?

   A. Fentanyl

   B. Meperidine

   C. Morphine sulfate

   D. Oxycodone

3. A postoperative client is given morphine sulfate 10 mg intramuscularly and then develops respiratory depression. Naloxone is prescribed to reverse the respiratory depression. Which of the following actions should the nurse take? (Select all that apply.)

   _____ Administer 0.9% sodium chloride 500 mL fluid bolus

   _____ Continue to monitor respirations after the effects of the naloxone (Narcan) have worn off.

   _____ Titrate the naloxone (Narcan) slowly to achieve reversal of respiratory depression, without reversal of analgesia.

   _____ Prepare to insert an indwelling catheter for urinary retention.

   _____ Assess SaO_2 and apply oxygen if needed.

4. Agonist-antagonist opioids differ from pure opioid agonists in that they

   A. have a greater risk for abuse due to an increase in euphoria.

   B. cause a higher incidence of respiratory depression.

   C. may not be reversed with an opioid antagonist.

   D. may cause abstinence syndrome in clients physically dependent to opioids.

CHAPTER 36: OPIOID AGONISTS AND ANTAGONISTS

Application Exercises Answer Key

1. Which of the following opioids can result in the buildup of a toxic metabolite with repetitive dosing and should not be used for more than 48 hr?

    A. Dolophine (Methadone)

    B. Hydromorphone (Dilaudid)

    C. Meperidine (Demerol)

    D. Morphine sulfate

    Repeated use of meperidine can result in accumulation of normeperidine, which can result in seizures and neurotoxicity. Do not administer more than 600 mg/24 hr, and limit use to less than 48 hr. This does not occur with the other opioids.

NCLEX® Connection: Pharmacological and Parenteral Therapies, Adverse Effects/ Contraindications/Side Effects/Interactions

2. Which of the following opioids is available as a transdermal patch?

    A. Fentanyl

    B. Meperidine

    C. Morphine sulfate

    D. Oxycodone

    Fentanyl is available as a transdermal patch. None of the other opioids are available in this form.

NCLEX® Connection: Pharmacological and Parenteral Therapies, Medication Administration

3. A postoperative client is given morphine sulfate 10 mg intramuscularly and then develops respiratory depression. Naloxone is prescribed to reverse the respiratory depression. Which of the following actions should the nurse take? (Select all that apply.)

_____ Administer 0.9% sodium chloride 500 mL fluid bolus

__X__ **Continue to monitor respirations after the effects of the naloxone have worn off.**

__X__ **Titrate the naloxone slowly to achieve reversal of respiratory depression, without reversal of analgesia.**

_____ Prepare to insert an indwelling catheter for urinary retention.

__X__ **Assess SaO_2 and apply oxygen if needed.**

Half-life of an opioid analgesic may exceed the half-life of naloxone (60 to 90 min). Monitor respirations for up to 2 hr after use to assess for reoccurrence of respiratory depression and the need for repeat dosage of naloxone. Titrate dosage to achieve reversal of respiratory depression without full reversal of pain management effects. Rapid infusion of naloxone may cause hypertension, tachycardia, nausea, and vomiting. The nurse should assess the client for respiratory depression, apply oxygen if needed, and have intubation equipment ready. It is not necessary to administer a fluid bolus and there is no indication for insertion of an indwelling urinary catheter.

NCLEX® Connection: Pharmacological and Parenteral Therapies, Medication Administration

4. Agonist-antagonist opioids differ from pure opioid agonists in that they

A. have a greater risk for abuse due to an increase in euphoria.

B. cause a higher incidence of respiratory depression.

C. may not be reversed with an opioid antagonist.

D. may cause abstinence syndrome in clients physically dependent to opioids.

Clients physically dependent on opioids may develop abstinence syndrome with the use of an agonist-antagonist opioid. Symptoms include abdominal pain, fever, and anxiousness. Agonist-antagonist opioids produce less respiratory depression and have a lower potential for abuse due to less euphoria. They may be reversed or partially reversed with an opioid antagonist, such as naloxone.

NCLEX® Connection: Pharmacological and Parenteral Therapies, Expected Actions/ Outcomes

UNIT 9 MEDICATIONS FOR PAIN AND INFLAMMATION

Chapter 37 Adjuvant Medications for Pain

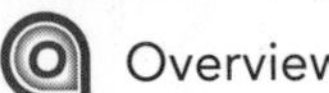

Overview

- Adjuvant medications for pain are used with a primary pain medication, usually an opioid agonist, to increase pain relief while reducing the dosage of the opioid agonist.
- Reduced dosage of the opioid results in reduced adverse reactions, such as respiratory depression, sedation, and constipation. Targeting pain stimulus using different types of medications often provides improved pain reduction.
- Categories of medications in this section include tricyclic antidepressants, anticonvulsants, CNS stimulants, antihistamines, glucocorticoids, bisphosphonates, and nonsteroidal anti-inflammatory drugs (NSAIDs).

MEDICATION CLASSIFICATION: ADJUVANT MEDICATIONS FOR PAIN

- Select Prototype Medication:
  - Tricyclic antidepressants: amitriptyline (Elavil) – oral/IM
  - Anticonvulsants: carbamazepine (Tegretol) – gabapentin (Neurontin) oral
  - CNS stimulants: methylphenidate (Ritalin) – oral
  - Antihistamines: hydroxyzine (Vistaril) – oral/IM
  - Glucocorticoids: dexamethasone (Decadron) – oral, IV, IM
  - Bisphosphonates: etidronate (Didronel) – oral
  - NSAIDs: ibuprofen (Motrin) – oral
- Other Medications:
  - Tricyclic antidepressants: imipramine (Tofranil) – oral
  - Anticonvulsants: phenytoin (Dilantin) – oral, IV, IM
  - CNS stimulants: dextroamphetamine (Dexedrine) – oral
  - Glucocorticoids: prednisone (Deltasone) – oral
  - Bisphosphonates: pamidronate (Aredia) – IV
  - NSAIDs: ketorolac (Toradol)

Purpose

- Expected Pharmacological Action
  - Adjuvant medications for pain enhance the effects of opioids
- Therapeutic Uses
  - These medications are used in combination with opioids and cannot be used as a substitute for opioids.
  - NSAIDs are used to treat inflammation.
  - Tricyclic antidepressants are used to treat depression and neuropathic pain such as cramping, aching, burning, darting, and lancinating pain.
  - Anticonvulsants are used to relieve neuropathic pain.
  - CNS stimulants augment analgesia and decrease sedation.
  - Antihistamines decrease anxiety, prevent insomnia and relieve nausea.
  - Glucocorticoids decrease pain from intracranial pressure and spinal cord compression.
  - Bisphosphonates manage hypercalcemia and bone pain.

Complications

SIDE/ADVERSE EFFECTS	NURSING INTERVENTIONS/CLIENT EDUCATION
Tricyclic antidepressants: Amitriptyline	
Orthostatic hypotension	• Advise clients to sit or lie down if symptoms of lightheadedness or dizziness occur and to change positions slowly. • Provide assistance with ambulation as needed. • Monitor the client's blood pressure while the client is lying down, sitting, and standing.
Sedation	• Advise clients to avoid hazardous activities, such as driving or operating heavy machinery.
Anticholinergic effects such as dry mouth, urinary retention, constipation, blurred vision	• Advise clients to increase fluid intake, sip fluids throughout the day, chew gum, or suck on hard candy. • Instruct clients to increase physical activity by engaging in a regular exercise routine. • Administer a stimulant laxative, such as bisacodyl (Dulcolax) to counteract decreased bowel motility, and a stool softener, such as docusate sodium (Colace), to prevent constipation. • Advise clients to void every 4 hr and to report urinary retention. • Advise clients to report blurred vision. • Monitor the client's I/O, and assess the client's bladder for distention by palpating the lower abdomen area every 4 to 6 hr.

SIDE/ADVERSE EFFECTS	NURSING INTERVENTIONS/CLIENT EDUCATION
Anticonvulsants: Carbamazepine, gabapentin	
Bone marrow suppression	• Periodically monitor the client's complete blood count and platelets. • Advise clients to observe for signs of easy bruising and bleeding, fever, or sore throat and to notify the provider if they occur.
Gastrointestinal distress (nausea, vomiting and diarrhea)	• Advise clients to take the medication with food.
CNS stimulants: Methylphenidate	
Weight loss	• Monitor the client's weight. Encourage good nutrition.
Insomnia	• Instruct clients to take the last dose of the day no later than 4 p.m.
Antihistamines: Hydroxyzine	
Sedation	• Advise clients to avoid hazardous activities, such as driving or operating heavy machinery. Reduce dosage in older adult clients.
Dry mouth	• Advise clients to increase fluid intake, sip fluids throughout the day, chew gum, or suck on hard candy.
Glucocorticoids: Dexamethasone	
Adrenal insufficiency (hypotension, dehydration, weakness, lethargy, vomiting, diarrhea associated with prolonged use)	• Advise clients to observe for symptoms and to notify the provider if symptoms occur.
Osteoporosis	• Advise clients to take calcium supplements, vitamin D, and/or bisphosphonate (alendronate [Fosamax]) as prescribed.
Hypokalemia	• Monitor the client's potassium levels and administer potassium supplements as needed.
Glucose intolerance	• Monitor the client's blood glucose levels.
Peptic ulcer disease	• Advise clients to take the medication with meals. • Encourage prophylactic use of an H_2 antagonist such as ranitidine (Zantac).
Bisphosphonate: Etidronate	
Transient flu-like symptoms	• Monitor for fever. Advise clients to notify the provider if symptoms occur.
Venous irritation at injection site	• Monitor the injection site and infuse with sufficient IV fluids.
Renal failure, UTI	• Monitor creatinine levels. Advise clients to monitor for symptoms of UTI (pain and burning, discolored urine).

SIDE/ADVERSE EFFECTS	NURSING INTERVENTIONS/CLIENT EDUCATION
NSAIDs: Ibuprofen	
Bone marrow suppression	• Periodically monitor the client's complete blood count and platelets. • Advise clients to observe for signs of easy bruising and bleeding, fever or sore throat and to notify the provider if they occur.
Gastrointestinal distress, such as nausea, vomiting and diarrhea. or ulceration	• Advise client to take with food or meals. • Monitor for GI bleed (coffee-ground emesis; bloody, tarry stools; or abdominal pain).

 Contraindications/Precautions

MEDICATION	CONTRAINDICATIONS
Tricyclic antidepressants: Amitriptyline	• These medications are contraindicated in clients recovering from an MI and within 14 days of taking a MAOI. • Use caution with clients who have a seizure disorder, urinary retention, prostatic hypertrophy, angle-closure glaucoma, hyperthyroidism, and liver or kidney disease.
Anticonvulsants: Carbamazepine, gabapentin	• These medications are contraindicated in clients who have bone marrow suppression and within 14 days of taking a MAOI. • Use caution with and including those clients with a seizure disorder.
CNS stimulants: Methylphenidate	• Methylphenidate is contraindicated in clients with hyperthyroidism and hypertension and within 14 days of taking a MAOI. • Use caution with clients who have agitation or tics.
Antihistamines: Hydroxyzine	• Hydroxyzine is contraindicated in clients who are hypersensitive to this medication. • Use caution with older adults.
Glucocorticoids: Dexamethasone	• Dexamethasone is contraindicated in clients who have fungal infection. • Use caution with clients who have a seizure disorder, peptic ulcer disease, hypertension, hypothyroidism, diabetes mellitus, or liver disease.
Bisphosphonate: Etidronate	• Etidronate is contraindicated in clients who are hypersensitive to this medication. • Use caution with clients who have kidney disease.
NSAIDs: Ibuprofen	• Ibuprofen is contraindicated in clients who have a history of bronchospasms with aspirin or NSAIDs. • Use caution with clients who have peptic ulcers, hypertension, and liver or kidney disease.

Interactions

MEDICATION/FOOD INTERACTIONS	NURSING INTERVENTIONS/CLIENT EDUCATION
Tricyclic antidepressants: Amitriptyline	
Barbiturates, CNS depressants, and alcohol may cause additive CNS depression.	• Do not use together.
Anticonvulsants: Carbamazepine, gabapentin	
Carbamazepine causes a decrease in the effects of oral contraceptives and warfarin (Coumadin) because of the stimulation of hepatic drug-metabolizing enzymes.	• Advise clients to increase dose of oral contraceptives. • Monitor for therapeutic effects of warfarin with PT and INR. • Dosages may need to be adjusted.
Grapefruit juice inhibits metabolism, and thus increases carbamazepine levels.	• Advise clients to avoid intake of grapefruit juice.
Phenytoin and phenobarbital decrease the effects of carbamazepine.	• Concurrent use is not recommended.
CNS stimulants: Methylphenidate	
Alkalizing medications may cause increase in reabsorption.	• Monitor for increase in amphetamine effects.
Acidifying medications may increase excretion of amphetamine.	• Monitor for decrease in amphetamine effects.
Insulin and oral diabetics may decrease glucose level.	• Monitor glucose.
MAOIs may cause severe hypertension.	• Avoid concurrent use.
Caffeine may increase stimulant effect.	• Advise clients to avoid caffeine.
OTC medications with sympathomimetic action may lead to increased CNS stimulation.	• Instruct clients to avoid use of OTC medications.
Antihistamines: Hydroxyzine	
Barbiturates, CNS depressants, and alcohol may cause additive CNS depression.	• Do not use together.
Glucocorticoids: Dexamethasone	
Glucocorticoids promote hyperglycemia, thereby counteracting the effects of insulin and oral hypoglycemics.	• The dose of hypoglycemic medications may need to be increased.
Concurrent use of salicylates and NSAIDs may increase the risk for GI bleed.	• Monitor for GI bleed. Use together cautiously.
Because of the risk for hypokalemia there is an increased risk of dysrhythmias caused by digoxin.	• Monitor potassium and cardiac rhythm. • Administer potassium supplements.
Diuretics that promote potassium loss increase the risk for hypokalemia.	• Monitor serum potassium level. • Encourage clients to eat potassium-rich foods. • Administer potassium supplements.

MEDICATION/FOOD INTERACTIONS	NURSING INTERVENTIONS/CLIENT EDUCATION
Bisphosphonates: Etidronate, pamidronate	
None significant	
NSAIDs: Ibuprofen	
NSAIDs may reduce effectiveness of antihypertensives, furosemide, and thiazide diuretics.	• Monitor for medication effectiveness.
Aspirin and corticosteroids may increase GI effects.	• Do not use together.
NSAIDs may increase levels of oral anticoagulants and lithium.	• Monitor medication levels.

Nursing Administration

- Clients should receive a pain management plan.
- Encourage clients who have cancer to voice fears and concerns about cancer, cancer pain, and pain treatment.
- Advise clients that pain medications should be given on a fixed schedule around the clock, and not as needed.
- Advise clients that physical dependence is not considered addiction.

Nursing Evaluation of Medication Effectiveness

- Depending on the therapeutic intent, effectiveness may be evidenced by:
    - Relief of depression, seizures, dysrhythmias, and other symptoms that aggravate the client's pain level
    - Decreased opioid side effects
    - Relief of neuropathic pain
    - Decreased cancer bone pain

CHAPTER 37: ADJUVANT MEDICATIONS FOR PAIN

Application Exercises

1. Adjuvant medications are used in conjunction with an opioid agonist to do which of the following? (Select all that apply)

   _____ Reduce the dosage of the opioid.

   _____ Reduce the side effects of the opioid.

   _____ Increase the analgesic effects.

   _____ Increase CNS stimulation.

   _____ Increase opioid tolerance.

2. Anticonvulsants are most effective as an adjuvant to pain medications when treating which of the following?

   A. Visceral pain

   B. Bone pain

   C. Neuropathic pain

   D. Muscle pain

3. Nursing care for a client who is on a glucocorticoid for pain control may include doing which of the following? (Select all that apply)

   _____ Monitoring for urinary retention

   _____ Monitoring serum glucose

   _____ Monitoring serum potassium level

   _____ Monitoring for gastric bleeding

   _____ Monitoring for respiratory depression

CHAPTER 37: ADJUVANT MEDICATIONS FOR PAIN

Application Exercises Answer Key

1. Adjuvant medications are used in conjunction with an opioid agonist to do which of the following? (Select all that apply)

    __X__ **Reduce the dosage of the opioid.**

    __X__ **Reduce the side effects of the opioid.**

    __X__ **Increase the analgesic effects.**

    _____ Increase CNS stimulation.

    _____ Increase opioid tolerance.

    Adjuvant medications for pain are used with an opioid to increase pain relief while reducing the dosage of the opioid agonist. Reduced dosage of the opioid agonist results in reduced adverse reactions, such as respiratory depression, sedation, and constipation. Targeting pain stimulus using different types of medications often provides increased pain reduction. Adjuvant medications do not increase CNS stimulation or opioid tolerance.

NCLEX® Connection: Pharmacological and Parenteral Therapies, Adverse Effects/Contraindications/Side Effects/Interactions

2. Anticonvulsants are most effective as an adjuvant to pain medications when treating which of the following?

    A. Visceral pain

    B. Bone pain

    C. Neuropathic pain

    D. Muscle pain

    Anticonvulsants are most effective in treating neuropathic pain, which is pain that stems from nerve injury. It may be described as sharp or burning. These medications are not effective for visceral, bone, or muscle pain.

NCLEX® Connection: Pharmacological and Parenteral Therapies, Pharmacological Pain Management

3. Nursing care for a client who is on a glucocorticoid for pain control may include doing which of the following? (Select all that apply)

_____ Monitoring for urinary retention
__X__ **Monitoring serum glucose**
__X__ **Monitoring serum potassium level**
__X__ **Monitoring for gastric bleeding**
_____ Monitoring for respiratory depression

Glucocorticoids may cause hyperglycemia, hypokalemia, peptic ulcer disease, decreased resistance to infection, osteoporosis, and adrenal insufficiency. They may be used to help control pain in spinal cord compression and other cancer-related pain.

NCLEX® Connection: Pharmacological and Parenteral Therapies, Expected Agents/Outcomes

UNIT 9 MEDICATIONS FOR PAIN AND INFLAMMATION

Chapter 38 Miscellaneous Pain Medications

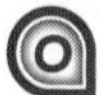

Overview

- Pain is subjective and may be indicative of tissue injury or impending tissue injury.
- Pain may result from the release of chemical mediators, inflammation, or pressure.
- Gout is caused by elevated levels of uric acid, which may accumulate and cause localized inflammation in synovial areas. Antigout medications act either by reducing inflammation or decreasing serum uric acid levels.
- Migraine headaches may be caused by the inflammation and vasodilation of cerebral blood vessels. Medications used to control migraine headaches may be used as needed to stop an oncoming migraine or to prevent a migraine from occurring.
- Local anesthetics block motor and sensory neurons to a specific area. They may be given topically, injected directly into an area, or given regionally, epidurally, or into the subarachnoid (spinal) space.

MEDICATION CLASSIFICATION: ANTIGOUT MEDICATION

MEDICATIONS	EXPECTED PHARMACOLOGICAL ACTION	THERAPEUTIC USES
	Anti-inflammatory agents	
• Select Prototype Medication: colchicine (Colgout) • Other Medications: ○ NSAIDs: Indomethacin (Indocin), naproxen (Naprosyn), diclofenac (Voltaren)	• These medications decrease inflammation. • Colchicine is only effective for inflammation of gout.	• Abort an acute gout attack if given in response to precursor symptoms • Treatment of acute attacks • Decrease in incidence of acute attacks for clients with chronic gout
○ Glucocorticoids: prednisone (Deltasone)		• Prednisone is used for clients with acute gout who are unable to take or unresponsive to NSAIDs.

MEDICATIONS	EXPECTED PHARMACOLOGICAL ACTION	THERAPEUTIC USES
	Agents for hyperuricemia	
• Select Prototype Medication: allopurinol (Zyloprim) • Other Medications: febuxostat (Uloric), probenecid	• Allopurinol inhibits uric acid production. • Probenecid inhibits uric acid reabsorption by renal tubules.	• Hyperuricemia due to chronic gout or secondary to cancer chemotherapy

Route of Administration

- Colchicine – Oral, IV rarely used
- Allopurinol – Oral, IV

Complications

SIDE/ADVERSE EFFECTS	NURSING INTERVENTIONS/CLIENT EDUCATION
Colchicine	
Mild GI distress which may progress to GI toxicity (abdominal pain, diarrhea, nausea, vomiting)	• Take oral medications with food. • Provide antidiarrheal agents as prescribed. • If severe symptoms occur, stop colchicine.
Thrombocytopenia, suppressed bone marrow	• Advise clients to notify the provider of bleeding, bruising or sore throat.
Hepatic necrosis	• Monitor liver enzymes.
Allopurinol	
Hypersensitivity reaction, fever, rash	• If giving IV, stop infusion. Severe reaction may require hemodialysis or glucocorticoids.
Renal injury	• Alkalinize the urine and encourage intake of 2 to 3 L of fluids/day. Monitor I&O, BUN, and creatinine.
Hepatitis	• Monitor liver enzymes.
GI distress (nausea and vomiting)	• Give with food.

Contraindications/Precautions

- Colchicine:
  - Avoid use during pregnancy (Pregnancy Risk Category C, if used orally; Category D, if used IV).

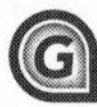

  - Use cautiously in older adults, clients who are debilitated, and clients who have renal, cardiac, and gastrointestinal dysfunction.

- Allopurinol:
  - Allopurinol is Pregnancy Risk Category C.
  - This medication is contraindicated in clients who have medication hypersensitivity or idiopathic hemochromatosis.

Interactions

MEDICATION/FOOD INTERACTIONS	NURSING INTERVENTIONS/CLIENT EDUCATION
Colchicine	
Salicylates may lessen the effectiveness of probenecid and may precipitate gout.	• Advise clients not to use salicylates during colchicine/probenecid therapy.
Loop diuretics may lessen the effectiveness of colchicine.	• Do not use together.
Phenylbutazamine may cause an increased risk for thrombocytopenia.	• Do not use together.
Alcohol use may lessen the effectiveness of colchicine.	• Do not use together.
Allopurinol	
Allopurinol slows the metabolism of warfarin within the liver, which places clients at risk for bleeding.	• Instruct clients to observe for signs of bleeding (bruising, petechiae, hematuria). • Monitor the client's prothrombin time and INR levels and adjust warfarin dosages accordingly.

Nursing Administration

- Monitor CBC and uric acid levels.
- Monitor IV infusion. This method may cause severe extravasation (leakage of fluid into outside tissue).
- Instruct clients to take the oral form with meals.
- Advise clients to report sore throat, fever or bleeding.
- Advise clients to avoid aspirin.
- Monitor BUN, creatinine, and urine output.
- If a rash develops, advise clients to stop the medication and report the occurrence to the provider.
- Instruct clients to concurrently take preventive measures such as avoiding alcohol and foods high in purine (red meat, scallops, cream sauces). Clients should ensure an adequate intake of water, exercise regularly, and maintain an appropriate body weight.

Nursing Evaluation of Medication Effectiveness

- Depending on the therapeutic intent, effectiveness may be evidenced by:
    - Improvement of pain caused by a gout attack (decrease in joint swelling, redness, and uric acid levels)
    - Decrease in number of gout attacks
    - Decrease in uric acid levels.

MEDICATION CLASSIFICATION: MIGRAINE MEDICATIONS

- Select Prototype Medications:
    - Ergot alkaloids: ergotamine (Ergostat)
    - Serotonin receptor agonists (Triptans):sumatriptan (Imitrex)
    - Beta-blockers: propranolol (Inderal)
    - Anticonvulsants: divalproex (Depakote ER)
    - Tricyclic antidepressants: amitriptyline (Elavil)
    - Calcium channel blockers: verapamil (Calan)
    - Estrogens: Estrogen gel and estrogen patches (Alora, Climara, and Estraderm)
- Other Medications:
    - Ergot alkaloids: ergotamine and caffeine (Cafergot)
    - Triptans: almotriptan (Axert), frovatriptan (Frova), naratriptan (Amerge), zolmitriptan (Zomig)

Purpose

- Expected Pharmacological Action
    - Migraine medications prevent the inflammation and dilation of the intracranial blood vessels, thereby relieving migraine pain.
- Therapeutic Uses
    - Stopping an acute migraine attacks
    - Prevention of migraine attacks
- Route of Administration
    - Ergotamine – Oral, sublingual, inhalation, rectal
    - Sumatriptan – Oral, sublingual, inhalation
    - Propranolol, divalproex, verapamil – Oral
    - Amitriptyline – Oral, IM

Complications

SIDE/ADVERSE EFFECTS	NURSING INTERVENTIONS/CLIENT EDUCATION
Ergot alkaloids: Ergotamine	
Gastrointestinal discomfort such as nausea and vomiting	• Administer metoclopramide (Reglan).
Ergotism (muscle pain; paresthesias in fingers and toes; cold, pale extremities)	• Stop medication, and immediately notify the provider if symptoms occur.
Physical dependence	• Advise clients not to exceed the prescribed dose. • Inform clients regarding symptoms of withdrawal (headache, nausea, vomiting, restlessness). • Instruct clients to notify the provider if symptoms occur.
Fetal abortion	• Avoid using this medication during pregnancy. • Use adequate contraception during therapy.
Serotonin receptor antagonists (Triptans): Sumatriptan	
Chest pressure (heavy arms or chest tightness)	• Warn clients about symptoms, and reassure clients that symptoms are self-limiting and not dangerous. • Advise clients to notify the provider for continuous or severe chest pain.
Coronary artery vasospasm/ angina	• Do not administer to a client who has, or is at risk for, coronary artery disease (CAD).
Dizziness or vertigo	• Advise client to avoid driving or operating machinery until medication effects are known.
Beta-blockers: Propranolol	
Extreme tiredness, fatigue, depression, and asthma exacerbation	• Advise clients to observe for symptoms and notify the provider if they occur.
Bradycardia, hypotension	• Monitor heart rate and blood pressure. Instruct client to take apical pulse prior to dosage. Notify the provider of significant change.
Anticonvulsants: Divalproex	
Neural tube defects	• Avoid use during pregnancy. • Use adequate contraception during therapy.
Liver toxicity	• Monitor liver enzymes. Notify the provider of lethargy or fever.
Pancreatitis	• Instruct clients to report abdominal pain, nausea, vomiting and anorexia. Medication should be discontinued.

SIDE/ADVERSE EFFECTS	NURSING INTERVENTIONS/CLIENT EDUCATION
Tricyclic antidepressants: Amitriptyline	
Anticholinergic effects (dry mouth, constipation, urinary retention, blurred vision, tachycardia)	• Increase fluid intake. • Increase physical activity by engaging in regular exercise. • Administer stimulant laxatives, such as bisacodyl (Dulcolax), to counteract reduced bowel motility, or stool softeners, such as docusate sodium (Colace), to prevent constipation. • Advise clients to void every 4 hr and to report urinary retention. • Advise clients to report blurred vision.
Drowsiness, dizziness	• Advise clients to avoid driving or operating machinery until medication effects are known.
Calcium channel blockers: Verapamil	
Orthostatic hypotension, bradycardia	• Advise clients to sit or lie down if symptoms of lightheadedness or dizziness occur and to change positions slowly. • Provide assistance with ambulation as needed. • Monitor heart rate.
Constipation	• Increase fluid intake. • Increase physical activity by engaging in regular exercise. • Administer stimulant laxatives, such as bisacodyl (Dulcolax) to counteract decreased bowel motility, or stool softeners, such as docusate sodium (Colace) to prevent constipation.

Contraindications/Precautions

- Ergotamine is contraindicated in clients with renal and/or liver dysfunction, sepsis, CAD, and during pregnancy.
  - Pregnancy Risk Category X
- Triptans are contraindicated in clients with liver failure, ischemic heart disease, a history of myocardial infarction, uncontrolled hypertension, and other heart diseases.
  - Pregnancy Risk Category C
- Propranolol is contraindicated in clients with greater than first degree heart block, bradycardia, bronchial asthma, cardiogenic shock or heart failure.
  - Use with caution in clients taking other antihypertensives, liver or renal impairment, diabetes mellitus, or Wolff-Parkinson-White syndrome.
  - Pregnancy Risk Category C
- Divalproex sodium (Depakote) is contraindicated in clients with liver disease.
  - Pregnancy Risk Category D

- Amitriptyline (Elavil) is contraindicated in clients with recent MI or within 14 days of a MAO inhibitor. Use with caution in clients with seizure history, urinary retention, prostatic hypertrophy, angle-closure glaucoma, hyperthyroidism and others.
  - Pregnancy Risk Category C
- Verapamil (Calan) Propranolol is contraindicated in clients with greater than first degree heart block, bradycardia, hypotension, left ventricle disease, atrial fibrillation or flutter or heart failure.
  - Use with caution in clients who have liver or renal impairment or increased intracranial pressure.
  - Pregnancy Risk Category C

Interactions

MEDICATION/FOOD INTERACTIONS	NURSING INTERVENTIONS/CLIENT EDUCATION
Ergotamine	
Sumatriptan can lead to spastic reaction of the blood vessels.	• Avoid concurrent use of these medications.
Some HIV protease inhibitors, antifungal medications, and macrolide antibiotics may increase ergotamine levels, causing increased vasospasm.	• Do not use together.
Sumatriptan	
Concurrent use of MAOIs can lead to MAO toxicity.	• Do not give triptans within 2 weeks of stopping MAOIs.
Ergotamine can lead to spastic reaction of the blood vessels.	• Avoid concurrent use of these medications.
SSRIs may cause weakness and hyper-reflexes.	• Monitor carefully.
Propranolol	
Verapamil (Calan) and diltiazem (Cardizem) have additive cardiosuppression effects.	• Monitor ECG, heart rate, and blood pressure.
Diuretics and antihypertensive medications have additive hypotensive effects.	• Monitor blood pressure.
Propranolol use can mask the hypoglycemic effect of insulin and prevent the breakdown of fat in response to hypoglycemia.	• Use with caution.
Divalproex	
Aspirin, chlorpromazine, and cimetidine may cause divalproex sodium toxicity.	• Monitor medication levels.
Benzodiazepines may cause CNS depression.	• Do not use together.
Divalproex may increase levels of phenobarbital and phenytoin.	• Monitor medication levels.

MEDICATION/FOOD INTERACTIONS	NURSING INTERVENTIONS/CLIENT EDUCATION
Amitriptyline	
Barbiturates may cause increased CNS depression.	• Do not use together.
Cimetidine may increase amitriptyline levels.	• Monitor medication effects.
MAOIs may increase CNS excitation or cause seizures.	• Do not give amitriptyline within 2 weeks of stopping MAOIs.
Verapamil	
Carbamazepine, digoxin may increase medication levels.	• Monitor medication levels.
Atenolol, esmolol, propranolol, and timolol may potentiate medication effects.	• Monitor medication effects. • Adjust dosage.

Nursing Administration

- Advise clients who have migraines to avoid trigger factors that cause stress such as consumption of alcohol, fatigue, and tyramine-containing foods (wine and aged cheese).
- Advise clients that lying down in a dark, quiet place may help ease symptoms.
- Advise clients to check apical pulse before dosage (propranolol).
- Clients may take dosage with food to reduce GI distress (Divalproex sodium, verapamil) and increase absorption (propranolol).
- Advise clients to protect skin from sun (amitriptyline) and avoid driving or operating machinery until medication effects are known (amitriptyline, verapamil).
- Use caution in case of orthostatic hypotension (amitriptyline).

Nursing Evaluation of Medication Effectiveness

- Depending on the therapeutic intent, effectiveness may be evidenced by:
    - Reduction in intensity and frequency of migraine attacks
    - Prophylaxis against migraine attacks
    - Termination of migraine headaches

MEDICATION CLASSIFICATION: LOCAL ANESTHETICS

- Select Prototype Medications:
  - Amide type: lidocaine (Xylocaine)
- Other Medications:
  - Ester type: Tetracaine (Pontocaine), procaine (Novocain)
  - Amide type: Eutectic mixture of 2.5% lidocaine/2.5% prilocaine (EMLA Cream)

Purpose

- Expected Pharmacological Action
  - These medications decrease pain by blocking conduction of pain impulses in a circumscribed area. Loss of consciousness does not occur.
- Therapeutic Uses
  - Parenteral administration includes:
    - Pain management for dental procedures, minor surgical procedures, labor and delivery, diagnostic procedures
    - Regional anesthesia (spinal, epidural)
  - Topical administration includes:
    - Skin and mucous membrane disorders
    - Minor procedures, such as IV insertion, injection (pediatric), wart removal

Complications

SIDE/ADVERSE EFFECTS	NURSING INTERVENTIONS/CLIENT EDUCATION
CNS excitation (seizures, followed by respiratory depression, leading to unconsciousness)	• Monitor for signs of seizure activity, sedation, change in mental status (decrease in level of consciousness). • Monitor the client's vital signs and respiratory status. • Have equipment ready for resuscitation. • Administer benzodiazepines such as midazolam (Versed) or diazepam (Valium) to treat seizures.
Hypotension, cardiosuppression as evidenced by bradycardia, heart block, and cardiac arrest (common in spinal anesthesia because of sympathetic block)	• Monitor the client's vital signs and ECG. • If symptoms occur, administer treatment accordingly as prescribed.

SIDE/ADVERSE EFFECTS	NURSING INTERVENTIONS/CLIENT EDUCATION
Allergic reactions (More likely with ester-type agents, such as procaine)	• Amide-type agents are less likely to cause allergic reactions, therefore are used for injection. • Observe for symptoms of allergy to anesthetics such as allergic dermatitis or anaphylaxis. • Treat with antihistamines or agency protocol.
Labor and delivery • Labor can be prolonged due to a decrease in uterine contractility. • Local anesthetics can cross the placenta and result in fetal bradycardia and CNS depression.	• Use cautiously in women who are in labor. • Monitor uterine activity for effectiveness. • Monitor fetal heart rate (FHR) for bradycardia and decreased variability.
Spinal headache	• Monitor clients for signs of severe headache. • Advise client to remain flat in bed for 12 hr postprocedure.
Urinary retention (May occur with spinal anesthesia)	• Monitor the client's urinary output. • Notify the provider if the client has not voided within 8 hr.

Contraindications/Precautions

- Local anesthetics are Pregnancy Risk Category B.
- These medications are contraindicated in clients with supraventricular dysrhythmias and/or heart block.
- Use cautiously in clients who have liver and kidney dysfunction, heart failure, and myasthenia gravis.

Interactions

MEDICATION/FOOD INTERACTIONS	NURSING INTERVENTIONS/CLIENT EDUCATION
Antihypertensive medications have additive hypotensive effects with parenteral administration of local anesthetics.	• Monitor heart rate and blood pressure.

Nursing Administration

- Advise clients to avoid hazardous activities when recovering from anesthesia.
- Maintain clients in a comfortable position during recovery.

- Injection of local anesthetic:
  - Vasoconstrictors, such as epinephrine (adrenaline), are often used in combination of local anesthetics to prevent the spread of the local anesthetic. Keeping the anesthetic contained prolongs the anesthesia and decreases the chance of systemic toxicity.
  - Prepare injection site for local anesthetic.
  - Maintain IV access for administration of emergency medications if necessary.
  - Have equipment ready for resuscitation.
  - For regional block, protect the area of numbness from injury.
- Spinal or epidural nerve blocks:

  - Monitor during insertion for hypotension, anaphylaxis, seizure, and dura puncture.
  - Monitor for respiratory depression and sedation.
  - Monitor insertion site for hematoma and signs of an infection.
  - Assess level of sensory block. Evaluate leg strength prior to ambulating.

  - Prepare IV fluids to administer to compensate for the sympathetic blocking effects of regional anesthetics.
- Client Education
  - Advise clients to notify the provider for signs of infection, such as fever, swelling and redness, increase in pain or severe headache, sudden weakness to lower extremities, or decrease in bowel or bladder control.
  - Notify the provider for signs of systemic infusion such as a metallic taste, ringing in ears, perioral numbness, and seizures.
- Topical cream (EMLA):
  - Apply to intact skin 1 hr before routine procedures or superficial puncture and 2 hr before more extensive procedures or deep puncture. Cover with occlusive dressing.
  - Prior to the procedure, remove the dressing and clean the skin with aseptic solution.
  - EMLA may be applied at home prior to coming to a health care facility for a procedure.

Nursing Evaluation of Medication Effectiveness

- Depending on the therapeutic intent, effectiveness may be evidenced by the following:
  - Client undergoes procedure without experiencing pain
  - Pain is relieved

CHAPTER 38: MISCELLANEOUS PAIN MEDICATIONS

Application Exercises

1. A nurse is providing teaching to a client who is to start Colchicine (Colgout) for acute gouty arthritis. The nurse should advise the client to do which of the following? (Select all that apply)

    _____ Decrease fluid intake.
    _____ Avoid alcohol use.
    _____ Take the medication on an empty stomach to increase absorption.
    _____ Notify the provider of bleeding, bruising, or sore throat.
    _____ Avoid aspirin or products containing salicylates.

2. Clients with migraine headaches should be instructed to do which of the following? (Select all that apply.)

    _____ Take ergotamine as a prophylaxis to prevent a migraine headache.
    _____ Try to identify and avoid trigger factors.
    _____ Lie down in a dark quiet room at the onset of a migraine.
    _____ Avoid foods that contain tyramine.
    _____ Avoid exercise that may increase heart rate.

3. A client is given a local anesthetic of lidocaine with epinephrine for the removal of a skin lesion. The nurse recognizes the epinephrine is used with the lidocaine to do which of the following?

    A. Reduce risk of systemic toxicity
    B. Reduce the risk of a seizure
    C. Cause localized vasodilation
    D. Cause additive anesthesia

4. A nurse recognizes toxic effects of a local anesthetic may cause

    A. coronary artery constriction.
    B. Stevens-Johnson syndrome.
    C. seizure activity.
    D. pulmonary edema.

CHAPTER 38: MISCELLANEOUS PAIN MEDICATIONS

Application Exercises Answer Key

1. A nurse is providing teaching to a client who is to start Colchicine (Colgout) for acute gouty arthritis. The nurse should advise the client to do which of the following? (Select all that apply)

_____ Decrease fluid intake.
X **Avoid alcohol use.**
_____ Take the medication on an empty stomach to increase absorption.
X **Notify the provider of bleeding, bruising, or sore throat.**
X **Avoid aspirin or products containing salicylates.**

Clients taking colchicine should be encouraged to avoid alcohol, notify the provider if bleeding, bruising or sore throat occur, and avoid aspirin or products containing salicylates. In addition clients should increase fluid intake and take the medication with food to avoid gastrointestinal distress.

NCLEX® Connection: Pharmacological and Parenteral Therapies, Medication Administration

2. Clients with migraine headaches should be instructed to do which of the following? (Select all that apply)

_____ Take ergotamine as a prophylaxis to prevent a migraine headache.
X **Try to identify and avoid trigger factors.**
X **Lie down in a dark quiet room at the onset of a migraine.**
X **Avoid foods containing tyramine.**
_____ Avoid exercise that may increase heart rate.

Ergotamine is only used at the onset of a migraine. It should not be given as a prophylaxis due to the risk of toxicity and dependence. Clients with migraine headaches should try to relieve stress with exercise, identify and avoid trigger factors, avoid foods that contain tyramine, and rest in a dark, quiet area.

NCLEX® Connection: Pharmacological and Parenteral Therapies, Medication Administration

3. A client is given a local anesthetic of lidocaine with epinephrine for the removal of a skin lesion. The nurse recognizes the epinephrine is used with the lidocaine to do which of the following?

   A. Reduce risk of systemic toxicity

   B. Reduce the risk of a seizure

   C. Cause localized vasodilation

   D. Cause additive anesthesia

   A vasoconstrictor, such as epinephrine, is often used along with a local anesthetic to prevent the spread of the local anesthetic. Keeping the anesthetic contained prolongs the anesthesia and decreases the chance of systemic toxicity.

NCLEX® Connection: Pharmacological and Parenteral Therapies, Adverse Effects/Contraindications/Side Effects/Interactions

4. A nurse recognizes toxic effects of a local anesthetic may cause

   A. coronary artery constriction.

   B. Stevens-Johnson syndrome.

   C. seizure activity.

   D. pulmonary edema.

   Toxicity of local anesthetics may cause seizure activity. Always aspirate when injecting a local anesthetic to prevent injecting into a vein or artery. IV access should be obtained prior to infusion of a local anesthetic. Monitor blood pressure, heart rate, respirations, and level of consciousness.

NCLEX® Connection: Pharmacological and Parenteral Therapies, Adverse Effects/Contraindications/Side Effects/Interactions

UNIT 10: MEDICATIONS AFFECTING THE ENDOCRINE SYSTEM

- Diabetes Mellitus
- Endocrine Disorders

NCLEX® CONNECTIONS

When reviewing the chapters in this unit, keep in mind the relevant sections of the NCLEX® outline, in particular:

CLIENT NEEDS: PHARMACOLOGICAL AND PARENTERAL THERAPIES

Relevant topics/tasks include:

- Adverse Effects/Contraindications/Side Effects/Interactions
  - Identify actual and potential incompatibilities of prescribed client medications.
- Dosage Calculation
  - Use clinical decision making/critical thinking when calculating dosages.
- Medication Administration
  - Mix medications from two vials when necessary.

UNIT 10 MEDICATIONS AFFECTING THE ENDOCRINE SYSTEM

Chapter 39 Diabetes Mellitus

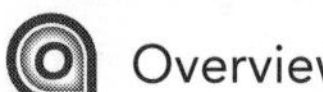

Overview

- Diabetes mellitus is a chronic illness that results from an absolute or relative deficiency of insulin.
    - Various insulins are available to manage diabetes. These medications differ in their onset, peak, and duration.
    - Oral hypoglycemic agents work in various ways to increase available insulin or modify carbohydrate metabolism.
    - Newer injectable medication are used to supplement insulin or oral agents to manage glucose control.

MEDICATION CLASSIFICATION: INSULIN

- Select Prototype Medications

CLASSIFICATION	GENERIC (TRADE NAME)	ONSET	PEAK	DURATION
Rapid-acting	Lispro insulin (Humalog)	Less than 15 min	0.5 to 1 hr	3 to 4 hr
Short-acting	Regular insulin (Humulin R)	0.5 to 1 hr	2 to 3 hr	5 to 7 hr
Intermediate-acting	NPH insulin (Humulin N)	1 to 2 hr	4 to 12 hr	18 to 24 hr
Long-acting	Insulin glargine (Lantus)	1 hr	None	10.4 to 24 hr

- Other Medications

CLASSIFICATION	GENERIC (TRADE NAME)
Rapid-acting	• Insulin aspart (NovoLog) • Insulin glulisine (Apidra)
Short-acting	• Regular insulin (Novolin R)
Intermediate-acting	• Insulin detemir (Levemir)

- Premixed insulins
  - 70% NPH and 30% Regular (Humulin 70/30) – mixture of intermediate acting and short-acting insulin
  - 75% insulin lispro protamine and 25% insulin lispro (Humalog 75/25) – mixture of intermediate acting and rapid-acting insulin

Purpose

- Expected Pharmacological Action
  - Promotes cellular uptake of glucose (decreases glucose levels)
  - Converts glucose into glycogen
  - Moves potassium into cells (along with glucose)
- Therapeutic Uses
  - Insulin is used for glycemic control of diabetes mellitus (type 1, type 2, gestational) to prevent complications.
  - Clients with type 2 diabetes mellitus may require insulin when:
    - Oral hypoglycemics, diet, and exercise are unable to control blood glucose levels.
    - Severe renal or liver disease is present.
    - Painful neuropathy is present.
    - Undergoing surgery or diagnostic tests.
    - Experiencing severe stress such as infection and trauma.
    - Undergoing emergency treatment of diabetes ketoacidosis (DKA) and hyperosmolar hyperglycemic nonketotic syndrome (HHNS).
    - Requiring treatment of hyperkalemia.

Complications

SIDE/ADVERSE EFFECTS	NURSING INTERVENTIONS/CLIENT EDUCATION
Risk for hypoglycemia (too much insulin)	• Monitor clients for signs of hypoglycemia. If abrupt onset, client will experience sympathetic nervous system (SNS) symptoms (tachycardia, palpitations, diaphoresis, shakiness). If gradual onset, client will experience parasympathetic (PNS) symptoms (headache, tremors, weakness). • Administer glucose. For conscious clients, administer a snack of 15 g of carbohydrate (4 oz orange juice, 2 oz grape juice, 8 oz milk, glucose tablets per manufacturer's suggestion to equal 15 g). • If the client is not fully conscious, do not risk aspiration. Administer glucose parenterally such as IV glucose, or SC/IM glucagon. • Encourage clients to wear a medical alert bracelet.
Lipohypertrophy	• Instruct clients to systematically rotate injection sites and to allow 1 inch between injection sites.

Interactions

MEDICATION/FOOD INTERACTIONS	NURSING INTERVENTIONS/CLIENT EDUCATION
Sulfonylureas, meglitinides, beta blockers, and alcohol have additive hypoglycemic effects with concurrent use.	• Monitor the client's serum glucose levels for hypoglycemia (less than 50 mg/dL) and adjust insulin or oral hypoglycemic dosages accordingly.
Concurrent use of thiazide diuretics and glucocorticoids may raise blood glucose levels and thereby counteract the effects of insulin.	• Monitor the client's serum glucose levels for hyperglycemia and adjust insulin doses accordingly. Higher insulin doses may be indicated.
Beta blockers may mask SNS response to hypoglycemia (tachycardia, tremors), making it difficult for clients to identify hypoglycemia	• Advise clients of the importance of monitoring glucose levels and not relying on SNS symptoms as an alert to developing hypoglycemia. • Instruct clients to maintain a regular eating schedule to ensure adequate glucose during times of hypoglycemic action.

Nursing Administration

- Adjust the client's insulin dosage to meet insulin needs.
    - The client's dosage may need to be increased in response to the client's increase in caloric intake, infection, stress, growth spurts, and in the second and third trimesters of pregnancy.
    - The client's dosage may need to be reduced in response to level of exercise or first trimester of pregnancy.
- Ensure adequate glucose is available at the time of onset of insulin and during all peak times.

- When mixing short-acting insulin with longer-acting insulin, draw the short-acting insulin up into the syringe first, then the longer-acting insulin. This prevents the possibility of accidentally injecting some of the longer-acting insulin into the shorter-acting insulin vial (this can pose a risk for unexpected insulin effects with subsequent uses of the vial).
- For insulin suspensions, the nurse should gently rotate the vial between his or her palms to disperse the particles throughout the vial prior to withdrawing insulin.
- Do not administer short-acting insulins if they appear cloudy or discolored.
- Insulin glargine and insulin detemir are both clear in color, not administered IV, and should not be mixed in a syringe with any other insulin.
- Administer lispro, aspart, glulisine, and regular insulin by subcutaneous injection, continuous subcutaneous infusion, and IV route.

- Administer NPH by subcutaneous route.
- Instruct clients to administer SC insulin in one general area to have consistent rates of absorption. Absorption rates from subcutaneous tissue increase from thigh to upper arm to abdomen.
- Use only insulin-specific syringes that correspond to the concentration of insulin being administered. Administer U-100 insulin with a U-100 syringe; administer U-500 insulin with a U-500 syringe.
- Select an appropriate needle length to ensure insulin is injected into subcutaneous tissue versus intradermal (too short) or intramuscular (too long).
- Encourage clients to enhance their diabetes medication therapy with a proper diet and consistent activity.
- Ensure proper storage of insulin.
  - Unopened vials of a single type of insulin may be stored in the refrigerator until their expiration date.
  - Vials of premixed insulins may be stored for up to 3 months.
  - Insulins premixed in syringes may be kept for 1 to 2 weeks under refrigeration. Keep the syringes in a vertical position, with the needles pointing up. Prior to administration, the insulin should be resuspended by gently moving the syringe.
  - Store the vial that is in use at room temperature, avoiding proximity to sunlight and intense heat. Discard after 1 month.

MEDICATION CLASSIFICATION: ORAL HYPOGLYCEMICS

MEDICATIONS	EXPECTED PHARMACOLOGICAL ACTION
Sulfonylureas • Select Prototype Medications: ○ 1st generation – tolbutamide (Orinase) ○ 2nd generation – glipizide (Glucotrol, Glucotrol XL) • Other Medications: ○ 1st generation – chlorpropamide (Diabinese) ○ 2nd generation – glyburide (DiaBeta, Micronase) glimepiride (Amaryl)	• Results in insulin release from the pancreas
Meglitinides • Select Prototype Medication: repaglinide (Prandin) • Other Medication: nateglinide (Starlix)	• Results in insulin release from the pancreas
Biguanides • Select Prototype Medication: metformin HCl (Glucophage)	• Reduces the production of glucose within the liver through suppression of gluconeogenesis • Increases muscles' glucose uptake and use
Thiazolidinediones (Glitazones) • Select Prototype Medication: rosiglitazone (Avandia) • Other Medication: pioglitazone (Actos)	• Increases cellular response to insulin by decreasing insulin resistance • Results in increased glucose uptake and decreased glucose production
Alpha glucosidase inhibitors • Select Prototype Medication: acarbose (Precose) • Other Medications: miglitol (Glyset)	• Slows carbohydrate absorption and digestion
Gliptins • Sitagliptin (Januvia)	• Augments naturally occurring incretin hormones, which promote release of insulin and decrease secretion of glucagon • Lowers fasting and postprandial blood glucose levels

- Therapeutic Uses
  - All classifications of oral hypoglycemic agents control blood glucose levels in clients with type 2 diabetes mellitus and are used in conjunction with diet and exercise lifestyle changes.
  - Metformin HCl is used to treat polycystic ovary syndrome (PCOS).

Complications

SIDE/ADVERSE EFFECTS	NURSING INTERVENTIONS/CLIENT EDUCATION
Glipizide and repaglinide	
Hypoglycemia	• Monitor clients for signs of hypoglycemia. If abrupt onset, the client will experience SNS symptoms, such as tachycardia, palpitations, diaphoresis, and shakiness. If gradual onset, the client will experience PNS symptoms, such as headache, tremors, and weakness. • Instruct clients to self-administer a snack of 15 g of carbohydrate (4 oz orange juice, 2 oz grape juice, 8 oz milk, glucose tablets per manufacturer's suggestion to equal 15 g). • Instruct clients to notify the provider if there is a recurrent problem. • If severe hypoglycemia occurs, IV glucose may be needed. • Encourage clients to wear a medical alert bracelet.
Metformin HCl	
Gastrointestinal effects (anorexia, nausea, vomiting, which frequently results in weight loss of 3 to 4 kg [6 to 8 lb])	• Monitor clients for severity of these effects. • Discontinue the client's medication if necessary.
Vitamin B_{12} and folic acid deficiency caused by altered absorption	• Provide supplements as needed.
Lactic acidosis (hyperventilation, myalgia, sluggishness, somnolence) – 50% mortality rate	• Instruct clients to discontinue medication if these symptoms occur, and to inform the provider immediately. • Severe lactic acidosis can be treated with hemodialysis.
Rosiglitazone	
Fluid retention	• Monitor clients for edema, weight gain, and/or signs of heart failure.
Elevations in low density lipoproteins (LDL) cholesterol	• Monitor the client's cholesterol levels.
Hepatotoxicity	• Perform baseline and periodic liver function tests. • Instruct clients to report any hepatotoxicity symptoms, such as jaundice or dark urine.

SIDE/ADVERSE EFFECTS	NURSING INTERVENTIONS/CLIENT EDUCATION
Acarbose	
Intestinal effects (abdominal distention and cramping, hyperactive bowel sounds, diarrhea, excessive gas)	• Monitor impact of these symptoms on the client. • Discontinue the medication if necessary.
Risk for anemia due to the decrease of iron absorption	• Monitor the client's hemoglobin and iron levels. • Discontinue the medication if necessary.
Hepatotoxicity with long-term use	• Check the client's baseline liver function and perform periodic liver function tests. • Discontinue the medication if elevations occur. • The client's liver function will return to normal after the medication is discontinued.
Sitagliptin – generally well tolerated	

Contraindications/Precautions

- Pregnancy Risk Category C: Glipizide, repaglinide, rosiglitazone
- Pregnancy Risk Category B: Metformin HCl (Glucophage), acarbose (Precose), sitagliptin (Januvia)
- These oral agents are generally avoided in pregnancy and lactation, but the provider may decide to prescribe them.
- Use cautiously in clients with renal failure, hepatic dysfunction, or heart failure because of the risk of medication accumulation and resulting hypoglycemia. Severity of disease may indicate contraindication.
- Contraindicated in the treatment of diabetic ketoacidosis (DKA)
- Metformin HCl is contraindicated for clients with severe infection, shock, and any hypoxic condition.
- Acarbose is contraindicated for clients with gastrointestinal disorders, such as inflammatory disease, ulceration, or obstruction.

Interactions

MEDICATION/FOOD INTERACTIONS	NURSING INTERVENTIONS/CLIENT EDUCATION
Glipizide	
Use of alcohol can result in disulfiram-like reaction (intense nausea and vomiting, flushing, palpitations).	• Inform clients about the risk and encourage them to avoid alcohol.
Alcohol, NSAIDs, sulfonamide antibiotics, ranitidine (Zantac), and cimetidine (Tagamet) have additive hypoglycemia effect.	• Inform clients of the risk and encourage clients to avoid alcohol. • Instruct clients to closely monitor glucose levels when these other agents are concurrently used. • If a client is taking a medication with an additive hypoglycemic effect, dosage adjustment of the oral hypoglycemic medication may be indicated.
Beta blockers may mask SNS response to hypoglycemia (tachycardia, tremors, palpitations, diaphoresis), making it difficult for clients to identify hypoglycemia.	• Advise clients of the importance of monitoring glucose levels and not relying on SNS symptoms as an alert to developing hypoglycemia. • Instruct client to maintain a regular eating schedule to ensure adequate glucose during times of hypoglycemic action.
Repaglinide and rosiglitazone	
Concurrent use of gemfibrozil (Lopid) results in inhibition of repaglinide metabolism, leading to an increased risk for hypoglycemia.	• Avoid concurrent use of repaglinide and gemfibrozil. • If used, closely monitor clients for signs of hypoglycemia.
Metformin HCl	
Alcohol increases the risk of lactic acidosis with concurrent use.	• Inform clients of the risks and encourage clients to avoid consuming alcohol.
Concurrent use of iodine-containing contrast media may result in acute renal failure.	• Clients taking metformin should discontinue medication 24 to 48 hr prior to procedure. They may resume medication 48 hr after test if lab results indicate normal renal function.
Acarbose	
Concurrent use of acarbose with sulfonylureas or insulin increase the risk for hypoglycemia.	• If acarbose is combined with a sulfonylurea or insulin, monitor clients carefully for hypoglycemia.
Concurrent use of metformin causes additive gastrointestinal effects and risk for hypoglycemia.	• If acarbose is combined with metformin, monitor clients carefully for gastrointestinal symptoms and hypoglycemia.
Sitagliptin – no significant interactions	

Nursing Administration

- Encourage clients to consistently exercise and to follow appropriate dietary guidelines.
- Encourage clients to maintain a log of glucose levels and to note patterns that impact glucose levels (increased dietary intake, infection).
- Consider referring clients to a registered dietician and/or diabetic nurse educator.
- Administer medications orally and at appropriate times:
    - Glipizide – Best taken 30 min prior to meal
    - Repaglinide – Instruct clients to eat within 30 min of taking a dose of the medication, 3 times/day
    - Metformin HCl – Instruct clients to take immediate release tablets 2 times/day with breakfast and dinner and to take sustained release tablets 1 time/day with dinner.
    - Rosiglitazone – Instruct clients to take once or twice a day, with or without food
    - Acarbose – Instruct clients to take with the first bite of food, 3 times/day. If a dose is missed, instruct the client to take the dose at the next meal but not to take 2 doses.
    - Sitagliptin – Instruct clients to take once a day with or without food.
- Instruct clients that formulations may combine two medications.
- Instruct clients who are also taking insulin to monitor for signs of hypoglycemia.

MEDICATION CLASSIFICATION: AMYLIN MIMETICS

- Select prototype medication: pramlintide (Symlin)

Purpose

- Expected Pharmacological Action
    - Pramlintide mimics the actions of the naturally occurring peptide hormone amylin, resulting in reduction of postprandial glucose levels from decreased gastric emptying time and inhibition of secretion of glucagon. There is also an increase in the sensation of satiety, which helps decrease caloric intake.
- Therapeutic Uses
    - Supplemental glucose control for clients with type 1 or type 2 diabetes
    - May be used in conjunction with insulin or an oral hypoglycemic agent, usually metformin or a sulfonylurea

Complications

SIDE/ADVERSE EFFECTS	NURSING INTERVENTIONS/CLIENT EDUCATION
Nausea	Instruct clients to report symptom to the provider. Dose may be decreased.
Reaction at injection sites	Generally self-limiting

Contraindications/Precautions

- Pramlintide is Pregnancy Risk Category C.
- This medication is contraindicated for clients who have renal failure or are receiving dialysis.
- Use cautiously in clients who have thyroid disease, osteoporosis, or alcoholism.

Interactions

MEDICATION/FOOD INTERACTIONS	NURSING INTERVENTIONS/CLIENT EDUCATION
Insulin increases risk for hypoglycemia.	Concurrent use may require a decrease in insulin dose, usually 50% of rapid- or short-acting insulin. Avoid use in clients unable to self-monitor blood glucose levels.
Concurrent use of pramlintide with medications that slow gastric emptying, such as opioids, or medications that delay food absorption, such as acarbose, may further slow gastric emptying time.	Avoid concurrent use.
Oral medication absorption is delayed.	Administer oral medications 1 hr before or 2 hr after injection of pramlintide.

Nursing Administration

- Administer subcutaneously prior to meals, using the thigh or abdomen.
- Instruct clients to keep unopened vials in the refrigerator and not to freeze. Opened vials may be kept cool or at room temperature but should be discarded after 28 days. Keep vials out of direct sunlight.
- Instruct clients not to mix medication with insulin in the same syringe.

MEDICATION CLASSIFICATION: INCRETIN MIMETICS

- Select Prototype Medication: Exenatide (Byetta)

Purpose

- Expected Pharmacological Action
  - Mimics the effects of naturally occurring glucagon-like peptide-1, and thereby promotes release of insulin, decreases secretion of glucagon, and slows gastric emptying. Fasting and postprandial blood glucose levels are lowered.
- Therapeutic Uses
  - Supplemental glucose control for clients with type 2 diabetes
  - May be used in conjunction with an oral hypoglycemic agent, usually metformin or a sulfonylurea

Complications

SIDE/ADVERSE EFFECTS	NURSING INTERVENTIONS/CLIENT EDUCATION
GI effects (nausea, vomiting, diarrhea)	Instruct client to notify provider if symptoms are intolerable.
Pancreatitis (severe and intolerable abdominal pain)	Instruct client to stop taking medication and to notify provider.

Contraindications/Precautions

- Pregnancy risk category C
- Contraindicated with clients with renal failure, ulcerative colitis, Crohn's disease

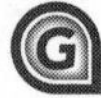

- Use cautiously in older adult clients and clients with renal impairment or thyroid disease.

Interactions

MEDICATION/FOOD INTERACTIONS	NURSING INTERVENTIONS/CLIENT EDUCATION
Oral medication absorption is delayed, especially oral contraceptives and antibiotics.	Administer oral medications 1 hr before or 2 hr after injection of exenatide.
Concurrent use of sulfonylurea increases risk of hypoglycemia.	Clients may require a lower dose of sulfonylurea. Instruct clients to monitor blood glucose levels.

Nursing Administration

- This medication is supplied in prefilled injector pens.
- Administer subcutaneously in the thigh, abdomen, or upper arms.
- Give injection within 60 min before the morning and evening meal. Never administer after a meal.
- Instruct clients to keep the injection pen in the refrigerator and to discard after 30 days.

Nursing Evaluation of Medication Effectiveness

- Depending on therapeutic intent, effectiveness may be evidenced by:
    - Preprandial glucose levels of 90 to 130 mg/dL and postprandial levels of less than 180 mg/dL
    - HgbA1c less than 7%

MEDICATION CLASSIFICATION: HYPERGLYCEMIC AGENT

- Select Prototype Medication: Glucagon

Purpose

- Expected Pharmacological Action
    - Increases blood glucose levels by increasing the breakdown of glycogen into glucose, decreasing glycogen synthesis enhances the synthesis of glucose
- Therapeutic Uses
    - Emergency management of hypoglycemic reactions, such as insulin overdose in clients who do not have IV glucose available or clients who are unable to take oral glucose
    - Decrease in gastrointestinal motility in clients undergoing radiological procedures of the stomach and intestines

Complications

SIDE/ADVERSE EFFECTS	NURSING INTERVENTIONS/CLIENT EDUCATION
GI distress (nausea, vomiting)	Turn clients onto the left side following administration to reduce the risk of aspiration if emesis occurs.

 Contraindications/Precautions

- Glucagon is ineffective for hypoglycemia resulting from inadequate glycogen stores (starvation).
- This medication is Pregnancy Risk Category B.
- Use cautiously in clients who have cardiovascular disease.

Nursing Administration

- Administer glucagon SC, IM, or IV immediately following reconstitution parameters.
- Provide food as soon as the client regains full consciousness and is able to swallow.
- Instruct clients to maintain access to a source of glucose and glucagon kit at all times.

Nursing Evaluation of Medication Effectiveness

- Depending on therapeutic intent, effectiveness may be evidenced by:
  - Elevation in blood glucose level to greater than 50 mg/dL

CHAPTER 39: DIABETES MELLITUS

Application Exercises

1. Fill in the following table by identifying the onset, peak and duration for each insulin.

CLASSIFICATION	GENERIC (TRADE NAME)	ONSET	PEAK	DURATION
Rapid-acting	Lispro insulin (Humalog)			
Short-acting	Regular insulin (Humulin R)			
Intermediate-acting	NPH insulin (Humulin N)			
Long-acting	Insulin glargine (Lantus)			

2. A nurse is providing teaching to a client who has type 2 diabetes mellitus and is starting repaglinide (Prandin). Which of the following statements made by the client indicates understanding of the administration of this medication?

    A. "I'll take this medicine with my meals."
    B. "I'll take this medicine 30 minutes before I eat."
    C. "I'll take this medicine just before I go to bed."
    D. "I'll take this medicine as soon as I wake up in the morning."

3. Clients taking metformin (Glucophage) should be monitored for which of the following?

    A. Lactic acidosis
    B. Hypertension.
    C. Hyperlipidemia.
    D. Respiratory alkalosis.

4. A client taking glipizide (Glucotrol) for control of type 2 diabetes mellitus should be cautioned against the use of which of the following?

    A. Magnesium hydroxide (Milk of Magnesia)
    B. Hydrocortisone acetate cream
    C. Calcium supplements
    D. Alcohol

5. Four clients need to receive morning insulin. Breakfast trays are due in 15 min. A nurse should first administer insulin to which of the following clients?

   A. Client with ac glucose level of 70 mg/dL, scheduled to receive NPH insulin (Humulin N) 3 units

   B. Client with ac glucose level of 90 mg/dL, scheduled to receive Regular insulin (Humulin R) 5 units

   C. Client with ac glucose level of 120 mg/dL, scheduled to receive NPH (Humulin N) 15 units insulin and Regular insulin 6 units

   D. Client with ac glucose level of 170 mg/dL, scheduled to receive lispro insulin (Humalog) 5 units

6. Which of the following should be included in a teaching plan for a client newly diagnosed with type 2 diabetes? (Select all that apply.)

   _____ "Check your blood glucose levels less frequently when not feeling well."
   _____ "Take an extra dose of the oral hypoglycemic agent the next day if you miss a dose."
   _____ "Carry a fast-acting glucose source."
   _____ "Eat a snack prior to planned exercise."
   _____ "Inspect feet surfaces daily."

7. A nurse is providing teaching to a client who is prescribed pramlintide (Symlin) for type 1 diabetes. Which of the following should the nurse include in the teaching?

   _____ "Take oral medications 1 hr before injection."
   _____ "Use upper arms as preferred injection sites."
   _____ "Mix medication with breakfast dose of insulin."
   _____ "Freeze unopened vials of medication."
   _____ "Discard open vials after 28 days."

CHAPTER 39: DIABETES MELLITUS

Application Exercises Answer Key

1. Fill in the following table by identifying the onset, peak and duration for each insulin.

CLASSIFICATION	GENERIC (TRADE NAME)	ONSET	PEAK	DURATION
Rapid-acting	Lispro insulin (Humalog)	**Less than 15 min**	**0.5 to 1 hr**	**3 to 4 hr**
Short-acting	Regular insulin (Humulin R)	**0.5 to 1 hr**	**2 to 3 hr**	**5 to 7 hr**
Intermediate-acting	NPH insulin (Humulin N)	**1 to 2 hr**	**4 to 12 hr**	**18 to 24 hr**
Long-acting-	Insulin glargine (Lantus)	**1 hr**	**None**	**10.4 to 24 hr**

NCLEX® Connection: Pharmacological and Parenteral Therapies: Expected Actions/ Outcomes

2. A nurse is providing teaching to a client who has type 2 diabetes mellitus and is starting repaglinide (Prandin). Which of the following statements made by the client indicates understanding of the administration of this medication?

    A. "I'll take this medicine with my meals."

    B. "I'll take this medicine 30 minutes before I eat."

    C. "I'll take this medicine just before I go to bed."

    D. "I'll take this medicine as soon as I wake up in the morning."

    Repaglinide causes a rapid, short-lived release of insulin. The client should take this medication within 30 min before each meal so that insulin is available when food is being digested.

NCLEX® Connection: Pharmacological and Parenteral Therapies: Medication Administration

3. Clients taking metformin (Glucophage) should be monitored for which of the following?

    A. Lactic acidosis

    B. Hypertension.

    C. Hyperlipidemia.

    D. Respiratory alkalosis.

    Lactic acidosis is a rare side effect, but if it occurs, it has a 50% mortality rate. Hypertension, hyperlipidemia, and respiratory alkalosis are not side effects of metformin.

NCLEX® Connection: Pharmacological and Parenteral Therapies: Adverse Effects/ Contraindications/Side Effects/Interactions

4. A client taking glipizide (Glucotrol) for control of type 2 diabetes mellitus should be cautioned against the use of which of the following?

    A. Magnesium hydroxide (Milk of Magnesia)

    B. Hydrocortisone acetate cream

    C. Calcium supplements

    D. Alcohol

    Alcohol taken currently with a sulfonylurea hypoglycemia agent can result in a disulfiram-like reaction. The client will experience intense nausea and vomiting, flushing, and palpitations. Clients taking glipizide can use magnesium hydroxide (Milk of Magnesia), but should not take it within 1 hr of taking glipizide. Topical hydrocortisone cream will not have any systemic effects and should not interfere with glipizide. There are no contraindications of calcium supplements with the use of glipizide.

NCLEX® Connection: Pharmacological and Parenteral Therapies: Adverse Effects/Contraindications/Side Effects/Interactions

5. Four clients need to receive morning insulin. Breakfast trays are due in 15 min. A nurse should first administer insulin to which of the following clients?

    A. Client with ac glucose level of 70 mg/dL, scheduled to receive NPH insulin (Humulin N) 3 units

    B. Client with ac glucose level of 90 mg/dL, scheduled to receive Regular insulin (Humulin R) 5 units

    C. Client with ac glucose level of 120 mg/dL, scheduled to receive NPH (Humulin N) 15 units insulin and Regular insulin 6 units

    D. Client with ac glucose level of 170 mg/dL, scheduled to receive lispro insulin (Humalog) 5 units

    This client's ac glucose level is already above pre-meal parameters. An onset of 15 min will coincide with food intake and may be helpful in avoiding post-meal hyperglycemia. The other clients' ac glucose levels are within normal range or low and a delay of a few minutes will not negatively impact their clinical outcomes.

NCLEX® Connection: Pharmacological and Parenteral Therapies: Expected Actions/Outcomes

6. Which of the following should be included in a teaching plan for a client newly diagnosed with type 2 diabetes? (Select all that apply.)

   _____ "Check your blood glucose levels less frequently when not feeling well."

   _____ "Take an extra dose of the oral hypoglycemic agent the next day if you miss a dose."

   X **"Carry a fast-acting glucose source."**

   X **"Eat a snack prior to planned exercise."**

   X **"Inspect feet surfaces daily."**

   A client with diabetes should always carry a fast-acting glucose source to treat unexpected hypoglycemia. Active muscle cells can take in glucose without insulin, and therefore prior to exercising the client should eat a snack to ensure enough glucose is available to prevent hypoglycemia. A client with diabetes should inspect his feet daily to monitor for skin breakdown and signs of infection. A client with newly diagnosed diabetes should check blood glucose levels at least before meals and at bedtime and more frequently when ill because acute illness can lead to hyperglycemia. The client should not take an extra dose of medication if a dose is missed.

 **NCLEX® Connection: Pharmacological and Parenteral Therapies: Medication Administration**

7. A nurse is providing teaching to a client who is prescribed pramlintide (Symlin) for type 1 diabetes. Which of the following should the nurse include in the teaching?

   X **"Take oral medications 1 hr before injection."**

   _____ "Use upper arms as preferred injection sites."

   _____ "Mix medication with breakfast dose of insulin."

   _____ "Freeze unopened vials of medication."

   X **"Discard open vials after 28 days."**

   Pramlintide delays oral medication absorption, so these medications should be taken 1 hr or 2 hr after an injection. Any opened vials of pramlintide should be discarded after 28 days. Pramlintide should only be injected into the thighs or abdomen and should not be mixed in a syringe with any type of insulin. Unopened vials should be refrigerated but not frozen.

 **NCLEX® Connection: Pharmacological and Parenteral Therapies: Medication Administration**

UNIT 10 MEDICATIONS AFFECTING THE ENDOCRINE SYSTEM

Chapter 40 Endocrine Disorders

Overview

- The endocrine system is made up of glands that secrete hormones, which act on specific receptor sites. Hormones target receptor sites to regulate response to stress, growth, metabolism, and homeostasis.
- An endocrine disorder usually involves the oversecretion or undersecretion of hormones or an altered response by the target area or receptor.
- Medications used to treat disorders of the thyroid, anterior and posterior pituitary, and adrenal glands are discussed in this chapter.

MEDICATION CLASSIFICATION: THYROID HORMONE

- Select Prototype Medication: levothyroxine (Synthroid, Levothroid)
- Other Medications:
    - Liothyronine (Cytomel)
    - Liotrix (Thyrolar)
    - Thyroid (Thyroid USP)

Purpose

- Expected Pharmacological Action
    - Thyroid hormones are a synthetic form of thyroxine (T_4) that increase metabolic rate, protein synthesis, cardiac output, renal perfusion, oxygen use, body temperature, blood volume, and growth processes.
- Therapeutic Uses
    - Thyroid hormone replacement is used for treatment of hypothyroidism (all ages, all forms).
    - Thyroid hormones are used for the emergency treatment of myxedema coma (IV route).
- Route of administration: oral, IV (myxedema coma)

Complications

SIDE/ADVERSE EFFECTS	NURSING INTERVENTIONS/CLIENT EDUCATION
Overmedication can result in signs of hyperthyroidism (anxiety, tachycardia, palpitations, altered appetite, abdominal cramping, heat intolerance, fever, diaphoresis, weight loss, and menstrual irregularities)	• Instruct clients to report signs of overmedication to the provider.

Contraindications/Precautions

- These medications are Pregnancy Risk Category A.
- Use cautiously in pregnancy and lactation.
- Use is contraindicated for clients with thyrotoxicosis.
- Because of cardiac stimulant effects, use is contraindicated following a MI.
- Use cautiously in clients who have cardiovascular problems (hypertension, angina pectoris, ischemic heart disease) because of cardiac stimulant effects.
- Thyroid hormone replacement is not for use in the treatment of obesity.

Interactions

MEDICATION/FOOD INTERACTIONS	NURSING INTERVENTIONS/CLIENT EDUCATION
Binding agents (cholestyramine, antacids, iron and calcium supplements) and sucralfate (Carafate) reduce levothyroxine absorption with concurrent use.	• Allow at least 3 hr between medication administration.
Many antiseizure and antidepressant medications, including carbamazepine (Tegretol), phenytoin (Dilantin), phenobarbital, and sertraline (Zoloft) can increase levothyroxine metabolism.	• Monitor clients for therapeutic effects of levothyroxine. The client's dosages of levothyroxine may need to be increased.
Levothyroxine can increase the anticoagulant effects of warfarin (Coumadin) by breaking down vitamin K.	• Monitor the client's prothrombin time (PT) and international normalized ratio (INR). • Instruct clients to report signs of bleeding (bruising, petechia). • Decreased dosages of warfarin may be needed.

Nursing Administration

- Obtain the client's baseline vital signs, weight, and height, and monitor periodically throughout treatment.
- Monitor and report signs of cardiac excitability (angina, chest pain, palpitations, dysrhythmias).

- Monitor the client's T_4 and TSH levels.
- Instruct clients to take daily on an empty stomach (before breakfast daily).
- Provide client education regarding the importance of lifelong replacement (even after improvement of symptoms). Advise clients not to discontinue the medication without checking with the provider.
- Instruct clients to check with the provider before switching to another brand of levothyroxine because some concerns regarding interchangeability of brands has been raised.

Nursing Evaluation of Medication Effectiveness

- Depending on therapeutic intent, evidence of effectiveness may include:
    - Decreased TSH levels
    - Normal T_4 levels
    - Absence of hypothyroidism symptoms (depression, weight gain, bradycardia, anorexia, cold intolerance, dry skin, menorrhagia)

MEDICATION CLASSIFICATION: ANTITHYROID MEDICATIONS

- Select Prototype Medication: propylthiouracil (PTU)
- Other Medications: methimazole (Tapazole)

Purpose

- Expected Pharmacological Action
    - Blocks the synthesis of thyroid hormones
    - Prevents the oxidation of iodide
    - Blocks conversion of T_4 into T_3
- Therapeutic Uses
    - Treatment of Graves' disease
    - Producing a euthyroid state prior to thyroid removal surgery
    - As an adjunct to irradiation of the thyroid gland
    - In the emergency treatment of thyrotoxicosis
- Route of administration: Oral

Complications

SIDE/ADVERSE EFFECTS	NURSING INTERVENTIONS/CLIENT EDUCATION
Overmedication can result in signs of hypothyroidism (drowsiness, depression, weight gain, edema, bradycardia, anorexia, cold intolerance, dry skin, menorrhagia)	• Instruct clients to report signs of overmedication to the provider. • Reduced dosages and/or temporary administration of thyroid supplements may be needed.
Agranulocytosis	• Monitor clients for early signs of agranulocytosis (sore throat, fever), and instruct clients to report them promptly to provider. • Monitor the client's blood counts at baseline and periodically. • If agranulocytosis occurs, stop treatment and monitor the client for reversal of agranulocytosis. • Neupogen may be indicated to treat agranulocytosis.

Contraindications/Precautions

- Use is contraindicated in pregnancy (Pregnancy Risk Category D) and during lactation because of the risk of neonatal hypothyroidism.
- Use cautiously in clients with bone marrow depression and/or immunosuppression.

Interactions

MEDICATION/FOOD INTERACTIONS	NURSING INTERVENTIONS/CLIENT EDUCATION
Concurrent use of antithyroid medications and anticoagulants may increase anticoagulation.	• Monitor the client's PT, INR, and activated partial thromboplastin time (aPTT), and adjust dosages of anticoagulants accordingly.
Concurrent use of antithyroid medications and digoxin (Lanoxin) may increase glycoside level.	• Monitor digoxin level and reduce digoxin dose as needed.

Nursing Administration

- Advise clients that therapeutic effects may take 1 to 2 weeks to be evident. Propylthiouracil does not destroy the thyroid hormone that is present, but rather prevents continued synthesis of TH.
- Monitor the client's vital signs, weight, and I&O at baseline and periodically.
- Instruct clients to take medication at consistent times each day and with meals to maintain a consistent therapeutic level and decrease gastric distress.

- Instruct clients not to discontinue the medication abruptly (risk of thyroid crisis due to stress response).
- Monitor clients for signs of hyperthyroidism (indicating inadequate medication).
- Clients with hyperthyroidism may be given a beta-adrenergic antagonist, such as propranolol (Inderal), to decrease tremors and tachycardia.
- Monitor for symptoms of hypothyroidism (indicating overmedication), such as drowsiness, depression, weight gain, edema, bradycardia, anorexia, cold intolerance and dry skin.
- Monitor CBC for leukopenia or thrombocytopenia.

Nursing Evaluation of Medication Effectiveness

- Depending on therapeutic intent, evidence of effectiveness may include:
    - Weight gain
    - Normal vital signs
    - Decreased T_4 levels
    - Absence of signs of hyperthyroidism (anxiety, tachycardia, palpitations, increased appetite, abdominal cramping, heat intolerance, fever, diaphoresis, weight loss, menstrual irregularities)

MEDICATION CLASSIFICATION: ANTITHYROID MEDICATIONS

- Select Prototype Medication: radioactive iodine (^{131}I)

Purpose:

- Expected Pharmacological Action
    - Radioactive iodine is absorbed by the thyroid and destroys some of the thyroid producing cells. At high doses, thyroid-radioactive iodine destroys thyroid cells.
- Therapeutic Uses
    - At high doses, thyroid-radioactive iodine is used for:
        - Hyperthyroidism
        - Thyroid cancer
    - At low doses, thyroid-radioactive iodine is used for:
        - Thyroid function studies (visualization of the degree of iodine uptake by the thyroid gland is helpful in the diagnosis of thyroid disorders)
- Route of administration: Oral

Complications

SIDE/ADVERSE EFFECTS	NURSING INTERVENTIONS/CLIENT EDUCATION
Radiation sickness	• Monitor clients for symptoms of radiation sickness (hematemesis, epistaxis, intense nausea, vomiting). • Stop treatment and notify the provider.
Bone marrow depression	• Monitor clients for anemia, leukopenia, and thrombocytopenia.
Hypothyroidism (intolerance to cold, edema, bradycardia, increase in weight, depression)	• Instruct clients to report signs of hypothyroidism to the provider.

Contraindications/Precautions

- Because of irradiating effects, use is contraindicated in pregnancy (Pregnancy Risk Category X), clients of childbearing age/intent, and during lactation.

Interactions

MEDICATION/FOOD INTERACTIONS	NURSING INTERVENTIONS/CLIENT EDUCATION
Concurrent use of other antithyroid medications reduces uptake of radioactive iodine.	• Discontinue use of other antithyroid medications for a week prior to therapy.

Nursing Administration

- Instruct clients regarding radioactivity precautions.
  - Encourage clients to void frequently to avoid irradiation of gonads.
  - Limit contact with clients to 30 min/day/person.
  - Encourage clients to increase fluid intake, usually 2 to 3 L/day.
  - Instruct clients to dispose of body wastes per protocol.
  - Instruct clients to avoid coughing and expectoration (source of radioactive iodine).

MEDICATION CLASSIFICATION: ANTITHYROID MEDICATIONS

- Select Prototype Medication: strong iodine solution (Lugol's Solution) – nonradioactive iodine
- Other Medications:
  - Sodium iodide
  - Potassium iodide

Purpose

- Expected Pharmacological Action
  - Thyroid-nonradioactive iodine creates high levels of iodide that will reduce iodine uptake (by the thyroid gland), inhibit thyroid hormone production, and block the release of thyroid hormones into the bloodstream.
- Therapeutic Uses
  - Thyroid-nonradioactive iodine is used for the development of euthyroid state and reduction of thyroid gland size prior to thyroid removal surgery.
  - Thyroid-nonradioactive iodine is used for the emergency treatment of thyrotoxicosis.
- Route of administration: Oral

Complications

SIDE/ADVERSE EFFECTS	NURSING INTERVENTIONS/CLIENT EDUCATION
Iodism symptoms due to corrosive property (metallic taste, stomatitis, sore teeth and gums, gastric distress, small bowel lesions)	• Take measures to prevent overdosage. • Instruct clients to drink through a straw to prevent tooth discoloration. • Instruct clients to take the medication with meals to reduce gastrointestinal distress.

Contraindications/Precautions

- Use in pregnancy is contraindicated (Pregnancy Risk Category D).

Interactions

MEDICATION/FOOD INTERACTIONS	NURSING INTERVENTIONS/CLIENT EDUCATION
Concurrent intake of foods high in iodine (iodized salt, seafood) increases risk for iodism.	• Monitor clients for signs of iodism (brassy taste in mouth, burning sensation in mouth, sore teeth). • Instruct clients regarding foods high in iodine.

Nursing Administration

- Thyroid-nonradioactive iodine can be used in conjunction with other therapy because effects are not usually complete or permanent.
- Obtain the client's baseline vital signs, weight, and I&O and monitor periodically.
- Instruct clients to dilute strong iodine solution (Lugol's Solution) with juice to improve taste.
- Instruct clients to take at the same time each day to maintain therapeutic levels.
- Encourage clients to increase fluid intake, unless contraindicated.

Nursing Evaluation of Medication Effectiveness

- Depending on therapeutic intent, effectiveness may be evidenced by the following:
    - Weight gain
    - Normal vital signs
    - Decreased T_4 levels
    - Reduction in size of thyroid gland
    - Client will be able to get adequate sleep, achieve and maintain appropriate weight, maintain blood pressure and heart rate within expected reference range, and be free of complications of hyperthyroidism.

MEDICATION CLASSIFICATION: ANTERIOR PITUITARY HORMONES/GROWTH HORMONES

- Select Prototype Medication: somatropin (Genotropin, Nutropin)
- Other Medication: somatrem (Protropin)

Purpose

- Expected Pharmacological Action
    - Anterior pituitary hormones/growth hormones stimulate overall growth and the production of protein, and decrease the use of glucose.
- Therapeutic Uses
    - Anterior pituitary hormones/growth hormones are used to treat growth hormone deficiencies (pediatric and adult growth hormone deficiencies, Turner's syndrome, Prader-Willi syndrome).
- Routes of administration: IM or subcutaneous.

Complications

SIDE/ADVERSE EFFECTS	NURSING INTERVENTIONS/CLIENT EDUCATION
Hyperglycemia	• Observe clients for signs of hyperglycemia (polyphagia, polydipsia, polyuria).
Hypothyroidism	• Monitor thyroid function.

Contraindications/Precautions

- These medications are Pregnancy Risk Category C.
- Use is contraindicated in clients who are severely obese or have severe respiratory impairment (sleep apnea) because of higher risk of fatality.
- Use cautiously in clients with diabetes because of the risk of hyperglycemia.
- Treatment should be stopped prior to epiphyseal closure.

Interactions

MEDICATION/FOOD INTERACTIONS	NURSING INTERVENTIONS/CLIENT EDUCATION
Concurrent use of glucocorticoids can counteract growth-promoting effects.	• Avoid concurrent use of glucocorticoids and somatrem if possible.

Nursing Administration

- Obtain the client's baseline height and weight.
- Monitor growth patterns during medication administration, usually monthly.
- Reconstitute medication per directions. Rotate gently, and do not shake, prior to administration.

Nursing Evaluation of Medication Effectiveness

- Depending on therapeutic intent, effectiveness may be evidenced by the following:
    - Client increases height.

MEDICATION CLASSIFICATION: POSTERIOR PITUITARY HORMONES/ANTIDIURETIC HORMONES

- Select Prototype Medication: vasopressin (Pitressin Synthetic)
- Other Medication: desmopressin (DDAVP, Stimate)

Purpose

- Expected Pharmacological Action
    - Posterior pituitary hormones/antidiuretic hormones promote reabsorption of water within the kidneys.
    - Posterior pituitary hormones/antidiuretic hormones cause vasoconstriction because of the contraction of vascular smooth muscle (Vasopressin).
- Therapeutic Uses
    - Posterior pituitary hormones/antidiuretic hormones are used to treat diabetes insipidus.
    - Posterior pituitary hormones/antidiuretic hormones are used during cardiac arrest (Vasopressin).
- Route of Administration
    - Desmopressin – oral, intranasal, subcutaneous, IV
    - Vasopressin – intranasal, subcutaneous, IM, IV

Complications

SIDE/ADVERSE EFFECTS	NURSING INTERVENTIONS/CLIENT EDUCATION
Reabsorption of too much water	• Monitor clients for symptoms of overhydration (sleepiness, pounding headache). • In general, clients should be instructed to reduce fluid intake during therapy. • Clients should use the smallest effective dose of desmopressin.
Myocardial ischemia from vasoconstriction.	• Monitor ECG and blood pressure. Advise clients to notify the provider of chest pain, tightness, diaphoresis.

Contraindications/Precautions

- These medications are Pregnancy Risk Category X.
- Use of vasopressin is contraindicated in clients who have coronary artery disease (risk for angina, MI) or with decreased peripheral circulation (risk for gangrene) and in clients with chronic nephritis.

Interactions

MEDICATION/FOOD INTERACTIONS	NURSING INTERVENTIONS/CLIENT EDUCATION
Carbamazepine and tricyclic antidepressants may increase the antidiuretic action.	• Use cautiously together.

Nursing Administration

- Monitor vital signs, central venous pressure, intake and output, specific gravity, and laboratory studies (potassium, sodium, BUN, creatinine, specific gravity, and osmolality).
- Monitor blood pressure and heart rate.
- Monitor for headache, confusion, or other signs of water intoxication.
- With IV administration of vasopressin, monitor the client's IV site carefully because extravasation can lead to gangrene.

Nursing Evaluation of Medication Effectiveness

- Depending on therapeutic intent, evidence of effectiveness may include:
  - A reduction in the large volumes of urine output associated with diabetes insipidus to normal levels of urine output
  - Cardiac arrest survival

MEDICATION CLASSIFICATION: ADRENAL HORMONE REPLACEMENT

- Select Prototype Medication: hydrocortisone (Hydrocortone, Solu-Cortef)
- Other Medications:
  - Prednisone (Deltasone) dexamethasone (Decadron)
  - Mineral corticoids: Fludrocortisone acetate (Florinef)

Purpose

- Expected Pharmacological Action
  - Mimic effect of natural hormones
- Therapeutic Uses
  - Acute and chronic replacement therapy for adrenocortical insufficiency (Addison's disease)
  - Nonendocrine disorders include cancer, inflammation, and allergic reactions.
- Route of administration: Oral, IV

Complications

SIDE/ADVERSE EFFECTS	NURSING INTERVENTIONS/CLIENT EDUCATION
Glucocorticoids: Hydrocortisone	
Osteoporosis	• Advise clients to take calcium supplements, vitamin D, and/or bisphosphonate (Etidronate).
Adrenal suppression	• Advise clients to observe for symptoms, and to notify the provider if symptoms occur. • Increase dose with stress. Do not stop the medication suddenly. Taper dose to discontinue.
Peptic ulcer, GI discomfort	• Advise clients to observe for signs and symptoms (coffee-ground emesis, bloody or tarry stools, abdominal pain), and to notify the provider if symptoms occur. • Administer prophylactic H_2 antagonists.
Infection	• Advise client to avoid contact with people who have a communicable disease. Monitor for any sign of infection, such as fever.
Mineralocorticoid: Fludrocortisone acetate	
Retention of sodium and water, which may lead to hypertension, edema, heart failure and hypokalemia	• Monitor weight, blood pressure and serum potassium. Monitor breath sounds and urine output.

Contraindications/Precautions

- Pregnancy Risk Category
  - Hydrocortisone is not rated.
  - Mineralocorticoid: Fludrocortisone acetate is Pregnancy Risk Category C.
- Use is contraindicated in clients with a systemic fungal infection.
- Use with caution in clients with a recent MI, gastric ulcer, hypertension, kidney disorder, osteoporosis, diabetes mellitus, hypothyroidism, myasthenia gravis and seizure disorder.

Interactions

MEDICATION/FOOD INTERACTIONS	NURSING INTERVENTIONS/CLIENT EDUCATION
NSAIDs or alcohol use may cause increased gastric distress or bleed.	Use together with caution.
Concurrent use with oral anticoagulants may increase or decrease anticoagulation.	Monitor coagulations studies and drug levels.
Concurrent use with potassium depleting agents may cause increased potassium loss.	Monitor serum potassium and ECG.
Concurrent use with vaccines and toxoids may reduce the antibody response.	Do not use together.
Fludrocortisone acetate	
Barbiturates and phenytoin may reduce effects of fludrocortisone acetate.	Monitor for reduced medication effects.

Nursing Administration

- Monitor weight, blood pressure and electrolytes.
- Give with food to reduce gastric distress.
- Advise clients to observe for signs and symptoms of peptic ulcer (coffee-ground emesis, bloody or tarry stools, abdominal pain) and to notify the provider if symptoms occur.
- Do not stop the medication suddenly. Taper off dosage if discontinuing.
- Instruct clients to notify the provider of symptoms of increased adrenal insufficiency (fever, muscle and joint pain, weakness and fatigue).

Nursing Evaluation of Medication Effectiveness

- Depending on therapeutic intent, evidence of effectiveness may include:
  - Relief of symptoms of adrenocortical deficiency, such as weakness, hypoglycemia hyperkalemia and fatigue, with minimal adverse effects

CHAPTER 40: ENDOCRINE DISORDERS

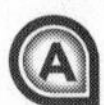

Application Exercises

1. A client tells a nurse that she has been taking her levothyroxine (Synthroid) every day for 9 days. She asks why there has been no improvement in her condition. Which of the following is the nurse's best response?

    A. "It may take several weeks for you to notice a therapeutic effect from the drug."

    B. "Your drug dose is probably too low."

    C. "Your body must be resistant to this drug."

    D. "Your doctor should be notified right away."

2. Propranolol (Inderal) may be prescribed to clients with hyperthyroidism to do which of the following?

    A. Increase the blood flow to the thyroid gland.

    B. Prevent thyroid hormone synthesis.

    C. Decrease tachycardia and tremors.

    D. Promote conversion of T_4 to T_3.

3. A client is starting on levothyroxine (Synthroid) for long-standing hypothyroidism. Which of the following dosage schedules should the nurse expect to administer?

    A. The client will start at a high dose and the dose will be tapered down as needed.

    B. The client's initial dosage will be based on body weight.

    C. The clients dosage will be adjusted daily based on blood levels.

    D. The client will start on a low dose, which will be gradually increased.

4. For which of the following clients would radioactive iodine (^{131}I) be contraindicated?

    A. A client who is over 40 years of age

    B. A client who is pregnant

    C. A client who has had a recent myocardial infarction

    D. A client who is scheduled for thyroid surgery

5. A nurse is caring for a client who is prescribed somatropin (Genotropin) to stimulate growth. The nurse should plan to monitor the client's urine for which of the following?

    A. RBCs

    B. Specific gravity

    C. Protein

    D. Glucose

6. A client is taking vasopressin (Pitressin) for diabetes insipidus. The nurse is assessing the client for vasopressin-related side effects. The nurse should monitor for

   A. hypovolemia.
   B. hypercalcemia.
   C. hyperglycemia.
   D. hypertension.

7. A client taking hydrocortisone for adrenocortical insufficiency (Addison's disease) is admitted to the hospital for a total hip arthroplasty. Which of the following actions is the highest priority?

   A. Administration of supplemental dose of hydrocortisone
   B. Instruction on coughing and deep breathing
   C. Insertion of an indwelling urinary catheter
   D. Requesting a referral for physical therapy

CHAPTER 40: ENDOCRINE DISORDERS

Application Exercises Answer Key

1. A client tells a nurse that she has been taking her levothyroxine (Synthroid) every day for 9 days. She asks why there has been no improvement in her condition. Which of the following is the nurse's best response?

   A. "It may take several weeks for you to notice a therapeutic effect from the drug."

   B. "Your drug dose is probably too low."

   C. "Your body must be resistant to this drug."

   D. "Your doctor should be notified right away."

   It may take several weeks to months to see the therapeutic effects of thyroid replacements. None of the other responses are appropriate.

NCLEX® Connection: Pharmacological and Parenteral Therapies: Expected Actions/ Outcomes

2. Propranolol (Inderal) may be prescribed to clients with hyperthyroidism to do which of the following?

   A. increase the blood flow to the thyroid gland.

   B. prevent thyroid hormone synthesis.

   C. decrease tachycardia and tremors.

   D. promote conversion of T_4 to T_3.

   Propranolol is a beta-adrenergic antagonist that decreases heart rate and controls tremors. Propranolol lowers blood pressure, but does not increase blood flow to the thyroid gland. Propranolol does not affect thyroid hormone synthesis.

NCLEX® Connection: Pharmacological and Parenteral Therapies: Expected Actions/ Outcomes

3. A client is starting on levothyroxine (Synthroid) for long-standing hypothyroidism. Which of the following dosage schedules should the nurse expect to administer?

   A. The client will start at a high dose and the dose will be tapered down as needed.

   B. The client's initial dosage will be based on body weight.

   C. The clients dosage will be adjusted daily based on blood levels.

   D. The client will start on a low dose, which will be gradually increased.

   This client will be very sensitive to thyroid replacement medications. Therapy should start at low doses and be increased gradually. None of the other dosage schedules are appropriate.

NCLEX® Connection: Pharmacological and Parenteral Therapies: Medication Administration

4. For which of the following clients would radioactive iodine (^{131}I) be contraindicated?

   A. A client who is over 40 years of age

   B. A client who is pregnant

   C. A client who has had a recent myocardial infarction

   D. A client who is scheduled for thyroid surgery

   Iodine (^{131}I) is in Pregnancy Risk Category X because of its irradiating effects that are harmful to the developing fetus. There are no contraindications for a client more than 40 years old or a client with a recent MI. Radioactive iodine can be used prior to thyroid surgery to produce a euthyroid state.

NCLEX® Connection: Pharmacological and Parenteral Therapies: Adverse Effects/ Contraindications/Side Effects/Interactions

5. A nurse is caring for a client who is prescribed somatropin (Genotropin) to stimulate growth. The nurse should plan to monitor the client's urine for which of the following?

   A. RBCs

   B. Specific gravity

   C. Protein

   D. Glucose

   Somatropin may increase glucose levels. The nurse should monitor the client for hyperglycemia. There is no indication to monitor the urine for RBCs, specific gravity, or protein.

NCLEX® Connection: Pharmacological and Parenteral Therapies: Adverse Effects/ Contraindications/Side Effects/Interactions

6. A client is taking vasopressin (Pitressin) for diabetes insipidus. The nurse is assessing the client for vasopressin-related side effects. The nurse should monitor for

   A. hypovolemia.

   B. hypercalcemia.

   C. hyperglycemia.

   D. hypertension.

   Vasopressin causes vasoconstriction and may increase blood pressure. It causes water retention, so fluid intake and output, and weight should be monitored. Headache and drowsiness may indicate fluid intoxication. Hypovolemia, hypercalcemia, and hyperglycemia are not side effects of vasopressin.

NCLEX® Connection: Pharmacological and Parenteral Therapies: Adverse Effects/ Contraindications/Side Effects/Interactions

7. A client taking hydrocortisone for adrenocortical insufficiency (Addison's disease) is admitted to the hospital for a total hip arthroplasty. Which of the following actions is the highest priority?

    A. Administration of supplemental dose of hydrocortisone

    B. Instruction on coughing and deep breathing

    C. Insertion of an indwelling urinary catheter

    D. Requesting a referral for physical therapy

    Adrenal crisis is the greatest risk to a client with Addison's disease who is taking a glucocorticoid and undergoing surgery. To prevent adrenal crisis, the client should receive supplemental doses during times of increased stress, such as infection or surgery. Instruction on coughing and deep breathing, insertion of an indwelling urinary catheter, and a referral for physical therapy are important but not the highest priority.

NCLEX® Connection: Pharmacological and Parenteral Therapies: Expected Actions/ Outcomes

UNIT 11: MEDICATIONS AFFECTING THE IMMUNE SYSTEM

- Immunizations
- Chemotherapy Agents

NCLEX® CONNECTIONS

When reviewing the chapters in this unit, keep in mind the relevant sections of the NCLEX® outline, in particular:

CLIENT NEEDS: PHARMACOLOGICAL AND PARENTERAL THERAPIES

Relevant topics/tasks include:

- Adverse Effects/Contraindications/Side Effects/Interactions
  - Identify a contraindication to the administration of a medication to the client.
- Expected Actions/Outcomes
  - Obtain information about prescribed medication for the client.
- Medication Administration
  - Administer and document medications given by parenteral routes.

UNIT 11 MEDICATIONS AFFECTING THE IMMUNE SYSTEM

Chapter 41 Immunizations

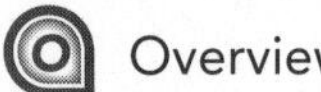

Overview

- Administration of a vaccine causes production of antibodies that prevent illness from a specific microbe.
- Active natural immunity develops when the body produces antibodies in response to exposure to a live pathogen. Active artificial immunity develops when an immunization is given and the body produces antibodies in response to exposure to a killed or attenuated virus.
- Passive natural immunity occurs when antibodies are passed from the mother to the newborn/infant through the placenta and then breast feeding. Passive artificial immunity is temporary, and occurs after antibodies in the form of immune globulins are administered to an individual who requires immediate protection against a disease after exposure has occurred.
- Immunizations may be made from killed viruses or live, attenuated or weakened viruses.

MEDICATION CLASSIFICATION: VACCINATIONS

- Childhood Vaccinations (See www.cdc.gov for updates)
  - Diphtheria and tetanus toxoids and acellular pertussis vaccine (DTaP) – Give doses at 2, 4, 6, 15 to 18 months, and at 4 to 6 years.
  - Tetanus and diphtheria toxoids and pertussis vaccine (Tdap) – Give one dose at 11 to 12 years.
  - Tetanus and diphtheria (Td) booster – Give one dose every 10 years following DTaP.
  - Haemophilus influenza Type B (Hib) – Give doses at 2, 4, 6, and at 12 to 15 months.
  - Rotavirus oral vaccine
    - Two formulations are available.
      - RotaTeq requires three doses beginning at age 6 weeks, with subsequent doses 4 to 10 weeks apart. RotaTeq vaccination should be completed before age 32 weeks. Vaccination should not be initiated for infants 15 weeks or older.
      - Rotarix requires two doses beginning at age 6 weeks with the next dose 4 weeks later.
    - All doses should be completed by age 8 months.

- Inactivated poliovirus vaccine (IPV) – Give doses at 2, 4, and 6 to 18 months, and at 4 to 6 years.
- Measles, mumps, and rubella vaccine (MMR) – doses at 12 to 15 months and at 4 to 6 years
- Varicella vaccine – Give one dose at 12 to 15 months and 4 to 6 years or 2 doses administered 4 weeks apart if administered after age 13.
- Pneumococcal conjugate vaccine (PCV) – Give doses at 2, 4, 6, and 12 to 15 months.
- Hepatitis A – Give two doses 6 months apart after age 12 months.
- Hepatitis B – Give within 12 hr after birth with additional doses at age 1 to 2 months and 6 to 18 months.
- Seasonal Influenza Vaccine
  - Annually, beginning at age 6 months, give trivalent inactivated influenza vaccine (TIV).
  - Starting at age 2 the live, attenuated influenza vaccine (LAIV) (nasal spray) may be used.
  - October through November is the ideal time, and December is acceptable.
- Meningococcal vaccine (MCV4) – Give one dose at age 11 to 12 years (earlier if specific risk factors are present).
- Human papillomavirus (HPV2 or HPV4) – Give three doses over a 6-month interval for girls at 9 to 12 years of age. HPV4 may be given to boys starting at age 9.

- Adult Vaccinations: 2010 CDC vaccination recommendations for adults 18 years of age and older (See www.cdc.gov for updates.)
  - Td booster – give at least one dose of tetanus, diphtheria, pertussis Tdap, and then Td every 10 years.
  - MMR – Give one or two doses at ages 19 to 49.
  - Varicella vaccine – Two doses should be given to adults who do not have evidence of previous infection. A second dose should be given for adults who had only one previous dose.
  - Pneumococcal polysaccharide vaccine (PPSV) – Vaccinate adults who are immunocompromised, who have a chronic disease, who smoke cigarettes, or who live in a long-term care facility. CDC guidelines should be followed for revaccination. If a client is not previously vaccinated or has no evidence of disease then one dose should be given at age 65.
  - Hepatitis A – Give two doses for high-risk individuals.
  - Hepatitis B – Give three doses for high-risk individuals.

- Seasonal Influenza Vaccine
    - One dose annually is recommended for all adults over age 50; health care providers including those who care for young children; individuals with chronic medical conditions such as cerebral palsy, asthma, and diabetes; individuals who are immunocompromised; and individuals living in long-term care settings.
    - Note that live, attenuated vaccine (LAIV), given as a nasal spray, is only indicated for adults under age 50 who are not pregnant or immunocompromised.
- Meningococcal conjugate vaccine (MCV4) – students entering college and living in college dormitories if not previously immunized. Meningococcal polysaccharide vaccine (MPSV4) is recommended for adults greater than 56 years of age. Revaccination may be recommended after 5 years for adults at high risk for infection.
- Human papilloma virus (HPV2 or HPV4) – Three doses are recommended for females up to age 26 who were not vaccinated as children. HPV4 may be given to males up to age 26.
- Herpes zoster vaccine – This is recommended for all adults over age 60 years.

Purpose

- Expected Pharmacological Action
    - Immunizations produce antibodies that provide active immunity. Immunizations may take months to have an effect but confer long-lasting protection against infectious diseases.
- Therapeutic Uses
    - Eradication of infectious diseases (polio, smallpox)
    - Prevention of childhood and adult infectious diseases and their complications (measles, diphtheria, mumps, rubella, tetanus, *H. influenza*)

Complications, Contraindications and Precautions

- Anaphylactic reaction to vaccine is a contraindication for further doses of that vaccine.
- Anaphylactic reaction to vaccine is a contraindication to use of other vaccines containing that substance.
- Moderate or severe illnesses with or without fever are contraindications. The common cold and other minor illnesses are not contraindications.
- Contraindications to vaccinations require the provider to analyze data and weigh the risks that come with vaccinating or not vaccinating.
- Immunocompromised individuals are defined by the CDC as those with hematologic or solid tumors, congenital immunodeficiency, or on long-term immunosuppressive therapy, including corticosteroids.

IMMUNIZATIONS	SIDE EFFECTS	CONTRAINDICATIONS/PRECAUTIONS
DTaP	• Local reaction at injection site • Fever and irritability • Crying that cannot be consoled, lasting up to 3 hours • Seizures • Rare: acute encephalopathy	• An occurrence of encephalopathy 7 days after the administration of the DTaP immunization • Seizures within 3 days of vaccination • History of uncontrollable crying or temperature of 40.5° C (105° F) or higher that occurs within 48 hr of vaccination
Haemophilus influenza type b conjugate vaccine	• Mild local reactions, low grade fever • Rarely fever, (temperature greater than 38.5° C [101.3° F]), vomiting, crying may occur	• Children less than 6 weeks of age
Rotavirus vaccine		• Infants with diarrhea and vomiting • Use caution with clients who are immunocompromised (with HIV infection or from medication administration).
IPV	• Local reaction at injection site • Allergic reaction possible in children allergic to streptomycin, neomycin, or bacitracin; these medications are contained in the vaccine in small amounts • Rare: vaccine-associated paralytic poliomyelitis	• Pregnancy
MMR	• Local reactions such as rash; fever; swollen glands in cheeks, neck and under the jaw • Possibility of joint pain lasting for days to weeks. • Risk for anaphylaxis and thrombocytopenia	• Pregnancy • Clients who are immunocompromised (with HIV infection or from medication administration). • Recent transfusion with blood products • History of thrombocytopenia
Varicella vaccine	• Varicella-like rash, local or generalized such as vesicles on the body	• Pregnancy • Pregnant women should avoid close proximity to children recently vaccinated. • Cancers of the blood and lymphatic system • Allergy to gelatin and neomycin • Clients who are immunocompromised (with HIV infection or from medication administration).

IMMUNIZATIONS	SIDE EFFECTS	CONTRAINDICATIONS/PRECAUTIONS
PCV	• Mild local reactions, fever, and no serious adverse effects	• Pregnancy
Hepatitis A and B vaccines	• Local reaction at injection site, mild fever • Anaphylaxis	• Hep A: ○ Pregnancy may be a contraindication • Hep B: ○ Allergy to baker's yeast
Seasonal influenza vaccine	• Inactivated: Mild local reaction, and fever • Live attenuated: headache, cough, fever • Rare: risk for Guillain-Barré syndrome manifested by ascending paralysis, beginning with weakness of lower extremities, and progressing to difficulty breathing	• LAIV, administered as nasal spray, is contraindicated for adults over 50 years and children under 2 years, for adults and children who are immunocompromised or who have a chronic disease. • History of Guillain-Barré syndrome
MCV4	• Mild local reaction • Rare: risk of allergic response	• History of Guillain Barré syndrome
HPV2 or HPV4 vaccine	• Mild local reaction and fever • Fainting has occurred shortly after receiving vaccination • Rare: risk for Guillain-Barré syndrome	• Pregnancy • Hypersensitivity to yeast
Herpes Zoster	• None	• Clients who are immunocompromised (with HIV infection or from medication administration).

Interactions

- None significant

Nursing Administration

- For infants and children:
  - Obtain parental consent for children.
  - Note the date, route, and site of vaccination on the child's immunization record at the time of immunization.
  - Give intramuscular vaccinations in the vastus lateralis muscle in infants and young children and into the deltoid muscle for older children and adolescents.

- Give subcutaneous injections in the outer aspect of the upper arm or anterolateral thigh.
- Use appropriate size needle for route, site, age, and amount of medication.
- Use strategies to minimize discomfort.
- Provide for distraction.
- Do not allow the child to delay the procedure.
- Encourage the parent to use comforting measures such as cuddling, pacifiers during procedure, and measures such as application of cool compresses to injection site or gentle movement of the involved extremity after the procedure.
- Provide praise afterward.
- Apply a colorful bandage if appropriate.
- Instruct parents to avoid administration of aspirin to children to treat fever or local reaction because of the risk of the development of Reye syndrome
- Instruct parents to premedicate infants and children with nonopioid analgesic/antipyretic prior to immunizations and for the following 24 hr. Use acetaminophen for infants 2 to 6 months. Parents may administer ibuprofen starting 6 months.
- Instruct parents to apply topical anesthetic prior to the injection.

- For adults:
  - Give subcutaneous vaccinations in the outer aspect of the upper arm or anterolateral thigh.
  - Give intramuscular vaccinations into the deltoid muscle.
- For clients of all ages:
  - Have emergency medications and equipment on standby in case the client experiences an allergic response such as anaphylaxis.
  - Follow storage and reconstitution directions. If reconstituted, use within 30 min.
  - Provide written vaccine information sheets and review the content with parents or clients.
  - Instruct parents and clients to observe for complications and to notify the provider if side effects occur.
  - Document administration of vaccines including date, route and site of vaccination; type, manufacturer, lot number and expiration of vaccine; and name, address, and signature.

Nursing Evaluation of Medication Effectiveness

- Depending on therapeutic intent, effectiveness may be evidenced by:
  - Improvement of local reaction to vaccination with absence of pain, fever, and swelling at the site of injection
  - Development of immunity

CHAPTER 41: IMMUNIZATIONS

Application Exercises

1. A nurse is caring for several clients who came to the clinic for a seasonal influenza vaccination. Which of the following clients could receive the vaccine via nasal spray rather than an injection?

    A. A 1 year old with no health problems

    B. A 17 year old who has a hypersensitivity to penicillin

    C. A 25 year old who is pregnant

    D. A 52 year old who takes a multivitamin supplement

2. A nurse is teaching a group of parents about immunizations. Which of the following vaccines should the nurse tell the parents is administered to children younger than 1 year of age and not to older children or adults?

    A. Pneumococcal vaccine

    B. Meningococcal vaccine

    C. Varicella vaccine

    D. Rotavirus vaccine

3. A 12-month-old child just received her first measles, mumps, and rubella (MMR) vaccine. For which of the following possible reactions to this vaccine should the nurse teach the parents to watch? (Select all that apply)

    _____ Rash

    _____ Redness and discomfort at injection site

    _____ Bruising on multiple areas of body

    _____ Fainting

    _____ Inconsolable crying

4. A nurse is caring for a group of clients who are not protected against varicella. Which of these clients should receive a varicella vaccination at this time?

    A. A 24-year-old woman in the third trimester of pregnancy

    B. A 3-year-old child with Wilms' tumor who is receiving chemotherapy

    C. A 2-month-old infant with no health problems

    D. A 32-year-old man with essential hypertension

CHAPTER 41: IMMUNIZATIONS

Application Exercises Answer Key

1. A nurse is caring for several clients who came to the clinic for a seasonal influenza vaccination. Which of the following clients could receive the vaccine via nasal spray rather than an injection?

   A. A 1 year old with no health problems

   B. A 17 year old who has a hypersensitivity to penicillin

   C. A 25 year old who is pregnant

   D. A 52 year old who takes a multivitamin supplement

   The adolescent can be vaccinated for influenza with the live vaccine (nasal spray); a hypersensitivity to eggs, not penicillin, is a contraindication for any influenza vaccination. The 1 year old client and the 52 year old client are not within the acceptable age range to receive the live vaccine via nasal spray, but both could receive the inactivated vaccine by IM injection. Women who are pregnant should not receive any live vaccine, but this client could receive the inactivated vaccine by IM injection.

NCLEX® Connection: Pharmacological and Parenteral Therapies: Adverse Effects/ Contraindications/Side Effects/Interactions

2. A nurse is teaching a group of parents about immunizations. Which of the following vaccines should the nurse tell the parents is administered to children younger than 1 year of age and not to older children or adults?

   A. Pneumococcal vaccine

   B. Meningococcal vaccine

   C. Varicella vaccine

   D. Rotavirus vaccine

   Rotavirus vaccine is administered to infants because the rotavirus causes gastroenteritis only in very young children. The other vaccines can all be administered to at-risk adults as well as children.

NCLEX® Connection: Pharmacological and Parenteral Therapies: Adverse Effects/ Contraindications/Side Effects/Interactions

3. A 12-month-old child just received her first measles, mumps, and rubella (MMR) vaccine. For which of the following possible reactions to this vaccine should the nurse teach the parents to watch for? (Select all that apply)

   ___X___ **Rash**

   ___X___ **Redness and discomfort at injection site**

   ___X___ **Bruising on multiple areas of body**

   _______ Fainting

   _______ Inconsolable crying

   Rash, redness, and discomfort at the injection site are usually transient. Bruising could be a sign of thrombocytopenia, which may subside without treatment, but should be reported because it could cause hemorrhage. Fainting is an adverse reaction that may occur with human papilloma virus vaccination. Inconsolable crying is a reaction that may occur after vaccination with diphtheria, tetanus, and acellular pertussis (DTaP) vaccination.

NCLEX® Connection: Pharmacological and Parenteral Therapies: Adverse Effects/ Contraindications/Side Effects/Interactions

4. A nurse is caring for a group of clients who are not protected against varicella. Which of these clients should receive a varicella vaccination at this time?

   A. A 24-year-old woman in the third trimester of pregnancy

   B. A 3-year-old child with Wilms' tumor who is receiving chemotherapy

   C. A 2-month-old infant with no health problems

   D. A 32-year-old man with essential hypertension

   The adult client with essential hypertension should receive a varicella vaccination at this time. Pregnant women should not receive varicella vaccine until after delivery. Immunocompromised clients and those with cancer who are receiving chemotherapy should not be immunized with this live vaccine. A 2-month-old infant is too young to receive this vaccine; the first dose is administered at 12 to 18 months of age.

NCLEX® Connection: Pharmacological and Parenteral Therapies: Expected Actions/ Outcomes

UNIT 11 MEDICATIONS AFFECTING THE IMMUNE SYSTEM

Chapter 42 Chemotherapy Agents

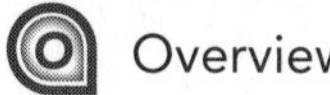

Overview

- Chemotherapy is used to cure some cancers, augment the treatment of other cancers, and attempt to increase a client's survival rate and time.
- Depending on the agent it can be given orally, parentally, intravenous, intracavitary, or intrathecal. Special training/certification is necessary for administration of some agents.
- Combination chemotherapy involves using more than one chemotherapy agent to treat the cancer. Medications used for combination chemotherapy should act in different phases of the cell cycle. Combination therapy is used to reduce medication resistance, increase effectiveness, and ideally reduce toxic effects with lower medication dosages.
- Personnel preparing and administering chemotherapeutic agents should follow safe handling procedures to prevent absorption through the skin.

- If a chemotherapy spill occurs, follow institutional procedures. Generally, small spills can be handled by following procedures and using supplies contained in a chemo spill kit (goggles, mask, protective clothing, shoe covers, absorbent pads, detergent cleansers, and chemo waste disposal bags). For large spills, contact the Occupational Safety and Health Administration.

CYTOTOXIC CHEMOTHERAPY AGENTS

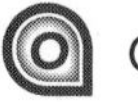

Overview

- Cytotoxic chemotherapy agents are toxic to cancer cells.
- Cytotoxic chemotherapy agents kill fast-growing cancer cells as well as healthy cells, including skin, hair, intestinal mucosa, and hematopoietic cells. Many of the adverse effects of chemotherapeutic agents are related to the unintentional harm done to normal, rapidly proliferating cells such as those found in the gastrointestinal (GI) tract, hair follicles, and bone marrow.
- Common adverse effects of cytotoxic chemotherapy agents include nausea and vomiting, myelosuppression, and alopecia. Many cytotoxic agents are vesicants and may cause severe damage if there is leakage into tissue. Extravasation of agents that are vesicants require special, immediate attention to minimize tissue damage. Selection of neutralizing solution is dependent on vesicant.

CYTOTOXIC CHEMOTHERAPY MEDICATIONS	EXPECTED PHARMACOLOGICAL ACTION
Antimetabolites	Kill cancer cells by interrupting a specific phase of cell reproduction
Antitumor antibiotics	Kill cancer cells by stopping the synthesis of RNA, DNA, or proteins
Antimitotics	Kill cancer cells by inhibiting mitosis and preventing cell division
Alkylating agents	Kill fast-growing cancer cells by altering DNA structure and preventing cell reproduction
Topoisomerase inhibitors	Kill cancer cells by interrupting DNA synthesis
Other	Kill cells by various mechanisms including interrupting DNA and RN synthesis in leukemia cells

MEDICATION CLASSIFICATION: ANTIMETABOLITES

MEDICATION	EXPECTED PHARMACOLOGICAL ACTION	THERAPEUTIC USES
Folic acid analog • Select Prototype Medication: ○ Methotrexate (Rheumatrex, Trexall) • Other Medications: ○ Pemetrexed (Alimta) • Route of administration – Oral, IV, IM, intrathecal	• Stops cell reproduction by inhibiting folic acid conversion • S-phase specific	• Choriocarcinoma, solid tumors, such as breast and lung, head and neck sarcomas, acute lymphocytic leukemia, non-Hodgkin's lymphoma
Pyrimidine analog • Select Prototype Medication: ○ Cytarabine (Cytosar-U) • Other Medications: ○ Fluorouracil (Adrucil) ○ Capecitabine (Xeloda) ○ Floxuridine (FUDR) • Route of administration – Subcut, IV, IM, intrathecal	• Inhibits RNA and DNA synthesis of cancer cells • S-phase specific	• Acute myelogenous leukemia • Solid tumors, such as breast and colon
Purine analogs: • Select Prototype Medication: ○ Mercaptopurine (Purinethol) • Other Medications: ○ Thioguanine (Tabloid) ○ Pentostatin Nipent) ○ Fludarabine (Fludara) • Route of administration – Oral, IV	• Interrupts RNA and DNA synthesis of cancer cells • S-phase specific	• Acute lymphocytic leukemia • Acute non-lymphocytic leukemias

Complications

SIDE/ADVERSE EFFECTS	NURSING INTERVENTIONS/CLIENT EDUCATION
All Antimetabolite Agents	
Bone marrow suppression (low WBC count or neutropenia, bleeding caused by thrombocytopenia or low platelet count, and anemia or low red blood cells)	• Monitor WBC, absolute neutrophil count, platelet count, Hgb, and Hct • Assess clients for bruising and bleeding gums. • Instruct clients to avoid crowds and contact with infectious individuals.
Gastrointestinal discomfort (nausea and vomiting)	• Administer antiemetic such as ondansetron (Zofran) in combination with dexamethasone, granisetron (Kytril), or metoclopramide (Reglan) before beginning chemotherapy.
Methotrexate	
Mucositis (GI tract), gastric ulcers, perforation	• Monitor for GI bleed (coffee-ground emesis or tarry black stools). Assess the client's mouth for sores. • Provide frequent oral hygiene using soft toothbrushes and avoid alcohol mouthwashes.
Reproductive toxicity (congenital abnormalities)	• Advise female clients against becoming pregnant while taking these medications and 6 months after.
Hyperuricemia or elevated levels of uric acid may cause renal damage.	• Monitor kidney function, BUN, creatinine, and I/O. • Encourage adequate fluid intake of 2 to 3 L/day. • Administer allopurinol if uric acid level is elevated.
Cytarabine	
Liver disease	• Monitor liver enzymes. Monitor for signs of jaundice.
Pulmonary edema	• Monitor breath sounds. Advise clients to notify the provider of shortness of breath.
Arachnoiditis (symptoms include nausea, headache and fever)	• Advise clients to notify the provider of nausea, vomiting, headache, or fever. Symptoms may be treated with dexamethasone (Decadron).
Mercaptopurine	
Liver toxicity	• Monitor liver enzymes. Monitor for signs of jaundice.
Mucositis (GI tract), gastric ulcers, perforation	• Monitor for GI bleed, such as coffee ground emesis or tarry black stools. Assess the client's mouth for sores. • Provide frequent oral hygiene using soft toothbrushes and avoiding alcohol mouthwashes.
Reproductive toxicity, such as congenital abnormalities	• Advise female clients against becoming pregnant while taking these medications and 6 months after.

 Contraindications/Precautions

MEDICATION	CONTRAINDICATIONS
Methotrexate	• Pregnancy Risk Category X • Contraindicated in clients with psoriasis, rheumatoid arthritis, liver failure, alcoholism, immunodeficiencies, or blood dyscrasias. • Use with caution in clients with liver or kidney dysfunction, suppressed bone marrow, leukopenia, thrombocytopenia, anemia or gastric ulcers.
Cytarabine	• Pregnancy Risk Category D • Use with caution in clients who have liver disease.
Mercaptopurine	• Pregnancy Risk Category D • Contraindicated in clients who are resistant to the medication

Interactions

MEDICATION/FOOD INTERACTIONS	NURSING INTERVENTIONS/CLIENT EDUCATION
Methotrexate	
Methotrexate may reduce digoxin (Lanoxin) level.	• Monitor digoxin level. Monitor ECG.
NSAIDs, salicylates and sulfonamides may cause methotrexate toxicity.	• Monitor methotrexate levels.
Methotrexate may reduce phenytoin (Dilantin) level.	• Monitor phenytoin level.
Procarbazine (Matulane) may cause increased nephrotoxicity.	• Monitor kidney function.
Food may decrease absorption.	• Take on an empty stomach.
Methotrexate may decrease vaccine strength.	• Use precautions against illness.
Alcohol use may increase risk of hepatotoxicity.	• Avoid use of alcohol
Cytarabine	
Cytarabine may reduce digoxin (Lanoxin) level.	• Monitor digoxin level and ECG.
Cytarabine may reduce gentamicin response to *Klebsiella* pneumoniae.	• Do not use together.
Mercaptopurine	
Allopurinol (Zyloprim) may reduce breakdown of mercaptopurine.	• Reduce medication dosage.
Use of mercaptopurine with hepatotoxic medications may increase risk for hepatotoxicity.	• Monitor liver functions.
Mercaptopurine may decrease the muscle relaxant effect of nondepolarizing neuromuscular medications, such as pancuronium.	• Alert anesthesiologist.
Mercaptopurine may reduce anticoagulant effect of warfarin.	• Monitor PT and INR.

Nursing Administration

- Reduce dosage in clients who have renal disease.
- Encourage 2 to 3 L of daily fluid intake from food and beverage sources.
- Give with sodium bicarbonate capsules to alkalinize urine.
- Advise female clients to use birth control during treatment.
- Advise clients to avoid use of alcohol during treatment.
- Monitor for bleeding (bruising) and/or infection (fever, sore throat).
- Monitor CBC and liver enzymes.
- Monitor intake and output. Monitor uric acid.
- Monitor the client's skin for jaundice. Advise clients to monitor for dark urine and clay-colored stools.
- Give an antiemetic for nausea and vomiting.
- Advise clients to practice good oral hygiene and to avoid mouthwash with alcohol.
- For methotrexate:
  - Administer with leucovorin rescue to reduce toxicity to healthy cells. Leucovorin is a folic acid derivative. It enters healthy cells and blocks methotrexate from damaging normal cells.
  - Instruct clients to take the medication on an empty stomach
  - Advise clients to protect the skin from sunlight.
- For cytarabine:
  - Monitor for signs of neurotoxicity, such as nystagmus.

MEDICATION CLASSIFICATION: ANTITUMOR ANTIBIOTICS

MEDICATION	EXPECTED PHARMACOLOGICAL ACTION	THERAPEUTIC USES

Anthracyclines
• Select Prototype Medication:
  ○ Doxorubicin (Adriamycin)
• Other Medications:
  ○ Liposomal doxorubicin (Doxil)
  ○ Daunorubicin (Cerubidine)
• Route of administration – IV
	• Binds to DNA, altering its structure
	• Cell cycle phase nonspecific
		• Includes solid tumors, such as lung, bone, stomach and breast cancers, Hodgkin's and non-Hodgkin's lymphomas

Nonanthracyclines
• Select Prototype Medication:
  ○ Dactinomycin (Actinomycin D)
• Other Medications:
  ○ Bleomycin (Blenoxane)
  ○ Mitomycin (Mutamycin)
• Route of administration – IV
	• Binds to DNA, altering its structure
	• Cell cycle phase nonspecific
		• Includes Wilms' tumor, rhabdomyosarcoma, choriocarcinoma, Ewing's sarcoma and Kaposi's sarcoma

Complications

SIDE/ADVERSE EFFECTS	NURSING INTERVENTIONS/CLIENT EDUCATION
All antitumor antibiotics	
Bone marrow suppression (low WBC or neutropenia, bleeding caused by thrombocytopenia or low platelet count, and anemia or low red blood cells)	• Monitor WBC, absolute neutrophil count, platelet count, Hgb and Hct. • Assess clients for bruising and bleeding gums. • Instruct clients to avoid crowds and contact with infectious individuals.
Gastrointestinal discomfort, such as nausea and vomiting	• Administer antiemetic such as ondansetron (Zofran) in combination with dexamethasone, granisetron (Kytril), or metoclopramide (Reglan) before beginning chemotherapy.
Extravasations of vesicants cause severe tissue damage.	• Stop chemotherapeutic medications if extravasation occurs. • Use central line for infusion. • Only clinically trained personnel should give these medications IV.
Alopecia	• Advise clients that hair loss will occur 7 to 10 days after the beginning of treatment and will last for a maximum of 2 months after the last administration of the chemotherapeutic agent. • Advise clients who want to do so to select a hairpiece before the occurrence of hair loss.

SIDE/ADVERSE EFFECTS	NURSING INTERVENTIONS/CLIENT EDUCATION
Doxorubicin	
Acute cardiac toxicity, dysrhythmias	• Monitor ECG and echocardiogram. • The client may be treated with dexrazoxane (Zinecard), but this medication may increase myelosuppression.
Cardiomyopathy, heart failure, may have delayed onset.	• Monitor ECG and echocardiogram. • The client may be treated with ACE inhibitors.

 Contraindications/Precautions

- Doxorubicin (Adriamycin)
  - Pregnancy Risk Category D
  - Contraindicated in clients with severe myelosuppression and those who have had a lifetime cumulative dose of 550 mg/m^2
- Dactinomycin (Actinomycin D)
  - Pregnancy Risk Category D
  - Contraindicated in clients with active chicken pox or herpes zoster

Interactions

MEDICATION/FOOD INTERACTIONS	NURSING INTERVENTIONS/CLIENT EDUCATION
Doxorubicin	
Calcium channel blockers may increase cardio-toxicity.	Monitor ECG and heart function.
Doxorubicin may reduce digoxin levels.	Monitor digoxin levels.
Phenobarbital may increase metabolism of doxorubicin.	Monitor clients for effectiveness of treatment.
Paclitaxel (Taxol) may decrease metabolism of doxorubicin.	Monitor clients for effectiveness of treatment.
Doxorubicin may reduce phenytoin (Dilantin) levels.	Monitor phenytoin level.
Dactinomycin	
None documented.	

Nursing Administration

- Reduce dose in liver disease.
- Monitor for bleeding (bruising) or infection (fever, sore throat).
- Monitor CBC and liver enzymes.

- Give an antiemetic for nausea and vomiting.
- Advise clients to practice good oral hygiene and to avoid mouthwash with alcohol. Stop chemotherapeutic medications if extravasation occurs.
- Advise clients that transient hair loss may occur 7 to 10 days after the beginning of treatment and will last for a maximum duration of 2 months after the last administration of the chemotherapeutic agent.
- Advise clients to select a hairpiece before the occurrence of hair loss.
- For doxorubicin:
    - Monitor ECG and cardiac function.
    - Advise clients to continue follow-up care after treatment is completed to monitor for delayed cardiac toxicity.
    - Advise clients to notify the provider if they experience chest pain and/or shortness of breath.

MEDICATION CLASSIFICATION: ANTIMITOTICS

MEDICATION	EXPECTED PHARMACOLOGICAL ACTION	THERAPEUTIC USES
Vinca Alkaloids • Select Prototype Medication: ○ Vincristine (Oncovin, Vincasar) • Other Medications: ○ Vinblastine (Velban) ○ Vinorelbine (Navelbine) • Route of administration – IV	• Useful in combination with other chemotherapy medications • Stops cell division during mitosis • Not bone marrow toxic • M-phase specific	Includes acute lymphocytic leukemia, Wilms tumor, rhabdomyosarcoma, solid tumors, such as bladder and breast cancers, Hodgkin's and non-Hodgkin's lymphomas.
Taxanes • Select Prototype Medication: ○ Paclitaxel (Taxol, Onxol) • Other Medications: ○ Docetaxel (Taxotere) • Route of administration – IV	• Stop cell division during mitosis	Includes ovarian, non-small cell lung tumors, and Kaposi's sarcoma

Complications

SIDE/ADVERSE EFFECTS	NURSING INTERVENTIONS/CLIENT EDUCATION
Vincristine	
Peripheral neuropathy symptoms may include weakness and paresthesia.	• Advise clients to report symptoms. Use caution to prevent injury.
Extravasations of vesicants cause severe tissue damage.	• Stop chemotherapeutic medications if extravasation occurs. • Only clinically trained personnel should give these medications intravenously. • Use a central line for infusion.
Alopecia	• Advise clients that hair loss will occur 7 to 10 days after the beginning of treatment and will last for a maximum duration of 2 months after the last administration of the chemotherapeutic agent. • Advise clients to select a hairpiece before the occurrence of hair loss.
Paclitaxel	
Anaphylaxis (findings include hypotension, dyspnea, rash)	• Monitor carefully during infusion. Premedicate with dexamethasone and diphenhydramine to prevent reaction.
Bone marrow suppression, such as low WBC count or neutropenia, bleeding caused by thrombocytopenia or low platelet count, and anemia or low red blood cells	• Monitor WBC, absolute neutrophil count, platelet count, Hgb, and Hct. • Assess clients for bruising and bleeding gums. • Instruct clients to avoid crowds and contact with infectious individuals.
Bradycardia, heart block, MI	• Monitor for cardiac symptoms. • Advise clients to inform the nurse of any chest pain or shortness of breath.
Alopecia	• Advise clients that hair loss will occur 7 to 10 days after the beginning of treatment and will last for a maximum duration of 2 months after the last administration of the chemotherapeutic agent. • Advise clients to select a hairpiece before hair loss occurs.

Contraindications/Precautions

- Vincristine
    - This medication is Pregnancy Risk Category D.
    - Use is contraindicated in clients with Charcot-Marie-Tooth syndrome.
    - Use with caution in clients with liver disease or neuromuscular disease.

- Paclitaxel
    - This medication is Pregnancy Risk Category D.
    - Use is contraindicated in clients with hypersensitivity to castor oil and those with a neutrophil count less than 1500/mm³. Use with caution in clients who have myelosuppression.

Interactions

MEDICATION/FOOD INTERACTIONS	NURSING INTERVENTIONS/CLIENT EDUCATION
Vincristine	
Asparaginase (Elspar) may reduce clearance of vincristine.	• Monitor for vincristine toxicity.
Calcium channel blockers, such as verapamil (Calan), may increase vincristine accumulation.	• Monitor for vincristine toxicity.
Vincristine may reduce effects of digoxin.	• Monitor digoxin level and ECG.
Mitomycin may increase risk for bronchospasm.	• Monitor breath sounds.
Vincristine may decrease level of phenytoin.	• Monitor phenytoin level.
Paclitaxel	
Cisplatin may increase myelosuppression.	• Use together with caution.
Cyclosporine, dexamethasone, diazepam, verapamil, quinidine, and vincristine may slow paclitaxel clearance.	• Use together with caution.
Phenobarbital and carbamazepine may speed metabolism of paclitaxel.	• Monitor effectiveness.

Nursing Administration

- Assess for signs of neuropathy, including weakness, numbness, tingling, foot drop, ataxia and paresthesia. Advise clients to use caution and report symptoms.
- Reduce dose for clients who have liver disease.
- Assess breath sounds for bronchospasm.
- Monitor carefully for hypersensitive reaction. Premedicate if needed.
- Monitor for bleeding (bruising) or infection (fever, sore throat).
- Monitor CBC and liver enzymes.
- Give an antiemetic for nausea and vomiting.
- Advise clients to use good mouth care.
- Stop chemotherapeutic medications if extravasation occurs.
- Advise clients to use birth control during treatment.

MEDICATION CLASSIFICATION: ALKYLATING AGENTS

MEDICATION	EXPECTED PHARMACOLOGICAL ACTION	THERAPEUTIC USES
Nitrogen Mustards • Select Prototype Medication: ○ Cyclophosphamide (Cytoxan, Neosar) – Oral, IV • Other Medications: ○ Mechlorethamine (Mustargen), Bendamustine (Treanda) – IV ○ Chlorambucil (Leukeran) – Oral	• Kills rapid growing cells by interrupting DNA and RNA synthesis • Cell cycle phase nonspecific	• Includes acute lymphomas, solid tumors, such as head, neck and breast cancers, Hodgkin's and non-Hodgkin's lymphomas
Nitrosoureas • Select Prototype Medication: ○ Carmustine (BiCNU) – IV, topical • Other Medications: ○ Lomustine (CCNU) – Oral ○ Streptozocin (Zanosar) – IV	• Kills rapid growing cells by interrupting DNA and RNA synthesis • Cell cycle phase nonspecific • Crosses the blood brain barrier.	• Includes brain tumors, Hodgkin's and non-Hodgkin's lymphomas, and multiple myeloma
Platinum Compounds • Select Prototype Medication: ○ Cisplatin (Platinol-AQ) – IV • Other Medications: ○ Carboplatin (Paraplatin) – IV	• Kills rapid growing cells by interrupting DNA and RNA synthesis • Cell cycle phase nonspecific.	• Includes bladder, testicular, and ovarian cancers

Complications

SIDE/ADVERSE EFFECTS	NURSING INTERVENTIONS/CLIENT EDUCATION
All alkylating agents	
Bone marrow suppression, such as low WBC count or neutropenia, bleeding caused by thrombocytopenia or low platelet count, and anemia or low red blood cells	• Monitor WBC, absolute neutrophil count, platelet count, Hgb, and Hct. • Assess clients for bruising and bleeding gums. • Instruct clients to avoid crowds and contact with infectious individuals.
Gastrointestinal discomfort, such as nausea and vomiting	• Administer antiemetic such as ondansetron (Zofran) in combination with dexamethasone, granisetron (Kytril), or metoclopramide (Reglan) before beginning chemotherapy.
Cyclophosphamide	
Acute hemorrhagic cystitis	• Increase fluids (3 L daily). • Monitor for blood in urine. • Mesna (Mesnex) may be given if needed. Mesna is a uroprotectant agent that detoxifies metabolites to reduce hematuria.
Alopecia	• Advise clients that hair loss will occur 7 to 10 days after the beginning of treatment and will last for a maximum duration of 2 months after the last administration of the chemotherapeutic agent. • Advise clients to select a hairpiece before the occurrence of hair loss.
Carmustine	
Pulmonary fibrosis	• Monitor lung function. The client may be treated with corticosteroids.
Liver and kidney toxicity	• Monitor liver and kidney function.
Reproductive toxicity, such as congenital abnormalities	• Advise female clients against becoming pregnant while taking these medications and 6 months after.
Cisplatin	
Renal toxicity	• Monitor kidney function. Increase fluids and give a diuretic if indicated.
Hearing loss	• Monitor for tinnitus and hearing loss.

Contraindications/Precautions

- Cyclophosphamide
  - Pregnancy Risk Category D
  - Contraindicated in clients with severe myelosuppression
  - Use with caution in clients who have kidney or liver disorders or leukopenia or thrombocytopenia.

- Carmustine
  - Pregnancy Risk Category D
- Cisplatin
  - Pregnancy Risk Category D
  - Contraindicated in clients who have severe myelosuppression, kidney disorders, or hearing loss

Interactions

MEDICATION/FOOD INTERACTIONS	NURSING INTERVENTIONS/CLIENT EDUCATION
Cyclophosphamide	
Barbiturates may cause increased effect of cyclophosphamide.	• Use together with caution.
Concurrent use of cyclophosphamide may increase cardiac toxicity of cardiotoxic medications.	• Do not use together.
Cyclophosphamide may reduce digoxin level.	• Monitor digoxin level.
Concurrent use of succinylcholine may cause increased neuromuscular blockage.	• Do not use together.
Carmustine	
Anticoagulants, aspirin, and NSAIDs may cause increased bleeding.	• Do not use together.
Concurrent use of carmustine and cimetidine (Tagamet) may increase bone marrow suppression.	• Do not use together.
Concurrent use of carmustine and mitomycin may increase the risk for corneal dysfunction.	• Monitor vision.
Cisplatin	
Concurrent use of cisplatin and aminoglycosides may increase risk for renal toxicity.	• Monitor kidney function.
Concurrent use of cisplatin and furosemide may increase hearing loss.	• Do not use together.
Cisplatin may reduce levels of phenytoin.	• Monitor phenytoin level.

Nursing Administration

- Encourage adequate fluid intake of 2 to 3 L/day
- Monitor for blood in urine. Mesna (Mesnex) may be indicated.
- Reduce dose for clients who have liver disease.

- Monitor for bleeding (bruising) or infection (fever, sore throat).
- Monitor CBC, uric acid level, and liver enzymes.
- Give antiemetic for nausea and vomiting.
- Advise clients to use good mouth care.
- Stop chemotherapeutic medications if extravasation occurs.
- Advise clients to use birth control during treatment.
- Monitor hearing prior to treatment with cisplatin

MEDICATION CLASSIFICATION: TOPOISOMERASE INHIBITORS

- Select Prototype Medication: topotecan (Hycamtin) – IV

Purpose

- Expected Pharmacological Action
  - Kills cancer cells by interrupting DNA synthesis
  - Cell cycle phase S-specific
- Therapeutic Uses
  - Includes ovary and small cell lung tumors

Complications

SIDE/ADVERSE EFFECTS	NURSING INTERVENTIONS/CLIENT EDUCATION
Bone marrow suppression, (low WBC count or neutropenia, bleeding caused by thrombocytopenia or low platelet count, and anemia or low red blood cells) – This may occur 4 to 6 weeks after infusion.	• Monitor WBC, absolute neutrophil count, platelet count, Hgb and Hct. • Assess clients for bruising and bleeding gums. • Instruct clients to avoid crowds and contact with infectious individuals. Advise clients to continue precautions after treatment is completed.
Gastrointestinal discomfort (nausea and vomiting)	• Administer antiemetic such as ondansetron (Zofran) in combination with dexamethasone, granisetron (Kytril), or metoclopramide (Reglan) before beginning chemotherapy.
Alopecia	• Advise clients that hair loss will occur 7 to 10 days after the beginning of treatment and will last for a maximum duration of 2 months after the last administration of the chemotherapeutic agent. • Advise clients to select a hairpiece before the occurrence of hair loss.

 Contraindications/Precautions

- Pregnancy Risk Category D
- Contraindicated in clients with severe myelosuppression

Interactions

- Cisplatin may increase myelosuppression. Use with caution.

Nursing Administration

- Monitor for bleeding (bruising) or infection (fever, sore throat).
- Monitor CBC.
- Give antiemetic for nausea and vomiting.
- Advise clients to perform good oral hygiene and avoid mouth wash with alcohol.
- Advise female clients to use birth control during treatment.

OTHER ANTINEOPLASTIC AGENTS

MEDICATION	EXPECTED PHARMACOLOGICAL ACTION	THERAPEUTIC USES
Asparaginase (Elspar) Route of administration – IV, IM.	• Kills cancer cells by interrupting DNA synthesis in leukemia cells • Cell cycle phase G1-specific.	Acute lymphocytic leukemia
Hydroxyurea (Hydrea, Mylocel) Route of administration – Oral	• Kills cancer cells by interrupting DNA synthesis • Cell cycle phase S-specific • May cross blood-brain barrier	Includes chronic myelogenous leukemia, ovarian and squamous cell cancers
Procarbazine (Matulane) Route of administration – Oral	• Kills cancer cells by interrupting DNA and RNA synthesis • Cell cycle phase non-specific • May cross blood-brain barrier	Includes brain tumors, Hodgkin's and non-Hodgkin's lymphomas

Complications

SIDE/ADVERSE EFFECTS	NURSING INTERVENTIONS/CLIENT EDUCATION
Asparaginase, hydroxyurea, procarbazine	
Gastrointestinal discomfort (nausea and vomiting)	• Administer antiemetic such as ondansetron (Zofran) in combination with dexamethasone, granisetron (Kytril), or metoclopramide (Reglan) before beginning chemotherapy.
Asparaginase	
Hypersensitivity reaction	• Premedicate if needed. Monitor for wheezing and/or rash. Give test dose. Monitor closely.
Alopecia	• Advise clients that hair loss will occur 7 to 10 days after the beginning of treatment and last for a maximum of 2 months after the last administration of the chemotherapeutic agent. • Advise clients to select a hairpiece before hair loss occurs.
Liver and pancreas toxicity	• Monitor liver enzymes. Monitor for signs of jaundice. Monitor pancreatic enzymes.
Renal toxicity	• Monitor kidney function. Increase fluids and give a diuretic if indicated.
Hydroxyurea and procarbazine	
Bone marrow suppression (low white blood cell count or neutropenia, bleeding caused by thrombocytopenia or low platelet count, and anemia or low red blood cells) – may occur 4 to 6 weeks after infusion.	• Monitor WBC, absolute neutrophil count, platelet count, hemoglobin, and hematocrit. • Assess clients for bruising and bleeding gums. • Instruct clients to avoid crowds and contact with infectious individuals. Advise clients to continue precautions after treatment is completed.
Procarbazine	
Peripheral neuropathy symptoms may include weakness and paresthesia.	Advise clients to report symptoms. Use caution to prevent injury.

Contraindications/Precautions

- Asparaginase
  - Pregnancy Risk Category C
  - Contraindicated in clients who have pancreatitis
  - Use with caution in clients with liver disease.
- Hydroxyurea
  - Pregnancy Risk Category D
  - Contraindicated in clients with severe myelosuppression or anemia
  - Use with caution in clients who have kidney disease.

- Procarbazine
  - Pregnancy Risk Category D
  - Contraindicated in clients with severe myelosuppression
  - Use with caution in clients who have liver or kidney disease.

Interactions

MEDICATION/FOOD INTERACTIONS	NURSING INTERVENTIONS/CLIENT EDUCATION
Asparaginase	
Asparaginase may decrease effects of methotrexate.	Use with caution. Monitor for medication effect.
Prednisone and vincristine may increase asparaginase toxicity.	Use with caution.
Hydroxyurea	
Cytotoxic medications may increase hydroxyurea.	Use with caution together.
Procarbazine	
Procarbazine may increase depressant effects of CNS depressants.	Use with caution.
Procarbazine may decrease digoxin level.	Monitor digoxin level.
Opioids may cause hypotension.	Do not use together.

Nursing Administration

- Asparaginase
  - Monitor for allergic reaction. Give a test dose. Have resuscitation equipment on hand.
  - Give an antiemetic for nausea and vomiting.
  - Advise clients to use good mouth care.
  - Advise clients to use birth control during treatment.
- Hydroxyurea
  - Monitor for bleeding (bruising) or infection (fever, sore throat).
  - Monitor CBC.
  - Give an antiemetic for nausea and vomiting.
  - Advise clients to use good mouth care.
  - Advise clients to use birth control during treatment.
- Procarbazine
  - Monitor for neuro effects, such as confusion or paresthesia.

NON-CYTOTOXIC CHEMOTHERAPY AGENTS

Overview

- Noncytotoxic chemotherapy medications are nontoxic to cells.
  - Hormonal agents are effective against tumors that are supported or suppressed by hormones.
    - Hormone agonists cause an increase in a hormone and may be effective against tumors that require a particular hormone for support. The use of androgenic hormones in a client with estrogen-dependent cancer can suppress growth of this type of cancer. Conversely, the use of estrogenic hormones for a testosterone-dependent cancer can suppress growth of this type of cancer.
    - Hormone antagonists block certain hormones and may be effective against tumors that require a particular hormone for support. The use of an anti-estrogen hormone in a client with estrogen-dependent cancer can suppress growth of this type of cancer. The same is true for anti-testosterone hormones.
  - Biological response modulators act as immunostimulants to enhance the immune response and reduce proliferation of cancer cells.
  - Targeted antineoplastic agents are antibodies or small molecules that attach to specific target sites to stop cancer growth without injuring healthy tissue.

MEDICATION CLASSIFICATION: HORMONAL AGENTS: PROSTATE CANCER MEDICATIONS

MEDICATION	EXPECTED PHARMACOLOGICAL ACTION	THERAPEUTIC USES
Gonadotropin-Releasing Hormone Agonists • Select Prototype Medication: ○ Leuprolide (Eligard, Lupron) • Other Medications: ○ Triptorelin (Trelstar Depot) • Route of administration – Subcutaneous, IM.	• The testes stop producing testosterone.	• Includes prostate cancer
Androgen Receptor Blockers • Select Prototype Medication: ○ Flutamide (Eulexin) • Other Medications: ○ Bicalutamide (Casodex) • Route of administration – Oral	• Blocks testosterone at receptor site • Used in conjunction with gonadotropin-releasing hormone agonists, to block androgen receptors and suppress the growth of prostate cancer	• Treatment of prostate cancer

Complications

SIDE/ADVERSE EFFECTS	NURSING INTERVENTIONS/CLIENT EDUCATION
Leuprolide	
Hot flushes, decreased libido	• Warn clients about adverse effects. Adverse reactions may be transient.
Decreased bone density	• Advise clients to increase calcium and vitamin D intake. • Advise clients to increase bone mass with weight-bearing exercises.
Arrhythmias, pulmonary edema	• Monitor for arrhythmias and assess breath sounds.
Flutamide	
Thrombocytopenia, leukopenia (rare)	• Advise clients to notify the provider of sore throat or bruising.
Gynecomastia	• Warn clients of side effects of medication.
Nausea, vomiting, diarrhea	• Monitor intake and output.
Hepatitis	• Monitor liver enzymes.

 Contraindications/Precautions

- Leuprolide
  - Pregnancy Risk Category X
  - Contraindicated in clients hypersensitive to gonadotropin-releasing agonists
- Flutamide
  - Pregnancy Risk Category D
  - Contraindicated in clients with severe liver disease

Interactions

MEDICATION/FOOD INTERACTIONS	NURSING INTERVENTIONS/CLIENT EDUCATION
Leuprolide	
None noted.	
Flutamide	
Concurrent use of flutamide and warfarin may increase anticoagulation.	Monitor PT and INR.

Nursing Administration

- Leuprolide
  - Advise clients to increase calcium and vitamin D intake. Advise clients to increase bone mass with weight-bearing exercises.
  - Monitor for arrhythmias and assess breathe sounds.
  - Warn clients that prostate symptoms may worsen at beginning of treatment.
- Flutamide
  - Administer with a gonadotropin-releasing hormone agonist.
  - Warn clients of side effects of the medication, such as gynecomastia.

MEDICATION CLASSIFICATION: HORMONAL AGENTS: BREAST CANCER MEDICATIONS

MEDICATION	EXPECTED PHARMACOLOGICAL ACTION	THERAPEUTIC USES
Estrogen Receptor Blockers • Select Prototype Medication: ○ Tamoxifen (Nolvadex) – Oral • Other Medications: ○ Raloxifene (Evista) – Oral ○ Fulvestrant (Faslodex) – IM	Stops growth of breast cancer cells, which are estrogen-dependent cancers	• Used to treat or prevent breast cancer
Aromatase Inhibitors • Select Prototype Medication: ○ Anastrozole (Arimidex) • Other Medications: ○ Letrozole (Femara) ○ Exemestane (Aromasin) • Route of administration – Oral	Stops growth of breast cancer cells by blocking estrogen production	• Used to treat breast cancer in postmenopausal women
Monoclonal Antibody • Select Prototype Medication: ○ Trastuzumab (Herceptin) • Route of administration – IV	Targets breast cancer cells, prevents cell growth and causes cell death	• Used to treat metastatic breast cancer • May be used alone or in conjunction with paclitaxel

Complications

SIDE/ADVERSE EFFECTS	NURSING INTERVENTIONS/CLIENT EDUCATION
Tamoxifen	
Endometrial cancer	Monitor for abnormal bleeding. Advise clients to have a yearly gynecological exam and PAP smear.
Hypercalcemia	Monitor calcium level.
Nausea and vomiting	Monitor fluid status. Administer fluids and antiemetics as prescribed.
Pulmonary embolus	Assess breath sounds. Advise clients to report chest pain or shortness of breath.
Hot flushes	Warn clients about adverse effects.
Vaginal discharge or bleeding	Monitor bleeding and discharge.
Anastrozole	
Muscle and joint pain, headache	Treat pain with a mild analgesic as prescribed.
Nausea	Monitor fluid status. Administer fluids and antiemetics as prescribed.
Vaginal bleeding	Monitor bleeding and CBC.
Increased risk for osteoporosis.	Advise clients to take calcium and vitamin D supplements and perform weight-bearing exercises.
Hot flushes	Warn clients about adverse effects.
Trastuzumab	
Cardiac toxicity, tachycardia, heart failure	Monitor ECG, Obtain baseline ECG. Monitor for dyspnea and edema. Advise clients to report chest pain or shortness of breath.
Hypersensitivity reaction	Monitor closely during infusion. Have resuscitation equipment nearby.
Nausea and vomiting.	Monitor fluid status.

Contraindications/Precautions

- Tamoxifen
  - Pregnancy Risk Category D
  - Contraindicated in clients taking warfarin and in clients with a history of blood clots or pulmonary embolism
- Anastrozole
  - Pregnancy Risk Category D
  - Contraindicated in clients hypersensitive to medication
  - Use with caution in clients who have liver disease.

- Trastuzumab
  - Pregnancy Risk Category B
  - Contraindicated in clients hypersensitive to the medication
  - Use with caution in clients who have heart disease.

Interactions

MEDICATION/FOOD INTERACTIONS	NURSING INTERVENTIONS/CLIENT EDUCATION
Tamoxifen	
Tamoxifen may increase the anticoagulation action of warfarin.	• Monitor PT and INR. • Warfarin doses may need to be adjusted.
Antacids may alter absorption.	• Allow 2 hr between doses.
Anastrozole	
Tamoxifen and estrogen-like medications may reduce anastrozole effects.	• Avoid using together.
Concurrent use of anastrozole and anthracyclines may increase the risk for cardiac effects.	• Monitor for cardiac effects.

Nursing Administration

- Advise clients to increase calcium and vitamin D intake. Advise clients to increase bone mass with weight-bearing exercises.
- Monitor for arrhythmias and assess breathe sounds.
- Encourage clients to perform monthly breast self-examination and schedule annual gynecologic and breast examinations and mammogram with the provider.
- Monitor CBC and calcium levels.
- Monitor fluid status.
- Advise female clients to use birth control during therapy.

MEDICATION CLASSIFICATION: BIOLOGIC RESPONSE MODIFIERS

- Select Prototype Medication: interferon Alfa-2a, interferon al-fa-2b
- Other Medications: aldesleukin (Interleukin-2), BCG vaccine (TheraCys)
- Route of administration – IV, IM and subcutaneous

Purpose

- Expected Pharmacological Action
  - Increases immune response and decreases pro-duction of cancer cells

- Therapeutic Uses
  - Used to treat or prevent hairy cell leukemia, chronic myelogenous leukemia, malignant melanoma, and AIDS-related Kaposi's sarcoma

Complications

SIDE/ADVERSE EFFECTS	NURSING INTERVENTIONS/CLIENT EDUCATION
Flu-like symptoms (fever, fatigue, headache, chills, myalgia)	• Administer acetaminophen as prescribed.
Bone marrow suppression, alopecia, cardiotoxicity, and neurotoxicity (with prolonged therapy)	• Monitor CBC, fatigue level, and signs of cardiotoxicity (arrhythmias, palpitations, MI, heart failure) and neurotoxicity, (confusion, ataxia, inability to concentrate). • Monitor clients for signs of infection. • Instruct clients to report dizziness or tingling/numbness of the hands or feet. • Monitor for bruising, bleeding, and blood in stools, urine, sputum, and/or emesis.
Hypotension	• Assess baseline blood pressure prior to administration. • Monitor blood pressure following administration. • Encourage clients to change positions slowly.

Contraindications/Precautions

- Pregnancy Risk Category C
- Contraindicated in clients who have hypersensitivity to the medication, liver or kidney failure, seizure or cardiac history, or compromised immune systems

Interactions

MEDICATION/FOOD INTERACTIONS	NURSING INTERVENTIONS/CLIENT EDUCATION
Concurrent use with theophylline (Theo-Dur) can lead to theophylline toxicity.	• Monitor clients for signs of toxicity. Decreased theophylline dosage may be indicated.
Zidovudine (Retrovir) may increase the risk of neutropenia.	• Monitor clients for neutropenia. Instruct clients to avoid crowds and contact with infectious individuals.
Concurrent use with antihypertensives can have an additive hypotensive effect.	• Monitor clients for additive hypotension.
Concurrent use with medications that are cardio or neurotoxic may increase cardio or neurotoxicity.	• Monitor for cardio or neurotoxicity.
Concurrent use with vaccines using a live virus may reduce antibody response.	• Avoid use together.

Nursing Administration

- Store the medication in the refrigerator and do not freeze. Administer at room temperature. Do not shake the vial.

- Monitor for flu symptoms. Pre-medicate with acetaminophen if prescribed.
- Advise clients to practice good oral hygiene.
- Monitor CBC, platelets and electrolytes.
- Monitor fluid status.

MEDICATION CLASSIFICATION: TARGETED ANTINEOPLASTIC MEDICATIONS

MEDICATION	EXPECTED PHARMACOLOGICAL ACTION	THERAPEUTIC USES
EGFR-tyrosine Kinase Inhibitors • Select Prototype Medication: ○ Cetuximab (Erbitux) • Other Medications: ○ Panitumumab (Vectibix) • Route of administration – IV.	Antibody that stops cancer cell growth and increases cell death	Used to treat cancers that are EGFR positive, such as colorectal and solid tumors of the head and neck
BCR-ABL Tyrosine Kinase Inhibitors • Select Prototype Medication: ○ Imatinib (Gleevec) • Route of administration – Oral.	Stops cancer growth by inhibiting intracellular enzymes	Used to treat chronic myeloid leukemia
CD20-Directed Antibodies • Select Prototype Medication: ○ Rituximab (Rituxan) • Route of administration – IV.	Antibody that stops cancer cell growth and increases cell death	Used to treat non- Hodgkin's lymphoma
Angiogenesis Inhibitors • Select prototype: ○ Bevacizumab (Avastin) • Route of administration – IV.	Antibody that stops cancer cell growth and increases cell death	Used to treat colorectal and lung cancers

Complications

SIDE/ADVERSE EFFECTS	NURSING INTERVENTIONS/CLIENT EDUCATION
Cetuximab	
Infusion reaction, rash, hypotension, wheezing	• Monitor carefully for signs of a reaction. • Premedicate if needed with diphenhydramine or corticosteroids. • Stop treatment and administer antihistamines as prescribed.
Pulmonary emboli	• Monitor breath sounds. Monitor SaO_2.
Skin toxicity, rash	• Monitor for rash over 2 weeks of treatment. Treat with topical antibiotics if needed.

SIDE/ADVERSE EFFECTS	NURSING INTERVENTIONS/CLIENT EDUCATION
Imatinib	
Gastrointestinal discomfort, such as nausea and vomiting	• Administer antiemetic such as ondansetron (Zofran) in combination with dexamethasone, granisetron (Kytril), or metoclopramide (Reglan) before beginning chemotherapy. • Take with food.
Flu-like symptoms (fever, fatigue, headache, chills, myalgia)	• Administer acetaminophen as prescribed.
Edema	• Monitor for edema.
Hypokalemia	• Monitor potassium level.
Neutropenia, anemia	• Monitor CBC. Assess clients for bruising and bleeding gums. • Instruct clients to avoid crowds and contact with infectious individuals.
Rituximab	
Infusion reaction, rash, hypotension, wheezing	• Monitor carefully for signs of a reaction. Premedicate if needed with diphenhydramine or corticosteroids. Stop treatment and administer antihistamines as prescribed.
Flu-like symptoms (fever, fatigue, headache, chills, myalgia)	• Administer acetaminophen as prescribed.
Tumor lysis syndrome due to rapid cell death may lead to kidney failure, hypocalcemia and hyperuricemia.	• Monitor kidney function, dialyze if needed. Monitor fluids and electrolytes.
Bevacizumab	
Gastrointestinal discomfort, such as nausea and vomiting	• Administer antiemetic such as ondansetron (Zofran) in combination with dexamethasone, granisetron (Kytril), or metoclopramide (Reglan) before beginning chemotherapy.
Alopecia	• Advise clients that hair loss may occur 7 to 10 days after the beginning of treatment and will last for a maximum duration of 2 months after the last administration of the chemotherapeutic agent. • Advise clients to select a hairpiece before the occurrence of hair loss.
Mucositis (GI tract)	• Assess the client's mouth for sores. • Provide frequent oral hygiene using soft toothbrushes and avoiding alcohol mouthwashes.
Hypertension	• Monitor blood pressure.
Gastric perforation	• Advise clients to notify the provider if they experience abdominal pain.

 Contraindications/Precautions

- Cetuximab
  - Pregnancy Risk Category C
  - Contraindicated in clients who have hypersensitivity to the medication
- Imatinib
  - Pregnancy Risk Category D
  - Contraindicated in clients who have hypersensitivity to the medication
  - Use with caution in clients with liver disease.
- Rituximab
  - Pregnancy Risk Category C
  - Contraindicated in clients who have hypersensitivity to the medication
  - Use with caution in clients with liver or kidney failure.
- Bevacizumab
  - Pregnancy Risk Category C
  - Contraindicated in clients who have hypersensitivity to the medication, or have recent history of hemoptysis or surgery
  - Use with caution in clients with cardiac history.

Interactions

MEDICATION/FOOD INTERACTIONS	NURSING INTERVENTIONS/CLIENT EDUCATION
Cetuximab	
Sun may increase skin toxicity.	• Advise clients to use sunscreen and avoid exposure.
Imatinib	
Acetaminophen may increase chance of liver failure.	• Monitor liver enzymes.
Concurrent use with warfarin may increase anticoagulant effect.	• Monitor clients for signs of bleeding. • Monitor INR and PT and adjust warfarin dosage accordingly.
Clarithromycin, erythromycin, and ketoconazole may slow imatinib metabolism and cause toxicity.	• Monitor clients for toxicity.
Carbamazepine and phenytoin may increase imatinib metabolism.	• Monitor for effectiveness.

MEDICATION/FOOD INTERACTIONS	NURSING INTERVENTIONS/CLIENT EDUCATION
Rituximab	
Calcium channel blockers may alter medication effects.	• Use together with caution.
Bevacizumab	
Bevacizumab may increase irinotecan level.	• Monitor medication levels.

Nursing Administration

- Monitor for infusion reaction, and premedicate if prescribed.
- Advise clients to protect skin from the sun and assess for rash.
- Advise clients to notify the provider for shortness of breath.
- Advise clients to practice good oral hygiene.
- Monitor CBC, platelets, and electrolytes.
- Monitor fluid status.
- Assess for edema.
- Advise clients to report adverse reactions such as abdominal pain, skin lesions, and headache.

CHAPTER 42: CHEMOTHERAPY AGENTS

Application Exercises

1. A client with breast cancer is receiving a combination therapy of cyclophosphamide, methotrexate, and fluorouracil. Combination chemotherapy is used to do which of the following? (Select all that apply)

    _____ Decrease medication resistance.
    _____ Attack cancer cells at different stages of cell growth.
    _____ Block chemotherapy agent from entering healthy cells.
    _____ Stimulate immune system.
    _____ Reduce the dosage of each chemotherapy agent.

2. Hemorrhagic cystitis in a client taking nitrogen mustards may be minimized by administering which of the following?

    A. Uroprotectant agent, such as mesna (Mesnex)
    B. Glucocorticoid, such as dexamethasone (Decadron)
    C. Loop diuretic, such as furosemide (Lasix)
    D. H_1 receptor antagonist, such as diphenhydramine (Benadryl)

3. Leucovorin is given to a client who is taking methotrexate to

    A. reduce the risk of a transfusion reaction.
    B. increase production of platelets.
    C. potentiate the cytotoxic effects of methotrexate.
    D. protect healthy cells from the toxic effects of methotrexate.

4. A client is taking tamoxifen (Nolvadex), an estrogen receptor blocker, for treatment of breast cancer. Which of the following is an adverse effect of this medication for which the client should be alert?

    A. Chest pain or palpitations
    B. Abnormal uterine bleeding
    C. Yellow sclera or dark-colored urine.
    D. Shortness of breath.

5. A client is being treated with Interferon Alfa-2a for chronic myelogenous leukemia. Which of the following are common adverse reactions to biologic response modifiers? (Select all that apply.)

    _____ Tinnitus
    _____ Flu-like symptoms, such as fever, chills, myalgia
    _____ Peripheral neuropathy
    _____ Bone loss
    _____ Skin rashes

6. A client is receiving rituximab (Rituxan) for the treatment of non-Hodgkin's leukemia. Targeted anticancer medications may act to destroy cancer cells by

   A. blocking hormone receptors.

   B. increasing immune response.

   C. binding with specific antigens on tumor cells.

   D. stopping DNA replication during cell division.

CHAPTER 42: CHEMOTHERAPY AGENTS

Application Exercises Answer Key

1. A client with breast cancer is receiving a combination therapy of cyclophosphamide, methotrexate, and fluorouracil. Combination chemotherapy is used to do which of the following? (Select all that apply)

    __X__ **Decrease medication resistance.**

    __X__ **Attack cancer cells at different stages of cell growth.**

    _____ Block chemotherapy agent from entering healthy cells.

    _____ Stimulate immune system.

    __X__ **Reduce the dosage of each chemotherapy agent.**

    Medications used for combination chemotherapy should act in different phases of the cell cycle to increase cytotoxicity. Combination therapy is used to reduce medication resistance, increase effectiveness, and, ideally, reduce toxic effects with lower medication dosages. Combination therapy does not block chemotherapy agents from entering healthy cells. Biological response modifiers stimulate the immune system.

NCLEX® Connection: Pharmacological and Parenteral Therapies, Adverse Effects/Contraindications/Side Effects/Interactions

2. Hemorrhagic cystitis in a client taking nitrogen mustards may be minimized by administering which of the following?

    A. Uroprotectant agent such as mesna (Mesnex).

    B. Glucocorticoid, such as dexamethasone (Decadron).

    C. Loop diuretic such as furosemide (Lasix).

    D. H_1 receptor antagonist, such as diphenhydramine (Benadryl).

    A uroprotectant agent such as mesna (Mesnex) is used to prevent hemorrhagic cystitis, a severe adverse reaction to nitrogen mustards. Increasing daily fluid intake to 3 L may also prevent this reaction. The nurse should monitor for hematuria. Other adverse reactions may include immunosuppression, nausea and vomiting, and alopecia.

NCLEX® Connection: Pharmacological and Parenteral Therapies, Adverse Effects/Contraindications/Side Effects/Interactions

3. Leucovorin is given to a client who is taking methotrexate to

    A. reduce the risk of a transfusion reaction.

    B. increase production of platelets.

    C. potentiate the cytotoxic effects of methotrexate.

    D. protect healthy cells from the toxic effects of methotrexate.

Leucovorin rescue is given within 12 hr of high doses of methotrexate to protect healthy cells from the toxic effects of the methotrexate. High doses of methotrexate may kill healthy cells. Leucovorin is a folic acid derivative that enters healthy cells and blocks methotrexate from damaging normal cells. Administer methotrexate with leucovorin rescue to reduce toxicity to healthy cells. Leucovorin does not reduce the risk of transfusion reaction, increase platelet production or potentiate the cytotoxic effects of methotrexate.

NCLEX® Connection: Pharmacological and Parenteral Therapies, Expected Actions/ Outcomes

4. A client is taking tamoxifen (Nolvadex), an estrogen receptor blocker, for treatment of breast cancer. Which of the following is an adverse effect of this medication for which the client should be alert?

    A. Chest pain or palpitations.

    B. Abnormal uterine bleeding.

    C. Yellow sclera or dark-colored urine.

    D. Shortness of breath.

Endometrial cancer is a severe side effect to tamoxifen therapy. The client should be advised to have a gynecologic exam yearly and monitor for abnormal uterine bleeding. Other adverse effects may include hot flushes, nausea and vomiting, and blood clots. Chest pain or palpitations, yellow sclera or dark-colored urine, and shortness of breath are not adverse effects of tamoxifen.

NCLEX® Connection: Pharmacological and Parenteral Therapies, Adverse Effects/ Contraindications/Side Effects/Interactions

5. A client is being treated with Interferon Alfa-2a for chronic myelogenous leukemia. Which of the following are common adverse reactions to biologic response modifiers? (Select all that apply.)

_____ Tinnitus

__X__ **Flu-like symptoms, such as fever, chills, myalgia**

__X__ **Peripheral neuropathy**

_____ Bone loss

__X__ **Skin rashes**

Interferon Alfa-2a is a biologic response modifier that may cause flu-like symptoms, which may be treated with acetaminophen. Other adverse reactions may include edema, peripheral neuropathy, and skin reactions. Tinnitus is not a side effect of Interferon Alfa-2a Bone loss is associated with estrogen antagonists and may lead to osteoporosis.

NCLEX® Connection: Pharmacological and Parenteral Therapies, Adverse Effects/ Contraindications/Side Effects/Interactions

6. A client is receiving rituximab (Rituxan) for the treatment of non-Hodgkin's leukemia. Targeted anticancer medications may act to destroy cancer cells by

A. blocking hormone receptors.

B. Increasing immune response.

C. binding with specific antigens on tumor cells.

D. stopping DNA replication during cell division.

Some targeted antineoplastic medications like rituximab (Rituxan), are antibodies and destroy tumor cells by binding to specific antigens on the tumor cells. Targeted antineoplastic medications attach to specific target sites to stop cancer growth without injuring healthy tissue. Hormonal agents may block hormone receptors. Biologic response modifiers are immunostimulants. Many cytotoxic agents act during cell division.

NCLEX® Connection: Pharmacological and Parenteral Therapies, Expected Actions/ Outcomes

UNIT 12: MEDICATIONS FOR INFECTION

- Principles of Antimicrobial Therapy
- Antibiotics Affecting the Bacterial Cell Wall
- Antibiotics Affecting Protein Synthesis
- Urinary Tract Infections
- Mycobacterial, Fungal, and Parasitic Infections
- Viral Infections, HIV, and AIDS

NCLEX® CONNECTIONS

When reviewing the chapters in this unit, keep in mind the relevant sections of the NCLEX® outline, in particular:

CLIENT NEEDS: PHARMACOLOGICAL AND PARENTERAL THERAPIES

Relevant topics/tasks include:

- Adverse Effects/Contraindications/Side Effects/Interactions
  - Identify symptoms/evidence of an allergic reaction.
- Medication Administration
  - Evaluate the appropriateness/accuracy of a medication order for the client per institution policy, including reconciling orders.
- Parenteral/Intravenous Therapy
  - Evaluate the client's response to intermittent parenteral fluid therapy.

UNIT 12 MEDICATIONS FOR INFECTION

Chapter 43 Principles of Antimicrobial Therapy

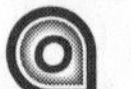

Overview

- Antimicrobial therapy (often termed "antibiotic therapy") is the use of medications to treat infections caused by bacteria, viruses, and fungi.
- Antimicrobials must use selective toxicity to kill or otherwise control microbes without destroying host cells. Methods of actions include:
  - Destroying the cell wall which is present in bacteria but not in mammals.
  - Preventing viral replication through reduction of enzymes needed by the virus to reproduce.
- New antimicrobials must be continually created due to changes in DNA of micro-organisms, called conjugation, which produces resistance to multiple existing drugs.
- Suprainfection is a type of resistance caused when normal flora are killed by use of an antibiotic, thus favoring the emergence of a new infection which is difficult to eliminate.
- Antimicrobial medications are classified by:
  - Defining which microbes are susceptible to each medication
  - The mechanism of action of each medication
- Antimicrobial medications are selected for clinical use based on multiple factors.

Selection of Antimicrobials

- Identification of the causative agent:
  - Laboratory testing is performed on body fluids, such as blood, urine, sputum, or wound drainage, to determine the micro-organism causing the infection.
    - Gram stain: an aspirate of the body fluid is examined under the microscope, where micro-organisms may be identified directly.
    - Culture of the fluid: the aspirate is applied to culture medium and colonies of the micro-organism are grown over several days. A culture may be preferable to gram stain in cases where positive identification cannot be made by the first method.
      - Culture should be obtained prior to treatment with antibiotics.
      - Fluid for culture should be carefully collected to prevent contamination and unnecessary antimicrobial treatment.

- Sensitivity of the micro-organism to the antimicrobial
    - For organisms where resistance is common, a test for sensitivity of the organism to various antimicrobials is performed.
        - Disk diffusion test (also called Kirby-Bauer test) is most common.
        - Broth dilution method is a quantitative method that helps determine the necessary amount of antibiotic for a specific infection.
- Host Factors
    - Immune System of Client
        - In a person with an intact immune system, the antibiotic works with host defense systems to suppress organisms, Antibiotics that are not bactericidal may be used.
        - An immunocompromised person needs strong bactericidal antibiotics.
    - Site of the Infection
        - Certain sites are difficult for antimicrobials to reach.
            - Infections in cerebral spinal fluid, where the blood-brain barrier must be crossed (meningitis)
            - Bacterial infiltration within the heart (endocarditis)
            - Purulent abscesses anywhere within the body, due to poor blood supply (Drainage through surgery increases the effect of antimicrobials.)
    - Age of the Client
        - Infants are at increased danger of antibiotic toxicity because of undeveloped renal and liver function.

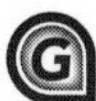

        - Older adult clients may also develop toxicity because of reduction in drug metabolism and excretion.
    - Pregnancy

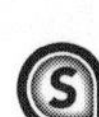

        - Antibiotics may harm the developing fetus.
        - Antimicrobials are generally avoided in breastfeeding mothers because of possible danger to the nursing infant.
    - Presence of a previous allergic reaction, especially with penicillin (Clients should not receive penicillin after an allergic reaction, narrowing the antibiotic choice for those clients)
    - Combination Therapy
        - Combining more than one antimicrobial may cause additive or potentiative effects. Indications include:
            - Severe infections
            - Infections caused by more than one micro-organism
            - Infections, such as tuberculosis, where combination therapy actually prevents bacterial resistance from developing

        - Where use of combinations can decrease chance of toxicity by reducing necessary dosage
        - Where use of multiple antibiotics produces more effective treatment than use of only one
    - Combining antimicrobials can sometimes cause adverse effects, such as:
        - Increased resistance to antimicrobials
        - Increased cost of therapy
        - More adverse or toxic reactions
        - Antagonistic effects among the various antibiotics

Prophylactic Use

- Indications for prophylactic use include prevention of:
    - Infections for clients undergoing surgery of the GI tract, cardiac or vascular surgery, orthopedic surgery, some gynecologic surgeries
    - Influenza with amantadine (Symmetrel)
    - Sexually transmitted diseases following sexual exposure
- Limit prophylactic use of antimicrobials to individuals with:
    - Prosthetic heart valves, prior to dental or other procedures because of the danger of bacterial endocarditis
    - Recurring urinary tract infection

Nursing Interventions

- Perform hand hygiene before and after each client contact to prevent the spread of infection.
- Recognize invasive procedures that increase the chance of infection, such as urinary or other catheters.
- Encourage health measures to prevent infections:
    - Maintaining up to date immunization status
    - Hand hygiene
- Teach clients to take the full course of antibiotics prescribed to prevent medication resistance and recurrence of infection.
- Use infection control procedures to prevent transmission of resistant micro-organisms.
    - Practice proper use of infection control principles, such as use of aseptic technique, isolation, and proper assignment of rooms within facilities.
- Evaluate effectiveness of treatment:
    - Check post-treatment culture to determine if it is negative for bacteria.
    - Monitor the client for clinical improvement, such as improved breath sounds.

CHAPTER 43: PRINCIPLES OF ANTIMICROBIAL THERAPY

 Application Exercises

1. A nurse is caring for a client just admitted with an infected wound on her arm. Which of the following admission prescriptions should the nurse implement first?

   A. Administer a prescribed antibiotic.

   B. Obtain a wound culture.

   C. Have blood drawn for CBC and electrolyte panel.

   D. Apply dry dressing to the wound.

2. A nurse is caring for a school-age child who has been diagnosed with viral bronchitis. The parent tells the nurse, "I'm upset that the doctor didn't order an antibiotic for my child. I think I'll start giving her the leftover antibiotics from her last ear infection." What should concern the nurse in this situation?

3. A nurse is caring for a client who has a suspected bacterial infection in her urine. Which of the following prescribed laboratory tests will identify antibiotics that could treat the infection?

   A. Gram stain

   B. Culture

   C. Sensitivity

   D. Specific gravity

4. A nurse should understand that prophylactic use of antibiotics is indicated for which of the following clients?

   A. An older adult client who has recovered from several bouts of severe pneumonia

   B. A toddler who had multiple ear infections last winter

   C. A school-age child who will be having his tonsils and adenoids removed tomorrow

   D. An adult client who is undergoing total hip replacement surgery today

CHAPTER 43: PRINCIPLES OF ANTIMICROBIAL THERAPY

Application Exercises Answer Key

1. A nurse is caring for a client just admitted with an infected wound on her arm. Which of the following admission prescriptions should the nurse implement first?

   A. Administer a prescribed antibiotic.

   B. Obtain a wound culture.

   C. Have blood drawn for CBC and electrolyte panel.

   D. Apply dry dressing to the wound.

   A wound culture should be obtained prior to beginning the antibiotic in order to identify the causative agent. This is the nurse's priority in this situation. Administering the prescribed antibiotic is important, having blood drawn by the lab, and applying a dry dressing to the wound are important but are not the first priority at this time.

NCLEX® Connection: Pharmacological and Parenteral Therapies, Medication Administration

2. A nurse is caring for a school-age child who has been diagnosed with viral bronchitis. The parent tells the nurse, "I'm upset that the doctor didn't order an antibiotic for my child. I think I'll start giving her the leftover antibiotics from her last ear infection." What should concern the nurse in this situation?

   The parent is promoting resistance toward antibiotics in the child by a) not giving the full dose of previously prescribed antibiotics; and b) giving antimicrobials meant for a bacterial infection to the child for a viral infection, although these medications will be of no use for viral bronchitis. This indicates the mother needs health teaching about the proper use of antibiotics.

NCLEX® Connection: Pharmacological and Parenteral Therapies, Medication Administration

3. A nurse is caring for a client who has a suspected bacterial infection in her urine. Which of the following prescribed laboratory tests will identify antibiotics that could treat the infection?

   A. Gram stain

   B. Culture

   C. Sensitivity

   D. Specific gravity

   A test for sensitivity tells which antibiotic(s) will be effective in treating a specific infection. A gram stain simply identifies the presence of micro-organisms through direct visualization under a microscope. A culture allows micro-organisms to reproduce over several days in order to better identify them. A test for specific gravity of urine simply tells the concentration of urine compared to water; a high or low specific gravity does not indicate the presence of micro-organisms.

NCLEX® Connection: Pharmacological and Parenteral Therapies, Expected Actions/Outcomes

4. A nurse should understand that prophylactic use of antibiotics is indicated for which of the following clients?

   A. An older adult client who has recovered from several bouts of severe pneumonia

   B. A toddler who had multiple ear infections last winter

   C. A school-age child who will be having his tonsils and adenoids removed tomorrow

   D. An adult client who is undergoing total hip replacement surgery today

   Prophylactic use of antibiotics is indicated for clients who undergo orthopedic, cardiac, peripheral vascular, gastrointestinal, and some gynecologic surgeries. Prophylactic use of antibiotics is not indicated for the other clients.

NCLEX® Connection: Pharmacological and Parenteral Therapies, Expected Actions/ Outcomes

UNIT 12 MEDICATIONS FOR INFECTION

Chapter 44 Antibiotics Affecting the Bacterial Cell Wall

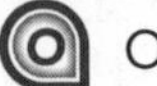

Overview

- Antibiotics that affect the cell wall are bactericidal. This group of antibiotics includes penicillins, cephalosporins, carbapenems, and monobactams.

MEDICATION CLASSIFICATION: PENICILLINS

- Select Prototype Medication: penicillin G (Bicillin LA)
- Other Medications:
  - Broad-spectrum
    - Amoxicillin-clavulanate (Augmentin)
    - Ampicillin (Principen)
  - Antistaphylococcal
    - Nafcillin (Unipen)
    - Methicillin
  - Antipseudomonas
    - Carbenicillin (Geocillin)
    - Ticarcillin-clavulanate (Timentin)
    - Piperacillin tazobactam (Zosyn)

Purpose

- Expected Pharmacological Action
  - Penicillins destroy bacteria by weakening the bacterial cell wall.
- Therapeutic Uses
  - Penicillins are the medication of choice for gram-positive cocci such as *Streptococcus pneumoniae* (pneumonia and meningitis), *Streptococcus viridans* (infectious endocarditis), and *Streptococcus pyogenes* (pharyngitis).
  - Penicillins are the medication of first choice for meningitis caused by gram–negative cocci *Neisseria meningitides*.

- Penicillins are the medication of choice for the treatment of syphilis caused by *Spirochete treponema pallidum*.
- Extended-spectrum penicillin (carbenicillin, piperacillin) is effective against organisms such as *Pseudomonas aeruginosa*, *Enterobacter species*, *Proteus*, *Bacteroides fragilis*, and *Klebsiella*.
- Penicillins are used as prophylaxis against bacterial endocarditis in at-risk clients prior to dental and other procedures.

Complications

SIDE/ADVERSE EFFECTS	NURSING INTERVENTIONS/CLIENT EDUCATION
• Allergies/Anaphylaxis	• Interview clients for prior allergy. • Advise clients to wear an allergy identification bracelet. • Observe clients for 30 min following administration of parenteral penicillin.
• Renal impairment	• Monitor the client's kidney function. • Monitor the client's intake and output.
• Hyperkalemia/dysrhythmias are possible with high doses of penicillin, penicillin G. • Hypernatremia may occur with IV carbenicillin and ticarcillin	• Monitor the client's cardiac status and electrolyte levels.

Contraindications/Precautions

- Penicillins are contraindicated for clients with a severe history of allergies to penicillin, cephalosporin, and/or imipenem.

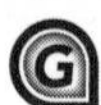

- Use cautiously in clients who have, or are at risk for, kidney dysfunction (clients who are acutely ill, older adults, or young children).
- Clients who are allergic to one penicillin should be considered cross allergic to other penicillins and at risk for a cross allergy to cephalosporin.

Interactions

MEDICATION/FOOD INTERACTIONS	NURSING INTERVENTIONS/CLIENT EDUCATION
Penicillin inactivates aminoglycosides when mixed in the same IV solution.	• Do not mix penicillin and aminoglycosides in the same IV solution.
Probenecid (Probalan) delays excretion of penicillin.	• Probenecid may be added to penicillin therapy to prolong action.

Nursing Administration

- Instruct clients that penicillin V, amoxicillin, and amoxicillin-clavulanate may be taken with meals. All others should be taken with a full glass of water 1 hr before meals or 2 hr after.
- Instruct clients to report any signs of an allergic response such as skin rash, itching, and/or hives.
- IM injection should be done cautiously to avoid injection into a nerve or an artery.
- Advise clients to complete the entire course of therapy regardless of presence of symptoms.

MEDICATION CLASSIFICATION: CEPHALOSPORINS

- Select Prototype Medication: cephalexin (Keflex) – 1st generation
- Other Medications:
  - 1st generation – Cephradine (Anspor, Velosef)
  - 2nd generation – Cefaclor (Ceclor), cefotetan (Cefotan)
  - 3rd generation – Ceftriaxone (Rocephin), cefotaxime (Claforan), cefoperazone (Cefobid)
  - 4th generation – Cefepime (Maxipime)

Purpose

- Expected Pharmacological Action
  - Cephalosporins are beta-lactam antibiotics, similar to penicillins that destroy bacterial cell walls causing destruction of micro-organisms.
  - Cephalosporins are grouped into four generations. Each generation of cephalosporins is:
    - More likely to reach cerebrospinal fluid.
    - Less likely to be destroyed by beta-lactamase.
    - More effective against gram-negative organisms and anaerobes.
- Therapeutic Uses
  - Cephalosporins are broad-spectrum bactericidal medications with a high therapeutic index that treat urinary tract infections, postoperative infections, pelvic infections, and meningitis.

Complications

SIDE/ADVERSE EFFECTS	NURSING INTERVENTIONS/CLIENT EDUCATION
• Allergic/hypersensitivity/anaphylaxis • Possible cross-sensitivity to penicillin	• If signs of allergy appear (urticaria, rash, hypotension, and/or dyspnea) stop cephalosporin immediately, and notify the provider. • Question client carefully regarding past history of allergy to a penicillin or other cephalosporin and notify the provider if present.
• Bleeding tendencies with use of cefotetan	• Cefotetan should be avoided in clients with bleeding disorders and those taking anticoagulants. • Observe clients for signs of bleeding. • Monitor clients for prothrombin time and bleeding time. Abnormal levels may require discontinuation of medication. • Administer parenteral vitamin K.
• Thrombophlebitis with IV infusion	• Rotate injection sites. • Administer as a diluted intermittent infusion or, if a bolus dose is prescribed, administer slowly over 3 to 5 min and in a dilute solution.
• Pain with IM injection	• Administer IM injection deep in large muscle mass.
• Antibiotic-associated pseudomembranous colitis	• Observe clients for diarrhea and notify the provider. • Medication should be discontinued.

Contraindications/Precautions

- Cephalosporins should not be given to clients who have a history of severe allergic reactions to penicillins.
- Use cautiously in clients who have renal impairment or bleeding tendencies.

Interactions

MEDICATION/FOOD INTERACTIONS	NURSING INTERVENTIONS/CLIENT EDUCATION
Disulfiram reaction (intolerance to alcohol) occurs with combined use of cefotetan and alcohol.	• Instruct clients not to consume alcohol while taking these cephalosporins.
Probenecid delays renal excretion.	• Monitor the client's I&O.

Nursing Administration

- Instruct clients to complete the prescribed course of therapy, even though symptoms may resolve before the full course of antimicrobial treatment is completed.
- Advise clients to take oral cephalosporins with food.
- Instruct clients to store oral cephalosporin suspensions in a refrigerator.

MEDICATION CLASSIFICATION: CARBAPENEMS

- Select Prototype Medication: imipenem (Primaxin)
- Other Medications: meropenem (Merrem IV)

Purpose

- Expected Pharmacological Action
  - Carbapenems are beta-lactam antibiotics that destroy bacterial cell walls, causing destruction of micro-organisms.
- Therapeutic Uses
  - Broad antimicrobial spectrum is effective for serious infections such as pneumonia, peritonitis, and urinary tract infections caused by gram-positive cocci, gram-negative cocci, and anaerobic bacteria.
  - Resistance develops when imipenem is used alone to treat *Pseudomonas aeruginosa*. A combination of antipseudomonal medications should be used to treat this micro-organism.

Complications

SIDE/ADVERSE EFFECTS	NURSING INTERVENTIONS/CLIENT EDUCATION
• Allergy/hypersensitivity • Possible cross-sensitivity to penicillin or cephalosporins	• Monitor clients for signs of allergic reactions, such as rashes or pruritus. • Question clients carefully regarding past history of allergy to a penicillin or other cephalosporin and notify provider if present.
• Gastrointestinal symptoms (nausea, vomiting, diarrhea)	• Observe clients for symptoms and notify the provider if they occur. • Monitor the client's I&O.
• Suprainfection	• Monitor clients for signs of colitis (diarrhea, oral thrush, and/or vaginal yeast infection).

Contraindications/Precautions

- Use cautiously in clients who have renal impairment.

Nursing Administration

- Instruct clients to complete the prescribed course of antimicrobial therapy, even though symptoms may resolve before the full course is completed.

MEDICATION CLASSIFICATION: OTHER INHIBITORS

- Select Prototype Medications:
  - Vancomycin (Vancocin)
  - Aztreonam (Azactam): classified as a monobactam
  - Fosfomycin (Monurol)

Purpose

- Expected Pharmacological Action
  - This group of antibiotics destroys bacterial cell walls, causing destruction of micro-organisms.
- Therapeutic Uses
  - They are the antimicrobials of choice for:
    - Serious infections caused by methicillin resistant *Staphylococcus aureus, E. Coli*, or *Staphylococcus epidermidis*
    - Antibiotic-associated pseudomembranous colitis caused by *Clostridium difficile*

Complications

SIDE/ADVERSE EFFECTS	NURSING INTERVENTIONS/CLIENT EDUCATION
Ototoxicity	• Assess clients for signs of hearing loss. • Instruct clients to notify the provider if changes in hearing acuity develop. • Monitor vancomycin levels.
Infusion reactions (rashes, flushing, tachycardia, and hypotension)	• Administer vancomycin slowly over 60 min.
Thrombophlebitis	• Rotate injection sites. • Monitor the infusion site for redness, swelling, and inflammation.

Interactions

MEDICATION/FOOD INTERACTIONS	NURSING INTERVENTIONS/CLIENT EDUCATION
• Increased risk for ototoxicity when vancomycin is used concurrently with another medication that also produces ototoxicity (loop diuretics).	• Assess for hearing loss.

Contraindications/Precautions

- Use cautiously in clients who have renal impairment.

Nursing Administration

- Vancomycin peak blood levels should be collected 1 to 2 hr after completion of IV infusion.

Nursing Evaluation of Medication Effectiveness

- Depending on therapeutic intent, effectiveness may be evidenced by:
  - Reduction of signs and symptoms such as fever, pain, inflammation, and adventitious breath sounds
  - Resolution of infection

CHAPTER 44: ANTIBIOTICS AFFECTING THE BACTERIAL CELL WALL

Application Exercises

Scenario: A client comes to a community clinic reporting a fever, sore throat, and cough. The client's posterior pharynx is reddened with patches of purulent exudate, and the client states that she experiences pain with swallowing. Her cervical lymph nodes are enlarged and tender to touch. The client's vital signs are: temperature 38.5° C (101.4° F) orally; pulse 96/min; respirations 22/min; and blood pressure 122/84 mm Hg. Based on the symptoms and physical examination, the primary care provider suspects a streptococcal infection, which is confirmed by a quick strep test performed in the clinic. The client is started on amoxicillin/clavulanate (Augmentin) 500 mg orally every 8 hr for 10 days.

1. Before administering the first dose of amoxicillin/clavulanate, what additional assessment data should the nurse collect?

2. When instructing the client on the use of amoxicillin/clavulanate, what should the nurse tell the client is most important?

3. After the first two doses, the client calls and states that she is experiencing an itchy rash. What should the nurse tell the client?

4. The client returns to the clinic and the provider discontinues amoxicillin/clavulanate and starts the client on cephalexin (Keflex), 250 mg orally every 6 hr for 10 days. The provider provides samples so the client can begin taking the medication immediately. What nursing intervention should the nurse follow? Explain.

CHAPTER 44: ANTIBIOTICS AFFECTING THE BACTERIAL CELL WALL

Application Exercises Answer Key

Scenario: A client comes to a community clinic complaining of a fever, sore throat, and cough. The client's posterior pharynx is reddened with patches of purulent exudate, and the client states that she experiences pain with swallowing. Her cervical lymph nodes are enlarged and tender to touch. The client's vital signs are: temperature 38.5° C (101.4° F) orally; pulse 96/min; respirations 22/min; and blood pressure 122/84 mm Hg. Based on the symptoms and physical examination, the primary care provider suspects a streptococcal infection, which is confirmed by a quick strep test performed in the clinic. The client is started on amoxicillin/clavulanate (Augmentin) 500 mg orally every 8 hr for 10 days.

1. Before administering the first dose of amoxicillin/clavulanate, what additional assessment data should the nurse collect?

   The nurse should inquire if the client has ever had a reaction to a previous antibiotic, especially if the antibiotic was a penicillin product.

NCLEX® Connection: Pharmacological and Parenteral Therapies, Medication Administration

2. When instructing the client on the use of amoxicillin/clavulanate, what should the nurse tell the client is most important?

   The client should be sure to take the medication with food to avoid gastrointestinal discomfort, and finish taking all of the medication as prescribed, even if the condition improves. Failure to complete a course of antibiotics can result in development of resistant strains of organisms. The client should be advised to never share this medication because some individuals may be allergic to penicillin and may develop a serious reaction. The client should report any signs or symptoms of allergic reaction to the provider.

NCLEX® Connection: Pharmacological and Parenteral Therapies, Medication Administration

3. After the first two doses, the client calls and states that she is experiencing an itchy rash. What should the nurse tell the client?

   The nurse should first assess if the client has any other adverse symptoms or is experiencing any difficulty breathing. If so, advise the client to call 9-1-1 immediately. If symptoms are not life-threatening, advise the client to stop taking the medication immediately and come to the clinic for further evaluation.

NCLEX® Connection: Pharmacological and Parenteral Therapies, Adverse Effects/Contraindications/Side Effects/Interactions

4. The client returns to the clinic and the primary care provider discontinues amoxicillin/clavulanate and starts the client on cephalexin (Keflex), 250 mg orally every 6 hr for 10 days. The provider provides samples so the client can begin taking the medication immediately. What nursing intervention should the nurse follow? Explain.

    The client should take the first dose and then sit in the waiting room for approximately 30 min. After 30 min, the nurse can assess the client for any possible allergic responses. Cephalosporins have a cross-sensitivity with penicillin medications, so the nurse should ensure that the client is safe. The nurse should carefully document the client's condition prior to sending her home and consider making a follow-up call to see how she is doing. Instruct the client to report any further signs or symptoms of allergic reaction immediately to the provider.

NCLEX® Connection: Pharmacological and Parenteral Therapies, Medication Administration

UNIT 12 MEDICATIONS FOR INFECTION

Chapter 45 Antibiotics Affecting Protein Synthesis

Overview

- Antibiotics affecting protein synthesis may be bacteriostatic, such as tetracyclines and macrolides, or bactericidal, such as aminoglycosides.
- Uses include infections of the respiratory, gastrointestinal, urinary and reproductive tract and infections caused by rickettsia.

MEDICATION CLASSIFICATION: TETRACYCLINES

- Select Prototype Medication: tetracycline hydrochloride (Sumycin)
- Other Medications: doxycycline (Vibramycin), minocycline (Minocin)

Purpose

- Expected Pharmacological Action
  - Tetracyclines are broad-spectrum antibiotics that inhibit micro-organism growth by preventing protein synthesis (bacteriostatic).
- Therapeutic Uses
  - Administered topically and orally to treat acne vulgaris and topically for periodontal disease
  - Used as first-line medication for
    - Rickettsial infections, such as typhus fever or Rocky Mountain spotted fever
    - Infections of the urethra or cervix caused by *Chlamydia trachomatis*
    - Brucellosis
    - Pneumonia caused by *Mycoplasma pneumonia*
    - Lyme disease
    - Anthrax
    - Gastrointestinal infections caused by *Helicobacter pylori*

Complications

SIDE/ADVERSE EFFECTS	NURSING INTERVENTIONS/CLIENT EDUCATION
Gastrointestinal discomfort (cramping, nausea, vomiting, diarrhea, and esophageal ulceration)	• Monitor clients for nausea, vomiting, and diarrhea. • Monitor the client's I&O. • Doxycycline and minocycline may be taken with meals. • Avoid taking at bedtime to reduce esophageal ulceration.
Yellow/brown tooth discoloration and/or hypoplasia of tooth enamel	• Avoid administration to children less than 8 years of age.
Hepatotoxicity (lethargy, jaundice)	• Avoid administration of high daily doses IV.
Photosensitivity (exaggerated sunburn)	• Advise clients to take precautions when out in the sun such as wearing protective clothing and using sunscreen.
Suprainfection of the bowel – antibiotic-associated pseudomembranous colitis (diarrhea, yeast infections of the mouth, pharynx, vagina, and bowels)	• Instruct clients to observe for symptoms of diarrhea and notify the provider.
Dizziness, lightheadedness, with minocycline	• Instruct clients to report these symptoms. Medication should be discontinued.

Contraindications/Precautions

- Use of tetracycline during pregnancy after the fourth month can cause staining of the deciduous teeth, but will not have a permanent effect on permanent teeth. In general, tetracyclines should not be given to women who are pregnant or to young children.
- Use cautiously in clients with liver and renal disease. Doxycycline and minocycline may be used in clients with renal disease.

Interactions

MEDICATION/FOOD INTERACTIONS	NURSING INTERVENTIONS/CLIENT EDUCATION
Interaction with milk products, calcium or iron supplements, laxatives containing magnesium such as magnesium hydroxide (Milk of Magnesia), and antacids causes formation of nonabsorbable chelates.	• Tetracycline should be taken on an empty stomach with a full glass of water. • Doxycycline and minocycline may be taken with meals. • Administer tetracyclines at least 1 hr before and 2 hr after taking food and supplements containing calcium and magnesium.
Tetracycline decreases the efficacy of oral contraceptives.	• Advise client to use an alternative form of birth control.

Nursing Administration

- Instruct clients to take tetracycline on an empty stomach, with a full glass of water. Doxycycline and minocycline may be taken with meals.
- Instruct clients to maintain a 2 hr interval between ingestion of chelating agents and medications.
- Instruct clients to complete the prescribed course of antimicrobial therapy, even though symptoms may resolve before the full course is completed.

Nursing Evaluation of Medication Effectiveness

- Depending on therapeutic intent, effectiveness may be evidenced by:
  - Improvement of infection symptoms, such as clear breath sounds
  - Resolution of yeast infections of the mouth, vagina, and bowels
  - Resolution of acne vulgaris facial lesions

MEDICATION CLASSIFICATION: MACROLIDES

- Select Prototype Medication: erythromycin (E-Mycin)
- Other medication: azithromycin (Zithromax)

Purpose

- Expected Pharmacological Action
  - Erythromycin slows the growth of micro-organisms by inhibiting protein synthesis (bacteriostatic) but can be bactericidal if given for susceptible bacteria at high enough doses.
- Therapeutic Uses
  - Used to treat infections in clients with a penicillin allergy, such as for prophylaxis against rheumatic fever and bacterial endocarditis
  - Used for clients with Legionnaires' disease, whooping cough (pertussis), and acute diphtheria (eliminates the carrier state of diphtheria)
  - Used for chlamydia infections (urethritis and cervicitis; pneumonia caused by *Mycoplasma pneumoniae*; respiratory tract infections caused by *Streptococcus pneumoniae*, and group A *Streptococcus pyogenes*)

Complications

SIDE/ADVERSE EFFECTS	NURSING INTERVENTIONS/CLIENT EDUCATION
Gastrointestinal discomfort (nausea, vomiting, epigastric pain)	• Administer erythromycin with meals. • Observe for GI symptoms and notify the provider.
Hepatotoxicity (abdominal pain, lethargy, jaundice)	• Instruct clients to notify the provider because the medication should be discontinued.
Prolonged QT interval causing dysrhythmias and possible sudden cardiac death	• Use in clients with prolonged QT intervals is not recommended. • Avoid concurrent use with maledictions that affect hepatic drug metabolizing enzymes.

Contraindications/Precautions

- Bacteriostatic inhibitors are contraindicated in clients with pre-existing liver disease.

Interactions

MEDICATION/FOOD INTERACTIONS	NURSING INTERVENTIONS/CLIENT EDUCATION
Erythromycin inhibits metabolism of antihistamines, theophylline, carbamazepine, and warfarin, which can lead to toxicity of these medications.	• To minimize toxicity, avoid using erythromycin with antihistamines, asthma medication, anticonvulsants, and anticoagulants.
Verapamil and diltiazem, HIV protease inhibitors, antifungal medications, and nefazodone inhibit hepatic drug-metabolizing enzymes, which can lead to erythromycin toxicity, causing a tachydysrhythmia and possible cardiac arrest.	• Concurrent use is not recommended.

Nursing Administration

- Administer oral preparation on an empty stomach (1 hr before meals or 2 hr after) with a full glass of water, unless GI upset occurs.
- Azithromycin may be administered with food.
- Intravenous route is rarely used.
- Instruct clients to complete the prescribed course of antimicrobial therapy, even though symptoms may resolve before the full course is completed.

Nursing Evaluation of Medication Effectiveness

- Depending on therapeutic intent, effectiveness may be evidenced by:
  - Improvement of infection symptoms (clear lung sounds; improvement of sore throat, cough, urinary tract symptoms; and resolution of bacterial endocarditis with negative blood cultures).

MEDICATION CLASSIFICATION: AMINOGLYCOSIDES

- Select Prototype Medication: gentamicin (Garamycin)
- Other Medications:
  - Amikacin (Amikin)
  - Tobramycin sulfate (Nebcin)
  - Neomycin (Mycifradin)
  - Streptomycin
  - Paromomycin (oral)

Purpose

- Expected Pharmacological Action
  - Aminoglycosides are bactericidal antibiotics that destroy micro-organisms by disrupting protein synthesis.
- Therapeutic Uses
  - Aminoglycosides are the medication of choice against aerobic gram-negative bacilli, such as *Escherichia coli, Klebsiella pneumoniae, Proteus mirabilis,* and *Pseudomonas aeruginosa*.
  - Paromomycin (oral aminoglycoside) is used for intestinal amebiasis and tapeworm infections.
  - Oral neomycin is often used prior to surgery of the GI tract to suppress normal flora.

Complications

SIDE/ADVERSE EFFECTS	NURSING INTERVENTIONS/CLIENT EDUCATION
Ototoxicity – Cochlear damage (hearing loss) and vestibular damage (loss of balance)	• Monitor clients for symptoms of tinnitus (ringing in the ears), headache, hearing loss, nausea, dizziness, and vertigo. • Instruct clients to notify the provider if tinnitus, hearing loss, or headaches occur. • Stop aminoglycoside if symptoms occur. Do baseline audiometric studies (hearing test).
Nephrotoxicity related to high total cumulative dose resulting in acute tubular necrosis (proteinuria, casts in the urine, dilute urine, elevated BUN, creatinine levels)	• Monitor I&O, BUN, and creatinine levels. • Instruct clients to report a significant decrease in the amount of urine output.
Intensified neuromuscular blockade resulting in respiratory depression	• Closely monitor use in clients with myasthenia gravis, clients taking skeletal muscle relaxants, and clients receiving general anesthetics.
Hypersensitivity (rash, pruritus, paresthesia of hands and feet, and urticaria)	• Monitor clients for allergic symptoms.
Streptomycin	
Neurologic disorder (peripheral neuritis, optic nerve dysfunction, tingling/numbness of the hands and feet)	• Instruct clients to promptly report any symptoms to the provider.

Contraindications/Precautions

- Use cautiously in clients with renal impairment, pre-existing hearing loss or myasthenia gravis.
- Use cautiously in clients taking ethacrynic acid (increases risk for ototoxicity), amphotericin B, cephalosporins, vancomycin (increases risk for nephrotoxicity), and neuromuscular blocking agents such as tubocurarine.
- Clients with renal impairment should receive reduced doses of aminoglycosides.

Interactions

MEDICATION/FOOD INTERACTIONS	NURSING INTERVENTIONS/CLIENT EDUCATION
Penicillin will inactivate aminoglycosides when mixed in the same IV solution.	• Do not mix aminoglycosides and penicillins in the same IV solution.
When administered concurrently with other ototoxic medications (such as loop diuretics), the risk for ototoxicity greatly increases.	• Assess frequently for hearing loss with concurrent medication use.

Nursing Administration

- Most aminoglycosides (such as gentamicin and amikacin) are administered only by IM or IV routes. Some others (such as neomycin) can be administered either orally or topically.
- Measure aminoglycoside levels based on dosing schedules.
    - Once a day dosing: only trough level needs to be measured. Take trough level 1 hr prior to the next dose.
    - Divided doses:
        - Peak – 30 min after administration of aminoglycoside intramuscularly or 30 min after an IV infusion has finished
        - Trough – Right before the next dose

Nursing Evaluation of Medication Effectiveness

- Depending on therapeutic intent, effectiveness may be evidenced by:
    - Improvement of infection symptoms (clear lung sounds, improvement of urinary tract symptoms, wound healing)

CHAPTER 45: ANTIBIOTICS AFFECTING PROTEIN SYNTHESIS

Application Exercises

1. A nurse is providing teaching to a client prescribed tetracycline hydrochloride (Sumycin) to treat a GI infection caused by *Helicobacter pylori*. Which of the following statements by the client indicates a need for further teaching?

   A. "I will be sure to wear long sleeves when out in the sun."

   B. "I will take this medication with a full glass of milk."

   C. "I will finish all the medicine even if I am feeling better."

   D. "I will take this medication first thing in the morning."

Scenario: A nurse plans to administer gentamicin (Garamycin) 50 mg intermittent IV bolus in 50 mL of 0.9% sodium chloride at 0900. The infusion will take 30 min.

---

2. When should the nurse plan for the peak serum level to be drawn

   A. 0930

   B. 1000

   C. 1030

   D. 1100

3. For which of the following side effects should the nurse monitor? (Select all that apply)

   _____ Proteinuria

   _____ Elevated BUN

   _____ Sedation

   _____ Reports of muscle weakness

   _____ Reports of headache

CHAPTER 45: ANTIBIOTICS AFFECTING PROTEIN SYNTHESIS

Application Exercises Answer Key

1. A nurse is providing teaching to a client prescribed tetracycline hydrochloride (Sumycin) to treat a GI infection caused by *Helicobacter pylori*. Which of the following statements by the client indicates a need for further teaching?

    A. "I will be sure to wear long sleeves when out in the sun."

    B. "I will take this medication with a full glass of milk."

    C. "I will finish all the medicine even if I am feeling better."

    D. "I will take this medication first thing in the morning."

    Tetracycline can form a nonabsorbable chelate when taken with dairy products and therefore should be taken with water. The client should wear long sleeves to protect against sun exposure. The client may feel better before the entire prescription is complete but should finish the entire dose to ensure eradication of the infection. Taking the medication in the morning will reduce esophageal ulceration, which can occur if the medication is taken just before lying down at night.

NCLEX® Connection: Pharmacological and Parenteral Therapies, Medication Administration

---

Scenario: A nurse plans to administer gentamicin (Garamycin) 50 mg intermittent IV bolus in 50 mL of 0.9% sodium chloride at 0900. The infusion will take 30 min.

---

2. When should the nurse plan for the peak serum level to be drawn?

    A. 0930

    B. 1000

    C. 1030

    D. 1100

    The peak serum level should be drawn at 1000, 30 min after the IV infusion is complete.

NCLEX® Connection: Pharmacological and Parenteral Therapies, Medication Administration

3. For which of the following side effects should the nurse monitor? (Select all that apply)

    __X__ **Proteinuria**

    __X__ **Elevated BUN**

    _____ Sedation

    _____ Reports of muscle weakness

    _____ Reports of headache

    Proteinuria and elevated BUN may indicate nephrotoxicity, a side effect of gentamicin. Sedation, muscle weakness, and headache are not side effects of gentamicin.

NCLEX® Connection: Pharmacological and Parenteral Therapies, Adverse Effects/Contraindications/Side Effects/Interactions

UNIT 12 MEDICATIONS FOR INFECTION

Chapter 46 Urinary Tract Infections

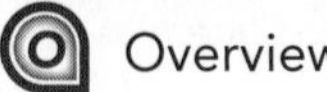

Overview

- Sulfonamides, trimethoprim, and urinary antiseptics are medications used to treat urinary tract infections.
- Other medications used include penicillins, aminoglycosides, cephalosporins, and fluoroquinolones.
- Medications are used to treat active infections and prophylaxis of recurrent infections for susceptible individuals.
- Regimens with these medications may be a single-dose, a short-course of 3 days, or the traditional course of 7 days.

MEDICATION CLASSIFICATION: SULFONAMIDES AND TRIMETHOPRIM

- Select Prototype Medications:
  - Trimethoprim-sulfamethoxazole (TMP-SMZ, Bactrim)
  - Co-trimoxazole (Cotrim, Septra)

Purpose

- Expected Pharmacological Action
  - Sulfonamides and trimethoprim inhibit bacterial growth by preventing the synthesis of folic acid. Folic acid is essential for the production of DNA, RNA, and proteins.
- Therapeutic Uses
  - TMP-SMZ is used to treat urinary tract infections.
    - Causative agents include *E. coli*, *Klebsiella*, *Proteus*, *Pseudomonas*, and *Candida* species.
    - Other infections include otitis media, bronchitis, shigellosis, and pneumonia caused by *Pneumocystis carinii*.

Complications

SIDE/ADVERSE EFFECTS	NURSING INTERVENTIONS/CLIENT EDUCATION
Hypersensitivity including Stevens-Johnson syndrome	• Do not administer TMP-SMZ to clients with allergies to: ○ Sulfonamides (sulfa) ○ Thiazide diuretics [hydrochlorothiazide (HCTZ)] ○ Sulfonylurea-type oral hypoglycemics [tolbutamide (Orinase)] ○ Loop diuretics [furosemide (Lasix)] • Stop TMP-SMZ at the first indication of hypersensitivity, such as rash.
Blood dyscrasias (hemolytic anemia, agranulocytosis, aplastic anemia)	• Draw the client's baseline and periodic CBC levels to detect any hematologic disorders. • Observe for any bleeding episodes, sore throat, or pallor. • If the above symptoms occur, instruct clients to notify the provider.
Crystalluria	• Maintain adequate oral fluid intake. • Instruct client to drink 2 to 3 L/day.
Kernicterus (jaundice, increased bilirubin levels)	• Avoid administering TMP-SMZ to women who are pregnant near term, breastfeeding mothers, and infants younger than 2 months. • Monitor the client's liver function.
Photosensitivity	• Avoid prolonged exposure to sunlight, use sunscreen, and wear appropriate protective clothing.

Contraindications/Precautions

- TMP-SMZ is contraindicated in clients who have folate deficiency (increases the risk of megaloblastic anemia).
- TMP-SMZ is contraindicated in clients with allergies to thiazide diuretics and sulfonylurea-type oral hypoglycemic agents.
- Avoid use in pregnancy and lactation (risk of kernicterus).
- Use cautiously in clients with renal dysfunction. Reduce dosage of TMP-SMZ by 50%.
- Do not use if creatinine clearance is less than 15 mL/min.

Interactions

MEDICATION/FOOD INTERACTIONS	NURSING INTERVENTIONS/CLIENT EDUCATION
Sulfonamides can increase the effects of warfarin (Coumadin), phenytoin (Dilantin), sulfonylurea oral hypoglycemics, and tolbutamide (Orinase) by inhibiting hepatic metabolism.	• Reduced dosages of these medications may be required during TMP-SMZ therapy.

Nursing Administration

- Instruct clients to take TMP-SMZ on an empty stomach with a full glass of water.
- Instruct clients to complete the prescribed course of antimicrobial therapy, even though symptoms may resolve before the full course is completed.

Nursing Evaluation of Medication Effectiveness

- Depending on therapeutic intent, effectiveness may be evidenced by:
  - Improvement of infection symptoms, such as improvement of urinary tract symptoms (decreased frequency, burning, and pain during urination) and negative urine cultures

MEDICATION CLASSIFICATION: URINARY TRACT ANTISEPTICS

- Select Prototype Medication: nitrofurantoin (Macrodantin)
- Other Medications: methenamine (Mandelamine), nalidixic acid (NegGram)

Purpose

- Expected Pharmacological Action
  - This medication is a broad-spectrum urinary antiseptic with bacteriostatic and bactericidal action. Bacterial injury occurs by damaging DNA.
- Therapeutic Uses
  - Acute urinary tract infections
  - Prophylaxis for recurrent lower urinary tract infections

Complications

SIDE/ADVERSE EFFECTS	NURSING INTERVENTIONS/CLIENT EDUCATION
Gastrointestinal discomfort (anorexia, nausea, vomiting, and diarrhea)	• Administer nitrofurantoin with milk or meals. • Reduce dosage and use the macrocrystalline tablet to reduce GI discomfort.
Hypersensitivity reactions with severe pulmonary manifestations (dyspnea, cough, and malaise)	• Advise clients to stop the medication and call the provider if this occurs. Pulmonary manifestations should subside within several days after nitrofurantoin is discontinued.
Blood dyscrasias (agranulocytosis, leukopenia, thrombocytopenia)	• Do baseline CBC and perform periodic blood tests • Monitor clients for easy bruising and epistaxis (nose bleeding) • Notify the provider if symptoms occur.
Peripheral neuropathy (numbness, tingling of the hands and feet, muscle weakness)	• Instruct clients to notify the provider if these symptoms occur.
Headache, drowsiness, dizziness	• Instruct clients to notify the provider if these symptoms occur.

Contraindications/Precautions

- Nitrofurantoin is contraindicated in clients with renal dysfunction and creatinine clearance less than 40 mL/min.
  - Impaired renal function will increase the risk of medication toxicity because of inability to excrete nitrofurantoin.

Nursing Administration

- Inform clients that urine will have a brownish discoloration.
- Administer with food if GI symptoms occur.
- Instruct clients to complete the prescribed course of antimicrobial therapy, even though symptoms may resolve before the full course is completed.

Nursing Evaluation of Medication Effectiveness

- Depending on therapeutic intent, effectiveness may be evidenced by:
  - Improvement of infection symptoms, such as improvement of urinary tract symptoms (decreased frequency, burning, and pain during urination) and negative urine cultures
  - Resolution of diarrhea, nausea, and vomiting

MEDICATION CLASSIFICATION: FLUOROQUINOLONES

- Select Prototype Medication: ciprofloxacin (Cipro)
- Other Medications: Ofloxacin (Floxin), lomefloxacin (Maxaquin)

Purpose

- Expected Pharmacological Action
  - Fluoroquinolones are bactericidal as a result of inhibition of the enzyme necessary for DNA replication.
- Therapeutic Uses
  - Broad-spectrum antimicrobials used for a wide variety of micro-organisms such as aerobic gram-negative bacteria, gram-positive bacteria, *Klebsiella*, and *Escherichia coli*
  - Alternative to parenteral antibiotics for clients with severe infections
  - Urinary, respiratory, and gastrointestinal tract infections; infections of bones, joints, skin, and soft tissues
  - Medication of choice for prevention of anthrax in clients who have inhaled anthrax spore

Complications

SIDE/ADVERSE EFFECTS	NURSING INTERVENTIONS/CLIENT EDUCATION
Gastrointestinal discomfort (nausea, vomiting, diarrhea)	• Administer medications accordingly.
Achilles tendon rupture	• Instruct clients to observe for signs and symptoms of pain, swelling, and redness at Achilles tendon site, and to notify the provider. • Ciprofloxacin should be discontinued. Clients should not exercise until inflammation subsides.
Suprainfection (thrush, vaginal yeast infection)	• Instruct clients to observe for signs and symptoms of yeast infection (cottage cheese/curd-like lesions on the mouth and genital area) and to notify the provider.

Contraindications/Precautions

- Ciprofloxacin should not be administered to children less than 18 years of age (due to risk of Achilles tendon rupture), unless the child is being treated for *Escherichia coli* infections of urinary tract or inhalational anthrax.

Interactions

MEDICATION/FOOD INTERACTIONS	NURSING INTERVENTIONS/CLIENT EDUCATION
Cationic compounds (aluminum-magnesium antacids, iron salts, sucralfate, milk and dairy products) decrease absorption of ciprofloxacin.	• Administer cationic compounds 6 hr before or 2 hr after ciprofloxacin.
Plasma levels of theophylline (Theolair) can be the increased with concurrent use of ciprofloxacin.	• Monitor levels and adjust dosage accordingly.
Plasma levels of warfarin (Coumadin) can be increased with concurrent use of ciprofloxacin	• Monitor prothrombin time and INR, and adjust the dosage of warfarin accordingly.

Nursing Administration

- Ciprofloxacin is available in oral and intravenous forms.
- Decrease doses of ciprofloxacin in clients with renal dysfunction.
- Intravenous ciprofloxacin should be administered slowly over 60 min.
- For inhalation anthrax infection, ciprofloxacin is administered every 12 hr for 60 days.
- Instruct clients to complete the prescribed course of antimicrobial therapy, even though symptoms may resolve before the full course is completed.

Nursing Evaluation of Medication Effectiveness

- Depending on therapeutic intent, effectiveness may be evidenced by:
    - Improvement of infection symptoms (improvement of urinary tract symptoms [decreased frequency, burning, and pain during urination], negative urine cultures)
    - No evidence of suprainfection such as absence of cottage cheese or curd-like lesions in the mouth and genital areas

CHAPTER 46: URINARY TRACT INFECTIONS

Application Exercises

Scenario: A client comes to the clinic stating that she has been taking trimethoprim-sulfamethoxazole (Bactrim) for a bladder infection. The client reports intense perineal itching and a whitish, cheese-like vaginal discharge.

1.The nurse should recognize that these findings are likely a result of

A. Suprainfection
B. Hypersensitivity reaction
C. Toxicity
D. Medication interaction

2. Which of the following are side effects of this medication for which the nurse should instruct the client to watch? (Select all that apply)

_____ Photosensitivity
_____ Dry mouth
_____ Rash
_____ Tinnitus
_____ Constipation

3. A nurse is providing teaching to a client who is prescribed nitrofurantoin. What teaching should the nurse include?

4. A nurse is teaching an adult client with a severe infection about her prescription for ciprofloxacin (Cipro). For which of the following adverse reactions should the nurse tell the client to watch? (Select all that apply)

_____ Achilles tendon rupture
_____ Vaginal yeast infection
_____ Irregular pulse rate
_____ Urinary hesitancy
_____ Achilles tendon pain

CHAPTER 46: URINARY TRACT INFECTIONS

Application Exercises Answer Key

Scenario: A client comes to the clinic stating that she has been taking trimethoprim-sulfamethoxazole (Bactrim) for a bladder infection. The client reports intense perineal itching and a whitish, cheese-like vaginal discharge.

1.The nurse should recognize that these findings are likely a result of

A. Suprainfection

B. Hypersensitivity reaction

C. Toxicity

D. Medication interaction

These findings indicate a suprainfection with a fungal infection as a result of the disruption of the body's normal flora. These findings do not indicate a hypersensitivity reaction, toxicity or medication interaction.

NCLEX® Connection: Pharmacological and Parenteral Therapies, Adverse Effects/ Contraindications/Side Effects/Interactions

2. Which of the following are side effects of this medication for which the nurse should instruct the client to watch? (Select all that apply.)

__X__ **Photosensitivity**

_____ Dry mouth

__X__ **Rash**

_____ Tinnitus

_____ Constipation

Side effects of TMP-SMZ include photosensitivity and rash. Dry mouth, tinnitus, and constipation are not side effects.

NCLEX® Connection: Pharmacological and Parenteral Therapies, Adverse Effects/ Contraindications/Side Effects/Interactions

3. A nurse is providing teaching to a client who is prescribed nitrofurantoin. What teaching should the nurse include?

Tell the client that the medication may cause the urine to appear a rust-brown color. Inform the client to report the following side effects: fever, sore throat, cough, dyspnea, unusual bleeding, and numbness and tingling of hands and feet.

NCLEX® Connection: Pharmacological and Parenteral Therapies, Medication Administration

4. A nurse is teaching an adult client with a severe infection about her prescription for ciprofloxacin (Cipro). For which of the following adverse reactions should the nurse tell the client to watch? (Select all that apply)

   __X__ **Achilles tendon rupture**
   __X__ **Vaginal yeast infection**
   _____ Irregular pulse rate
   _____ Urinary hesitancy
   __X__ **Achilles tendon pain**

   The client taking ciprofloxacin should be taught about adverse reactions including Achilles tendon rupture; suprainfection, which may cause vaginal yeast infection or yeast infection of the throat or mouth; and Achilles tendon pain, which could be a sign of impending tendon rupture. Cardiovascular symptoms, such as irregular pulse and urinary hesitancy, are not expected adverse reactions for a client taking ciprofloxacin.

NCLEX® Connection: Pharmacological and Parenteral Therapies, Adverse Effects/ Contraindications/Side Effects/Interactions

UNIT 12 MEDICATIONS FOR INFECTION

Chapter 47 Mycobacterial, Fungal, and Parasitic Infections

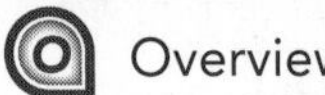

Overview

- *Mycobacterium tuberculosis* is a slow-growing pathogen that necessitates long-term treatment. Long-term treatment increases the risk for toxicity, poor patient adherence, and development of medication-resistant strains. Treatment for tuberculosis requires the use of at least two medications to which the pathogen is susceptible.
- Metronidazole (Flagyl) is the medication of choice for parasitic infections
- Antifungal medications belong to a variety of chemical families and are used to treat systemic and superficial mycoses

MEDICATION CLASSIFICATION: ANTIMYCOBACTERIAL (ANTITUBERCULOSIS)

- Select Prototype Medication: isoniazid (INH)
- Other Medications:
  - Pyrazinamide (PZA)
  - Ethambutol (Myambutol) bacteriostatic only to *M. tuberculosis*

Purpose

- Expected Pharmacological Action
  - This medication is highly specific for mycobacteria. Isoniazid inhibits growth of mycobacteria by preventing synthesis of mycolic acid in the cell wall.
- Therapeutic Uses
  - Indicated for active and latent tuberculosis
    - Latent: INH only – 6 to 9 months
    - Active: Multiple medication therapy including INH, for a minimum of 6 months
    - The initial phase (induction phase) focuses on irradiating the active tubercle bacilli, which will result in noninfectious sputum. The second phase (continuation phase) works toward eliminating any other pathogens in the body. Length of treatment varies and may be as short as 6 months for medication-sensitive tuberculosis (2 months for the initial phase and 4 months for the continuation phase) or as long as 24 months for medication-resistant infections.

Complications

SIDE/ADVERSE EFFECTS	NURSING INTERVENTIONS/CLIENT EDUCATION
Peripheral neuropathy (tingling, numbness, burning, and pain resulting from deficiency of pyridoxine, vitamin B_6).	• Instruct clients to observe for symptoms and to notify the provider if symptoms occur. • Administer 50 to 200 mg of vitamin B_6 daily.
Hepatotoxicity (anorexia, malaise, fatigue, nausea, and yellowish discoloration of skin and eyes).	• Instruct clients to observe for symptoms and notify the provider if symptoms occur. • Monitor liver function tests. • Instruct clients to avoid consumption of alcohol. • Medication may need to be discontinued if liver function test results are elevated.

Contraindications/Precautions

- INH is contraindicated for clients with liver disease.

Interactions

MEDICATION/FOOD INTERACTIONS	NURSING INTERVENTIONS/CLIENT EDUCATION
INH inhibits metabolism of phenytoin, leading to buildup of medication and toxicity. Ataxia and incoordination may indicate toxicity.	• Monitor the client's levels of phenytoin. Dosage of phenytoin may need to be adjusted based on phenytoin levels.
Concurrent use of alcohol, rifampin, and pyrazinamide increases the risk for hepatotoxicity.	• Instruct clients to avoid alcohol consumption. • Monitor liver function.

Nursing Administration

- Administer by oral route
- For active tuberculosis, direct observation therapy (DOT) is done to ensure adherence.
- Advise clients to take INH 1 hr before meals or 2 hr after. If gastric discomfort occurs, the client may take INH with meals.
- Instruct clients to complete the prescribed course of antimicrobial therapy, even though symptoms may resolve before the full course is completed.

MEDICATION CLASSIFICATION: ANTIMYCOBACTERIAL (ANTITUBERCULOSIS)

- Select Prototype Medication: rifampin (Rifadin)

Purpose

- Expected Pharmacological Action
  - Rifampin is bactericidal as a result of inhibition of protein synthesis
- Therapeutic Uses
  - Rifampin is a broad-spectrum antibiotic effective for gram-positive and gram-negative bacteria, *M. tuberculosis*, and *M. Leprae*.

Complications

SIDE/ADVERSE EFFECTS	NURSING INTERVENTIONS/CLIENT EDUCATION
Discoloration of body fluids.	• Inform clients of expected orange color of urine, saliva, sweat, and tears.
Hepatotoxicity (jaundice, anorexia, and fatigue)	• Monitor the client's liver function. • Inform clients regarding symptoms of anorexia, fatigue, and malaise, and instruct them to notify the provider if symptoms occur. • Avoid alcohol.
Mild gastrointestinal discomfort associated (anorexia, nausea, and abdominal discomfort.	• Abdominal discomfort is mild and usually does not require intervention.

Contraindications/Precautions

- Use cautiously in clients with liver dysfunction.

Interactions

MEDICATION/FOOD INTERACTIONS	NURSING INTERVENTIONS/CLIENT EDUCATION
Rifampin accelerates metabolism of warfarin (Coumadin), oral contraceptives, protease inhibitors, and NNRTIs (medications for HIV), resulting in diminished effectiveness.	• Increased dosages of HIV medications may be necessary. • Monitor PT and INR. • Clients may need to use alternative form of birth control.
Concurrent use with INH and pyrazinamide increases risk of hepatotoxicity.	• Instruct clients to avoid alcohol consumption. • Monitor liver function.

Nursing Evaluation of Medication Effectiveness

- Depending on therapeutic intent, effectiveness may be evidenced by:
  - Improvement of tuberculosis symptoms such as clear breath sounds, no night sweats, increased appetite, no afternoon rises of temperature
  - 3 negative sputum cultures for tuberculosis, usually taking 3 to 6 months to achieve

MEDICATION CLASSIFICATION: ANTIPROTOZOALS

- Select Prototype Medication: metronidazole (Flagyl)

Purpose

- Expected Pharmacological Action
  - Metronidazole is a broad-spectrum antimicrobial with bactericidal activity against anaerobic micro-organisms.
- Therapeutic Uses
  - Treatment of protozoal infections (intestinal amebiasis, giardiasis, trichomoniasis) and obligate anaerobic bacteria (*Bacteroides fragilis*, antibiotic-induced *Clostridium difficile*, *Gardnerella vaginalis)*
  - Prophylaxis for clients who will have surgical procedures and are high risk for anaerobic infection (vaginal, abdominal, colorectal surgery)
  - Treatment of *H. pylori* in clients who have peptic ulcer disease in combination with tetracycline and bismuth salicylate

Complications

SIDE/ADVERSE EFFECTS	NURSING INTERVENTIONS/CLIENT EDUCATION
Gastrointestinal discomfort (nausea, vomiting, dry mouth, and metallic taste)	• Advise clients to observe for symptoms and to notify the provider.
Darkening of urine.	• Advise clients that this is a harmless effect of metronidazole.
CNS symptoms (numbness of extremities, ataxia, and seizures)	• Advise clients to notify the provider if symptoms occur. • Stop metronidazole.

Contraindications/Precautions

- Use cautiously in clients with renal dysfunction to prevent accumulation of toxic levels with prolonged use.
- Avoid use during the first trimester of pregnancy and use with caution during the rest of pregnancy because metronidazole can pass through the placenta.

Interactions

MEDICATION/FOOD INTERACTIONS	NURSING INTERVENTIONS/CLIENT EDUCATION
Alcohol causes a disulfiram-like reaction/	• Advise clients to avoid alcohol consumption.
Metronidazole inhibits inactivation of warfarin.	• Monitor prothrombin time and INR, and adjust warfarin dosage accordingly.

Nursing Administration

- Administer by oral or IV route.
- Instruct clients to complete the prescribed course of antimicrobial therapy, even though symptoms may resolve before the full course is completed.

Nursing Evaluation of Medication Effectiveness

- Depending on therapeutic intent, effectiveness may be evidenced by:
  - Improvement of symptoms (resolution of bloody mucoid diarrhea, formed stools, negative stool results for ameba and *Giardia*, decrease or absence of watery vaginal/urethral discharge, negative blood cultures for anaerobic organisms in the CNS, blood, bones and joints, and soft tissues)

MEDICATION CLASSIFICATION: ANTIFUNGALS

- Select Prototype Medications:
  - Amphotericin B deoxycholate (Fungizone) a polyene antibiotic for systemic mycoses
  - Ketoconazole (Nizoral) an azole for treating both superficial and systemic mycoses
- Other Medications:
  - Flucytosine (Ancobon)
  - Nystatin (Mycostatin)
  - Miconazole (Monistat 3)
  - Clotrimazole (Lotrimin)
  - Terbinafine (Lamisil)
  - Fluconazole (Diflucan)
  - Griseofulvin (Grifulvin)

Purpose

- Expected Pharmacological Action
  - Amphotericin B deoxycholate is an antifungal agent that acts on fungal cell membranes to cause cell death. Depending on concentration, these agents can be fungistatic (slows growth on the fungus) or fungicidal (destroys the fungus).

- Therapeutic Uses
    - Antifungals are the treatment of choice for systemic fungal infection (*Candidiasis, Aspergillosis, Cryptococcosis, Mucormycosis)* and nonopportunistic mycoses, (*Blastomycosis, Histoplasmosis, Coccidioidomycosis)*.
    - Some antifungals treat superficial fungal infections: dermatophytic infections (tinea pedis [ringworm of the foot], tinea cruris [ringworm of the groin]); candida infections of the skin and mucous membranes; and fungal infections of the nails (*Onychomycosis*).

Complications

SIDE/ADVERSE EFFECTS	NURSING INTERVENTIONS/CLIENT EDUCATION
Infusion reactions (fever, chills, rigors, and headache) 1 to 3 hr after initiation	• Pretreat with diphenhydramine (Benadryl) and acetaminophen. • Meperidine (Demerol), dantrolene, or hydrocortisone may be given for rigors.
Thrombophlebitis	• Observe infusion sites for signs of erythema, swelling, and pain. • Rotate injection sites. • Administer in a large vein and administer heparin before infusing amphotericin B.
Nephrotoxicity	• Obtain baseline kidney function (BUN and creatinine) and do weekly kidney function tests. • Monitor I&O. • Infuse 1 L of saline on the day of amphotericin B infusion.
Hypokalemia	• Monitor electrolyte levels, especially potassium. • Administer potassium supplements accordingly.
Bone marrow suppression	• Obtain baseline CBC and hematocrit, and monitor weekly.
Ketoconazole	
Hepatotoxicity (anorexia, nausea, vomiting, jaundice, dark urine, and clay-colored stools)	• Obtain baseline liver function studies and monitor liver function monthly. • If symptoms occur, notify provider and discontinue medication.
Effects on sex hormones: • In males, gynecomastia (enlargement of breast), decreased libido, erectile dysfunction • In females, irregular menstrual flow	• Advise clients to observe for these symptoms and to notify the provider.

Contraindications/Precautions

- Antifungals are contraindicated in clients with renal dysfunction because of the risk for nephrotoxicity.

Interactions

MEDICATION/FOOD INTERACTIONS	NURSING INTERVENTIONS/CLIENT EDUCATION
Aminoglycosides (gentamicin, streptomycin, cyclosporine) have additive nephrotoxic risk when used concurrently with antifungal medications.	• Avoid use of these antimicrobials when clients are taking amphotericin B due to additive nephrotoxicity risk.
Antifungal effects of Flucytosine (Ancobon) are potentiated with concurrent use of amphotericin B.	• Potentiating the effects of flucytosine allows for a reduction in amphotericin B dosages.

Nursing Administration

- Amphotericin B is highly toxic and should be reserved for severe life-threatening fungal infections.
- Amphotericin B should be infused slowly over 2 to 4 hr by the IV route, because oral preparation is poorly absorbed in the GI tract. Observe solutions for precipitation and discard if precipitates are present. Renal damage can be lessened with administration of 1 L saline solution on the day of amphotericin B infusion.
- Instruct clients to complete the prescribed course of antimicrobial therapy, even though symptoms may resolve before the full course is completed.
- Antifungals for topical use to treat superficial vulvovaginal candidiasis may be applied as vaginal suppository or cream.

Nursing Evaluation of Medication Effectiveness

- Depending on therapeutic intent, effectiveness may be evidenced by:
  - Improvement of findings of systemic fungal infections, such as clear breath sounds and negative chest x-rays
  - Improvement of findings of superficial infections such as clear mucus membranes, clear nails, intact skin

CHAPTER 47: MYCOBACTERIAL, FUNGAL, AND PARASITIC INFECTIONS

Application Exercises

1. A nurse is caring for a client who has diabetes mellitus and pulmonary tuberculosis and has a new prescription for isoniazid (INH). Which of the following supplements should the nurse expect to administer to prevent an adverse effect of isoniazid?

   A. Ascorbic acid

   B. Pyridoxine

   C. Folic acid

   D. Cyanocobalamin

2. A nurse is infusing intravenous amphotericin B for a client who has a severe fungal infection. How soon after beginning the infusion should the nurse start to monitor for signs of an infusion reaction to begin?

   A. 5 to 10 min after beginning the infusion

   B. 20 to 30 min after beginning the infusion

   C. 1 to 3 hr after beginning the infusion

   D. 4 to 5 hr after beginning the infusion

3. A nurse is teaching a client who has been prescribed metronidazole (Flagyl) about important interactions that could occur when taking this medication. Which of the following could cause an adverse reaction to occur when taken along with metronidazole therapy?

   A. Smoking cigarettes or using nicotine

   B. Drinking a product containing alcohol

   C. Ingesting foods containing tyramine

   D. Taking a liquid antacid

CHAPTER 47: MYCOBACTERIAL, FUNGAL, AND PARASITIC INFECTIONS

Application Exercises Answer Key

1. A nurse is caring for a client who has diabetes mellitus and pulmonary tuberculosis and has a new prescription for isoniazid (INH). Which of the following supplements should the nurse expect to administer to prevent an adverse effect of isoniazid?

   A. Ascorbic acid

   B. Pyridoxine

   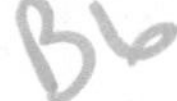

   C. Folic acid

   D. Cyanocobalamin

   Pyridoxine (Vitamin B_6) is frequently prescribed along with isoniazid to prevent peripheral neuropathy for clients who have increased risk factors such as diabetes or alcoholism. Ascorbic acid (vitamin C), folic acid, and cyanocobalamin (vitamin B_{12}) do not have the same action and are not prescribed to prevent this adverse effect.

NCLEX® Connection: Pharmacological and Parenteral Therapies: Adverse Effects/ Contraindications/Side Effects/Interactions

2. A nurse is infusing intravenous amphotericin B for a client who has a severe fungal infection. How soon after beginning the infusion should the nurse start to monitor for signs of an infusion reaction to begin?

   A. 5 to 10 min after beginning the infusion

   B. 20 to 30 min after beginning the infusion

   C. 1 to 3 hr after beginning the infusion

   D. 4 to 5 hr after beginning the infusion

   Signs and symptoms of infusion reaction may be seen 1 to 3 hr after beginning amphotericin B.

NCLEX® Connection: Pharmacological and Parenteral Therapies: Adverse Effects/ Contraindications/Side Effects/Interactions

3. A nurse is teaching a client who has been prescribed metronidazole (Flagyl) about important interactions that could occur when taking this medication. Which of the following could cause an adverse reaction to occur when taken along with metronidazole therapy?

   A. Smoking cigarettes or using nicotine

   B. Drinking a product containing alcohol

   C. Ingesting foods containing tyramine

   D. Taking a liquid antacid

   Drinking alcohol while taking metronidazole can cause a disulfiram-like reaction, including nausea, vomiting, headache, and flushing. Alcohol should be avoided for at least one day after metronidazole is discontinued to prevent the reaction. There are no interactions between metronidazole and nicotine, tyramine, or antacids.

NCLEX® Connection: Pharmacological and Parenteral Therapies: Adverse Effects/ Contraindications/Side Effects/Interactions

UNIT 12 MEDICATIONS FOR INFECTION

Chapter 48 Viral Infections, HIV, and AIDS

Overview

- Most antiviral medications act by altering viral reproduction. Antiviral medications are only effective during viral replication. Therefore, they are ineffective when the virus is dormant.
- The human immunodeficiency virus (HIV) is a retrovirus. A retrovirus must attach to a host cell in order to replicate. RNA is changed into DNA using the enzyme reverse transcriptase.
- Antiretroviral agents are used to treat HIV infections.
    - Antiretroviral agents may act by preventing the virus from entering the cells (fusion inhibitors). Others may act by inhibiting enzymes needed for HIV replication (nucleoside reverse transcriptase inhibitors [NRTIs], nonnucleoside reverse transcriptase inhibitors [NNRTIs], the protease inhibitors).
    - Biologic response modifiers, such as interleukin-2 (Interferon), act as immunostimulants to enhance the immune response. They are used in combination with antiretroviral agents to reduce the advancement of the virus.
- Highly active antiretroviral therapy (HAART) involves using 3 to 4 HIV medications in combination with other antiretroviral medications to reduce medication resistance, adverse effects, and dosages.

MEDICATION CLASSIFICATION: ANTIVIRAL

- Select Prototype Medications
    - Acyclovir (Zovirax): Oral, topical and IV
    - Ganciclovir (Cytovene): Oral, IV
- Other Medications:
    - Interferon alfa-2b
    - Lamivudine (Epivir)
    - Oseltamivir (Tamiflu)
    - Ribavirin (Rebetol)
    - Amantadine (Symmetrel)

Purpose

- Expected Pharmacological Action
  - Acyclovir prevents the reproduction of viral DNA and thus interrupts cell replication.
- Therapeutic Uses
  - Acyclovir is used to treat herpes simplex and varicella-zoster viruses
  - Ganciclovir is used for treatment and prevention of cytomegalovirus (CMV). Prevention therapy using ganciclovir is given for clients who have HIV/AIDS, organ transplants, and other immunocompromised states.
  - Interferon alfa-2b and lamivudine are used to treat hepatitis.
  - Oseltamivir is used to treat influenza A and B.
  - Ribavirin is used to treat respiratory syncytial virus (RSV) and influenza.

Complications

SIDE/ADVERSE EFFECTS	NURSING INTERVENTIONS/CLIENT EDUCATION
Acyclovir	
Phlebitis and inflammation at the site of infusion	• Rotate IV injection sites. • Monitor IV sites for swelling and redness.
Nephrotoxicity	• Administer acyclovir infusion slowly over 1 hr. • Ensure adequate hydration during infusion and 2 hr after to minimize nephrotoxicity by administering IV fluids and increasing oral fluid intake as prescribed.
Mild discomfort associated with oral therapy (nausea, headache, diarrhea)	• Observe for symptoms and notify the provider.
Ganciclovir	
Granulocytopenia and thrombocytopenia	• Obtain baseline CBC and platelet count. • Administer granulocyte colony-stimulating factors. • Monitor WBC, absolute neutrophil, and platelet counts.

Contraindications/Precautions

- Acyclovir should be used cautiously in clients with renal impairment or dehydration, and clients taking nephrotoxic medications.
- Ganciclovir is Pregnancy Risk Category C; contraindicated in clients with a neutrophil count below 500/mm^3 or platelet counts less than 25,000/mm^3, and should be used cautiously in clients with pre-existing low white and platelet counts.

Interactions

MEDICATION/FOOD INTERACTIONS	NURSING INTERVENTIONS/CLIENT EDUCATION
Acyclovir	
Probenecid may decrease elimination of acyclovir.	• Monitor for medication toxicity.
Concurrent use of zidovudine may cause drowsiness.	• Use with caution
Ganciclovir	
Cytotoxic medications may cause increased toxicity.	• Use together with caution.

Nursing Administration

- Acyclovir:
  - For topical administration, advise clients to put on rubber gloves to avoid transfer of virus to other areas of the body.
  - Administer IV infusion slowly over 1 hr or longer.
  - Inform clients to expect symptom relief but not cure.
  - Instruct clients to wash affected area with soap and water 3 to 4 times/day and to keep the lesions dry after washing.
  - Advise clients to refrain from sexual contact while lesions are present.
  - Clients with healed herpetic lesions should continue to use condoms to prevent transmission of the virus.
- Ganciclovir
  - Administer IV infusion slowly, with an infusion pump, over at least 1 hr.
  - Administer oral medication with food.
  - Administer intraocular for CMV retinitis.
- Instruct clients to complete the prescribed course of antimicrobial therapy, even though symptoms may resolve before the full course is completed.

Nursing Evaluation of Medication Effectiveness

- Depending on therapeutic intent, effectiveness may be evidenced by:
  - Improvement of findings such as healed genital lesions, decreased inflammation and pain, and improvement in vision

MEDICATION CLASSIFICATION: ENTRY/INFUSION INHIBITORS

- Select Prototype Medication: enfuvirtide (Fuzeon): subcutaneous

Purpose

- Expected Pharmacological Action
  - Decreases and limits the spread of HIV by blocking HIV from attaching to and entering CDC4 T cell.
- Therapeutic Uses
  - Treatment of HIV that is unresponsive to other antiretrovirals

Complications

SIDE/ADVERSE EFFECTS	NURSING INTERVENTIONS/CLIENT EDUCATION
Localized reaction at injection site.	• Rotate injection sites. Monitor for swelling and redness.
Bacterial pneumonia	• Assess breath sounds prior to start of therapy. Monitor for signs of pneumonia, such as fever, cough or shortness of breath.
Fever, chills, rash, hypotension	• Monitor for medication reaction. Discontinue and notify the provider.

Contraindications/Precautions

- Enfuvirtide is contraindicated in clients with medication hypersensitivity
- This medication is Pregnancy Risk Category B.

Interactions

- None significant

Nursing Administration

- Rotate injection sites and avoid areas with scars or bruising.
- Monitor for bacterial pneumonia.
- Monitor for medication reaction.
- Advise clients to notify the provider if they are pregnant or planning to become pregnant.

Nursing Evaluation of Medication Effectiveness

- Depending on therapeutic intent, effectiveness may be evidenced by the following:
  - The client will have a reduction of symptoms and remain free of opportunistic infection.

MEDICATION CLASSIFICATION: NUCLEOSIDE REVERSE TRANSCRIPTASE INHIBITORS (NRTIs)

- Select Prototype Medication: zidovudine (Retrovir)
- Other Medications:
  - Didanosine (Videx)
  - Stavudine (Zerit)
  - Lamivudine (Epivir)
  - Abacavir (Ziagen)
- Combination Medications:
  - Abacavir, lamivudine zidovudine (Trizivir)
  - Abacavir, lamivudine (Epzicom)
  - Lamivudine, zidovudine (Combivir)

Purpose

- Expected Pharmacological Action
  - Reduces HIV symptoms by inhibiting DNA synthesis and thus viral replication
- Therapeutic Uses
  - Used to treat HIV infection
- Route of Administration: Oral, IV

Complications

SIDE/ADVERSE EFFECTS	NURSING INTERVENTIONS/CLIENT EDUCATION
Suppressed bone marrow resulting in anemia, agranulocytosis (neutropenia) and thrombocytopenia	• Monitor CBC and platelets. Advise clients that transfusions may be needed.
Lactic acidosis	• Monitor for symptoms of lactic acidosis, such as hyperventilation, nausea, and abdominal pain. Pregnancy increases the risk of lactic acidosis.
Nausea, vomiting, diarrhea	• Clients may take the medication with food to reduce gastric irritation. Monitor fluids and electrolytes.
Hepatomegaly/fatty liver	• Monitor liver enzymes.

 Contraindications/Precautions

- These medications are Pregnancy Risk Category C. Pregnancy increases risk for lactic acidosis, liver enlargement, and fatty liver.
- These medications are contraindicated in clients with medication hypersensitivity.
- Use with caution in clients who have liver disease and bone marrow suppression.

Interactions

MEDICATION/FOOD INTERACTIONS	NURSING INTERVENTIONS/CLIENT EDUCATION
Probenecid, valproic acid, and methadone may increase zidovudine.	• Reduce dosage. Monitor for medication toxicity.
Ganciclovir or medications that decrease bone marrow production may further suppress bone marrow.	• Use together with caution.
Rifampin and ritonavir may reduce zidovudine levels.	• Adjust dosage if needed.
Phenytoin may alter both medication levels.	• Monitor medication levels.

Nursing Administration

- Monitor for bone marrow suppression. Obtain baseline CBC and platelets at the start of therapy and every 4 weeks.
- Anemia may be treated with epoetin alfa or transfusions.
- Neutropenia may be treated with colony-stimulating factors.
- Advise clients to monitor for fever, sore throat, increased bleeding, bruising or fatigue.

Nursing Evaluation of Medication Effectiveness

- Depending on therapeutic intent, effectiveness may be evidenced by the following:
    - The client will have a reduction of symptoms and remain free of opportunistic infection.

MEDICATION CLASSIFICATION: NON-NUCLEOSIDE REVERSE TRANSCRIPTASE INHIBITORS (NNRTIs)

- Select Prototype Medications: delavirdine (Rescriptor), efavirenz (Sustiva)
- Other Medications: nevirapine (Viramune), etravirine (Intelence)

Purpose

- Expected Pharmacological Action
    - NNRTIs act directly on reverse transcriptase to stop HIV replication.

- Therapeutic Uses
  - Primary HIV-1 infection
  - Often used in combination with other antiretroviral agents to prevent medication resistance
- Route of administration: Oral

Complications

SIDE/ADVERSE EFFECTS	NURSING INTERVENTIONS/CLIENT EDUCATION
Rash, which may become serious and lead to Steven's-Johnson syndrome	• Monitor for rash. Treat with diphenhydramine (Benadryl), if prescribed. • Notify the provider for fever or blistering.
Flu-like symptoms, headache, fatigue	• Monitor for adverse reactions. • Encourage rest and adequate oral fluid intake.

Contraindications/Precautions

- NNRTIs are Pregnancy Risk Category C.
- These medications are contraindicated in clients with medication hypersensitivity.
- Use with caution in clients who have liver disease.

Interactions

MEDICATION/FOOD INTERACTIONS	NURSING INTERVENTIONS/CLIENT EDUCATION
Antacids may decrease absorption of delavirdine.	• Allow 1 hr between medications.
NNRTIs may increase effects of amphetamines, antihistamines, calcium channel blockers, ergot alkaloids, quinidine, warfarin, and others.	• Monitor for medication toxicity.
Rifampin and phenytoin may cause decrease in levels of delavirdine.	• Do not use together.
Didanosine may reduce both medications' absorption.	• Allow 1 hour between medications.
NNRTIs may cause increase in sildenafil level.	• Monitor for hypotension and changes in vision. Use together with caution.

Nursing Administration

- Give with another antiretroviral to reduce risk of medication resistance.
- Monitor for rash.
- Efavirenz may be given with a high-fat meal to increase absorption.

Nursing Evaluation of Medication Effectiveness

- Depending on therapeutic intent, effectiveness may be evidenced by the following:
  - The client will have a reduction of symptoms and remain free of any opportunistic infection.

MEDICATION CLASSIFICATION: PROTEASE INHIBITORS

- Select Prototype Medication: ritonavir (Norvir)
- Other Medications:
  - Saquinavir (Invirase)
  - Indinavir (Crixivan)
  - Amprenavir (Agenerase)
  - Nelfinavir (Viracept)

Purpose

- Expected Pharmacological Action
  - Protease inhibitors act against HIV-1 and HIV-2 to alter and inactivate the virus by inhibiting enzymes needed for HIV replication.
- Therapeutic Uses
  - Used to treat HIV infections
  - Should be used with another antiretroviral medication to reduce medication resistance
- Route of administration: Oral

Complications

SIDE/ADVERSE EFFECTS	NURSING INTERVENTIONS/CLIENT EDUCATION
Diabetes mellitus/hyperglycemia	• Monitor serum glucose. Adjust diet and administer anti-diabetic medications as prescribed. Advise clients to monitor for increased thirst and urine output.
Hypersensitivity reaction.	• Monitor for rash. Notify the provider if rash develops.
Nausea and vomiting	• Take medication with food to reduce GI effects and increase absorption.
Elevated serum lipids	• Monitor for hyperlipidemia. Adjust diet.
Thrombocytopenia, leukopenia	• Monitor CBC. Monitor for signs of infection (fever, sore throat). Monitor for bleeding, (blood in stool, bruising).

 Contraindications/Precautions

- Protease inhibitors are Pregnancy Risk Category B.
- Use with caution in clients who have liver disease.

Interactions

MEDICATION/FOOD INTERACTIONS	NURSING INTERVENTIONS/CLIENT EDUCATION
Ritonavir may cause these medications to accumulate to toxic levels: Bupropion, carbamazepine, diazepam, lidocaine, prednisone clozapine, lovastatin, simvastatin, alprazolam, and ergotamine.	• Avoid concurrent use.
Ritonavir may increase medication levels of sildenafil, tadalafil, and vardenafil.	• Use with caution. Dosages of these medications may need to be reduced.
Ritonavir decreases levels of ethynyl estradiol in oral contraceptives.	• Instruct clients to use an alternative form of birth control.

Nursing Administration

- Instruct clients to report all other medications including over-the-counter and herbal medications to the provider.
- Give with food to increase absorption.
- Give along with another antiretroviral to reduce risk of medication resistance.

Nursing Evaluation of Medication Effectiveness

- Depending on therapeutic intent, effectiveness may be evidenced by the following:
  - The client will have a reduction of symptoms and remain free of any opportunistic infection.

CHAPTER 48: VIRAL INFECTIONS, HIV, AND AIDS

 Application Exercises

1. Antiviral medications act by interrupting which of the following?

   A. Cell membrane permeability

   B. Cell wall synthesis

   C. Prostaglandin synthesis

   D. Cell replication

2. A client with HIV is receiving combination medication therapy (HAART therapy) of abacavir, zidovudine, and lamivudine. HAART is used to do which of the following? (Select all that apply.)

   _____ Decrease medication resistance.

   _____ Reduce adverse medication effects.

   _____ Block antiretroviral agents from entering healthy cells.

   _____ Stimulate the immune system.

   _____ Reduce the medication dosages.

3. A client is taking zidovudine, a nucleotide reverse transcriptase inhibitor (NRTI), to treat HIV. The nurse instructs the client to be alert for which of the following that may indicate an adverse effect of NRTIs? (Select all that apply.)

   _____ Nausea and vomiting

   _____ Ataxia

   _____ Hyperventilation

   _____ Fatigue

   _____ Visual disturbance

4. A nurse is providing teaching to a client who is prescribed ritonavir to treat HIV. The nurse should include which of the following in the instructions?

   A. Change positions slowly to prevent dizziness.

   B. Use sunscreen and protective clothing to prevent sunburn.

   C. Report abdominal pain or anorexia, which may indicate lactic acidosis.

   D. Report polydipsia or polyuria, which may indicate hyperglycemia.

5. A client is taking enfuvirtide (Fuzeon) a fusion inhibitor, to treat HIV. For which of the following adverse reactions should the nurse monitor? (Select all that apply.)

_____ Stools or emesis for bleeding

_____ Breath sounds for pneumonia

_____ Level of consciousness for cerebral edema

_____ Injection site for infection

_____ Blood pressure for hypersensitive reaction

6. A client who is taking acyclovir (Zovirax) is advised to increase fluid intake in order to prevent

A. nephrotoxicity.

B. hepatomegaly.

C. lactic acidosis.

D. hyperlipidemia.

CHAPTER 48: VIRAL INFECTIONS, HIV, AND AIDS

Application Exercises Answer Key

1. Antiviral medications act by interrupting which of the following?

    A. Cell membrane permeability

    B. Cell wall synthesis

    C. Prostaglandin synthesis

    D. Cell replication

    Most antiviral medications act by interrupting cell replication. Antiviral medications need to be started during cell replication or within 2 days of the start of symptoms. They do not affect cell membrane permeability, cell wall synthesis, or prostaglandin synthesis.

NCLEX® Connection: Pharmacological and Parenteral Therapies: Expected Actions/Outcomes

2. A client with HIV is receiving combination medication therapy (HAART therapy) of abacavir, zidovudine, and lamivudine. HAART is used to do which of the following? (Select all that apply.)

    __X__ **Decrease medication resistance.**

    __X__ **Reduce adverse medication effects.**

    _____ Block antiretroviral agents from entering healthy cells.

    _____ Stimulate the immune system.

    __X__ **Reduce the medication dosages.**

    Highly active antiretroviral therapy (HAART) involves using 3 to 4 HIV medications in combination with other antiretroviral medications to reduce medication resistance, adverse effects, and dosages. Some of these agents are available together in one pill to reduce the amount of pills the client must take. HAART does not block antiretroviral agents from entering healthy cells. Biologic response modifiers stimulate the immune system.

NCLEX® Connection: Pharmacological and Parenteral Therapies: Adverse Effects/ Contraindications/Side Effects/Interactions

3. A client is taking zidovudine, a nucleotide reverse transcriptase inhibitor (NRTI), to treat HIV. The nurse instructs the client to be alert for which of the following that may indicate an adverse effect of NRTIs? (Select all that apply.)

    X **Nausea and vomiting**
    _____ Ataxia
    X **Hyperventilation**
    X **Fatigue**
    _____ Visual disturbance

    Monitor and report any symptoms of lactic acidosis, such as hyperventilation, nausea, abdominal pain, and fatigue. An arterial blood sample must be taken to diagnose lactic acidosis. NRTIs may also cause suppressed bone marrow resulting in anemia, agranulocytosis (neutropenia), and thrombocytopenia. Ataxia and visual disturbances are not related to lactic acidosis.

 **NCLEX® Connection: Pharmacological and Parenteral Therapies: Adverse Effects/Contraindications/Side Effects/Interactions**

4. A nurse is providing teaching to a client who is prescribed ritonavir to treat HIV. The nurse should include which of the following in the instructions?

    A. Change positions slowly to prevent dizziness.
    B. Use sunscreen and protective clothing to prevent sunburn.
    C. Report abdominal pain or anorexia, which may indicate lactic acidosis.
    D. Report polydipsia or polyuria, which may indicate hyperglycemia.

    Protease inhibitors such as ritonavir may cause hyperglycemia or diabetes mellitus. Advise the client to monitor for increased thirst and urine output, which could indicate hyperglycemia. Monitor serum glucose. The client may need to adjust his or her diet and take insulin or an oral hypoglycemic agent. Changing positions slowly, preventing sunburn, and lactic acidosis are not side effects of this medication.

 **NCLEX® Connection: Pharmacological and Parenteral Therapies: Medication Administration**

5. A client is taking enfuvirtide (Fuzeon) a fusion inhibitor, to treat HIV. For which of the following adverse reactions should the nurse monitor? (Select all that apply.)

_____ Stools or emesis for bleeding

X **Breath sounds for pneumonia**

_____ Level of consciousness for cerebral edema

X **Injection site for infection**

X **Blood pressure for hypersensitive reaction**

Bacterial pneumonia is an adverse reaction to fusion inhibitors. Assess breath sounds prior to the start of therapy. Monitor for signs of pneumonia, such as fever, cough, or shortness of breath. Monitor for swelling and redness at the injection site, which may indicate cellulitis. Rotate injection sites. Monitor for hypersensitivity medication reaction, such as fever, rash, or hypotension. If a reaction occurs, discontinue medication and notify the provider. Bleeding and cerebral edema are not adverse reactions related to this medication.

NCLEX® Connection: Pharmacological and Parenteral Therapies: Adverse Effects/ Contraindications/Side Effects/Interactions

6. A client who is taking acyclovir (Zovirax) is advised to increase fluid intake in order to prevent

A. nephrotoxicity.

B. hepatomegaly.

C. lactic acidosis.

D. hyperlipidemia.

Dehydration may cause acyclovir to precipitate and cause nephrotoxicity. Increase fluid intake and monitor kidney function. Use with caution in clients who have renal disease or dehydration. Increased fluid intake will not prevent hepatomegaly, and lactic acidosis and hyperlipidemia are not adverse effects of acyclovir.

NCLEX® Connection: Pharmacological and Parenteral Therapies: Adverse Effects/ Contraindications/Side Effects/Interactions

References

Berman, A., Snyder, S. J., Kozier, B., & Erb, G. (2008). *Fundamentals of nursing: Concepts, process, and practice* (8th ed.). Upper Saddle River, NJ: Pearson Prentice Hall.

Dudek, S. G. (2010). *Nutrition essentials for nursing practice* (6th ed.). Philadelphia, PA: Lippincott Williams & Wilkins.

Ignatavicius, D. D., & Workman, M. L. (2010). *Medical-surgical nursing* (6th ed.). St. Louis, MO: Saunders.

Lehne, R. A. (2010). *Pharmacology for nursing care* (7th ed.). St. Louis, MO: Saunders.

Lilley, L. L., Harrington, S., & Snyder, J. S. (2007). *Pharmacology and the nursing process* (5th Ed.). St. Louis, MO: Mosby.

Potter, P. A., & Perry, A. G. (2009). *Fundamentals of nursing* (7th ed.). St. Louis, MO: Mosby.

Roach, S. S., & Ford, S. M. (2008). *Introductory clinical pharmacology.* Philadelphia, PA: Lippincott Williams & Wilkins.

Smeltzer, S. C., Bare, B. G., Hinkle, J. L., & Cheever, K. H. (2008). *Brunner and Suddarth's textbook of medical-surgical nursing* (11th ed.). Philadelphia, PA: Lippincott Williams & Wilkins.

Wilson, B. A., Shannon, M. T., & Shields, K. M. (2010). *Pearson nurse's drug guide 2010.* Upper Saddle River, NJ: Prentice-Hall.